# Bacterial and Parasitic Diseases

*Guest Editor*

LAURA WADE, DVM, Dipl. ABVP–Avian

# VETERINARY CLINICS OF NORTH AMERICA: EXOTIC ANIMAL PRACTICE

www.vetexotic.theclinics.com

*Consulting Editor*
AGNES E. RUPLEY, DVM, Dipl. ABVP–Avian

September 2009 • Volume 12 • Number 3

SAUNDERS an imprint of ELSEVIER, Inc.

## W.B. SAUNDERS COMPANY

*A Division of Elsevier Inc.*

1600 John F. Kennedy Boulevard • Suite 1800 • Philadelphia, Pennsylvania 19103-2899

http://www.vetexotic.theclinics.com

**VETERINARY CLINICS OF NORTH AMERICA: EXOTIC ANIMAL PRACTICE Volume 12, Number 3**
**September 2009 ISSN 1094-9194, ISBN-13: 978-1-4377-1282-7, ISBN-10: 1-4377-1282-7**

Editor: John Vassallo; j.vassallo@elsevier.com

*Veterinary Clinics of North America: Exotic Animal Practice* (ISSN 1094-9194) is published in January, May, and September by Elsevier, Inc., 360 Park Avenue South, New York, NY 10010-1710. Subscription prices are $180.00 per year for US individuals, $323.00 per year for US institutions, $94.00 per year for US students and residents, $213.00 per year for Canadian individuals, $381.00 per year for Canadian institutions, $240.00 per year for international individuals, $381.00 per year for international institutions and $120.00 per year for Canadian and foreign students/residents. To receive student/resident rate, orders must be accompanied by name of affiliated institution, date of term, and the *signature* of program/residency coordinator on institution letterhead. Orders will be billed at individual rate until proof of status is received. Foreign air speed delivery is included in all *Clinics* subscription prices. All prices are subject to change without notice. **POSTMASTER:** Send address changes to *Veterinary Clinics of North America: Exotic Animal Practice*, Elsevier Health Sciences Division, Subscription Customer Service, 3251 Riverport Lane, Maryland Heights, MO 63043. **Customer Service: Telephone: 1-800-654-2452** (U.S. and Canada); **1-314-447-8871** (outside U.S. and Canada). **Fax: 1-314-447-8029. E-mail: journalscustomerservice-usa@elsevier.com** (for print support); **journalsonlinesupport-usa@elsevier.com** (for online support).

*Reprints.* For copies of 100 or more of articles in this publication, please contact the Commercial Reprints Department, Elsevier Inc., 360 Park Avenue South, New York, New York 10010-1710. Tel.: (212)-633-3813; Fax: (212)-633-1935; E-mail: reprints@elsevier.com.

*Veterinary Clinics of North America: Exotic Animal Practice* is covered in *MEDLINE/PubMed (Index Medicus)*.

Printed and bound by CPI Group (UK) Ltd, Croydon, CR0 4YY

Transferred to Digital Print 2011

# Contributors

## CONSULTING EDITOR

**AGNES E. RUPLEY, DVM**
Diplomate, American Board of Veterinary Practitioners–Avian Practice; and Director and Chief Veterinarian, All Pets Medical Center, College Station, Texas

## GUEST EDITOR

**LAURA WADE, DVM, DABVP–Avian**
Diplomate, American Board of Veterinary Practitioners–Avian; Specialized Care for Avian and Exotic Pets, Broadway Veterinary Clinic, PC, Lancaster, New York

## AUTHORS

**LORI ARENT, MS**
The Raptor Center, College of Veterinary Medicine, University of Minnesota, St. Paul, Minnesota

**SATHYA K. CHINNADURAI, DVM, MS**
Department of Clinical Sciences, North Carolina State University, College of Veterinary Medicine, Raleigh; and The North Carolina Zoological Park, Asheboro, North Carolina

**LUIS CRUZ-MARTINEZ, DVM**
The Raptor Center, College of Veterinary Medicine, University of Minnesota, St. Paul, Minnesota

**OLGA NICOLAS DE FRANCISCO, DVM**
The Raptor Center, College of Veterinary Medicine, University of Minnesota, St. Paul, Minnesota

**RYAN S. DEVOE, DVM, DACZM, DABVP–Avian**
Diplomate, American College of Zoological Medicine; Diplomate, American Board of Veterinary Practitioners–Avian; and Senior Veterinarian, The North Carolina Zoological Park, Asheboro, North Carolina

**ROBERT J.T. DONELEY, BVSc, FACVSc (Avian Medicine)**
West Toowoomba Veterinary Surgery, Toowoomba, Queensland, Australia

**GERRY M. DORRESTEIN, DVM, PhD, DRDCVP**
Diplomate, Royal Dutch College of Veterinary Pathology; and Diagnostic Pathology Laboratory, Dutch Research Institute for Avian and Exotic Animals (NOIVBD), Veldhoven, The Netherlands

**ROGER HARLIN, DVM**
Southside Dog, Cat and Bird Hospital, Oklahoma City, Oklahoma

**CATHY A. JOHNSON-DELANEY, DVM, DABVP–Avian**
Diplomate, American Board of Veterinary Practitioners–Avian, Eastside Avian and Exotic Animal Medical Center, Kirkland, Washington

**SUSAN KELLEHER, DVM**
Broward Avian and Exotic Animal Hospital, Coral Springs, Florida

**ERIC KLAPHAKE, DVM, DACZM, DABVP–Avian**
Diplomate, American College of Zoological Medicine; Diplomate, American Board of Veterinary Practitioners–Avian; Animal Medical Center, Bozeman; and ZooMontana, Billings, Montana

**ANGELA M. LENNOX, DVM, DABVP–Avian**
Diplomate, American Board of Veterinary Practitioners–Avian; and Avian and Exotic Animal Clinic of Indianapolis, Indianapolis, Indiana

**GLENN H. OLSEN, DVM, MS, PhD**
United States Geological Survey, Patuxent Wildlife Research Center, Laurel, Maryland

**IRENE BUENO PADILLA, DVM**
The Raptor Center, College of Veterinary Medicine, University of Minnesota, St. Paul, Minnesota

**BRIAN PALMEIRO, VMD, DACVD**
Diplomate, American College of Veterinary Dermatology; Pet Fish Doctor, Philadelphia; and Veterinary Referral Center, Malvern, Pennsylvania

**JULIA PONDER, DVM**
The Raptor Center, College of Veterinary Medicine, University of Minnesota, St. Paul, Minnesota

**LAUREN V. POWERS, DVM, DABVP–Avian**
Diplomate, American Board of Veterinary Practitioners–Avian; and Carolina Veterinary Specialists, Avian and Exotic Pet Service, Huntersville, North Carolina

**PATRICK REDIG, DVM, PhD**
The Raptor Center, College of Veterinary Medicine, University of Minnesota, St. Paul, Minnesota

**HELEN E. ROBERTS, DVM**
Aquatic Veterinary Services of WNY, PC, 5 Corners Animal Hospital, Orchard Park, New York

**MARCY J. SOUZA, DVM, MPH, DABVP–Avian**
Diplomate, American Board of Veterinary Practitioners–Avian; and Assistant Professor, Department of Comparative Medicine, University of Tennessee College of Veterinary Medicine, Knoxville, Tennessee

**LAURA WADE, DVM, DABVP–Avian**
Diplomate, American Board of Veterinary Practitioners–Avian; Specialized Care for Avian and Exotic Pets, Broadway Veterinary Clinic, PC, Lancaster, New York

**E. SCOTT WEBER III, VMD, MSc**
Companion Avian and Pet Exotic Animal Service, Department of Aquatic Animal Health, University of California, Medicine and Epidemiology, Davis, California

**MICHELLE WILLETTE, DVM**
The Raptor Center, College of Veterinary Medicine, University of Minnesota, St. Paul, Minnesota

# Contents

> Zoonoses are estimated to make up to 75% of today's emerging infectious diseases. Many of these diseases are carried and transmitted by exotic pets and wildlife. Exotic animal practitioners must be aware of these risks not only to protect their health but also to safeguard the health of staff and clients. This article reviews selected bacterial and parasitic zoonoses associated with exotic animals.

> As wild-caught birds become increasingly rare in aviculture, there is a corresponding decline in the incidence of bacterial and parasitic problems and an increase in the recognition of the importance of maintaining health through better nutrition and husbandry. Nevertheless, the relatively close confines of captivity mean an increased pathogen load in the environment in which companion and aviary parrots live. This increased pathogen load leads to greater exposure of these birds to bacteria and parasites, and consequently a greater risk of infection and disease. This article discusses bacterial and parasitic infections in companion and aviary parrots. It includes the origins, pathogens, diagnosis, treatment, and some of the associated risk factors.

> Many veterinarians are relatively unfamiliar with the passerines. The aviculture, diagnostic procedures, and common diseases, and their treatment have been discussed in several recent publications. Owners of passerines (songbirds) are using veterinary care in increasing numbers as aviculturists recognize the advances in avian medical and surgical treatment of these patients. This article discusses the bacterial and parasitic diseases of passerines.

> Bacterial and parasitic diseases are not uncommon in domestic doves and pigeons. Many of the bacteria and parasites found in columbids do not

cause disease unless the birds are immunocompromised. Often there are underlying viral infections that contribute to illness. This article focuses on some of the more common infections from a practical clinical point of view. Recent updates from the literature are included.

Several bacterial diseases are known to be major mortality factors of waterfowl (ducks, geese, and swans of the family *Anatidae*). Parasitic diseases of waterfowl are quite common but generally are not major mortality factors. However, parasites, if present during other disease outbreaks, can contribute to mortality. From a disease standpoint, the tendency of waterfowl to aggregate in large numbers during postbreeding molt, fall migration, and winter and spring migration can lead to the ready transfer of disease-causing organisms and can lead to high mortality from certain bacterial diseases.

Raptors are susceptible to a broad array of established and emerging bacterial and parasitic diseases, including babesiosis, chlamydiosis, clostridiosis, coccidiosis, cryptosporidiosis, malaria, mycobacteriosis, pasteurellosis, salmonellosis, trichomoniasis, and pododermatitis. Many of these conditions are opportunistic and can be easily managed or averted with proper preventive measures related to captive management, husbandry and diet, and veterinary care. Once infected, treatment must be prompt, appropriate, and judicious. This article examines the significance, diagnosis, management, and prevention of select bacterial and parasitic pathogens of raptors.

Bacterial disease is common in pet rabbits; parasitic disease occurs as well but at a much lower frequency. Of these, bacterial diseases of the respiratory tract and dental structures are seen most commonly in practice. Successful treatment depends on positive diagnosis of the disease process and causative agent. This article focuses on the more common bacterial and parasitic diseases encountered in clinical practice.

The domestic ferret, *Mustela putorius furo*, is a popular companion animal and is used in biomedical research. When compared with other companion mammals, primary bacterial and parasitic infections are less common in domestic ferrets. In countries such as the United States, pet ferrets are generally kept indoors, and the risk for exposure to primary bacterial and parasitic infectious agents is low. Companion, breeding, and working ferrets are commonly kept outdoors in other parts of the world, placing them at comparatively greater risk for exposure to infectious diseases. This article discusses clinical signs, diagnosis, and treatment of bacterial and parasitic diseases of ferrets.

Cathy A. Johnson-Delaney

Parasites of captive nonhuman primates generally are more limited than those reported for field studies and in wild-caught primates. Captive primates include those in zoos, laboratory animal facilities, and private collections or pets. Primates kept indoors generally have few parasites, and those are easily eliminated. Outdoor housing presents problems in breaking life cycles of parasites, particularly those with invertebrate intermediate hosts. Decontamination of soils and substrates also makes total elimination of parasites nearly impossible. For outdoor-housed primates and those in social settings, control can be achieved through regular examination and appropriate administration of antiparasite medication. Because many of the parasites have zoonotic potential, practitioners must be vigilant and educate caretakers about the parasite life cycle and sanitation procedures.

Sathya K. Chinnadurai and Ryan S. DeVoe

Bacterial, fungal, and parasitic diseases in reptiles are occasionally caused by primary pathogens, but often are the result of an immunocompromising condition, such as inappropriate temperatures, humidity, or enclosure hygiene. Treating bacterial and fungal diseases usually requires addressing the predisposing husbandry deficiency. Recent comprehensive publications list many reported bacterial, fungal, and parasitic pathogens. This article discusses general methods for diagnosing and treating infectious diseases, and discusses certain diseases in relation to body systems. Special attention is given to recently reported diseases.

Eric Klaphake

Whether in private practice or in a zoologic setting, veterinarians of the exotic animal persuasion are asked to work on amphibians. Veterinarians are able to evaluate amphibians thoroughly for medical issues, with infectious diseases at the forefront. Until quite recently, many infectious diseases were unknown or even misdiagnosed as being caused by opportunistic secondary organisms. Although *Batrachochytrium dendrobates* and viral diseases are in the forefront of research for amphibians, parasitic and bacterial diseases often present secondarily and, occasionally, even as the primary cause. Full diagnostic workups, when possible,

## THE CLINICS ARE NOW AVAILABLE ONLINE!

Access your subscription at:
**www.theclinics.com**

# Preface

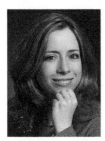

Laura Wade, DVM, DABVP–Avian
*Guest Editor*

Ever since *Veterinary Clinics of North America: Exotic Animal Practice* began publishing the year after I graduated from veterinary school, I have looked forward to each issue, which I read cover-to-cover and referenced often over the years. Back in 1998, I was already on track to work with exotic species, and I remember being especially pleased that the publishers of *Veterinary Clinics of North America* decided to devote a whole new burgundy series to exotics rather than an occasional article in the robin egg blue small animal series. Since that first issue on critical care, a new edition has been published every 4 months, and there remain topics still not covered. So, 33 issues later, and with 21 inches (53 cm) of shelf space already devoted to my growing burgundy library, I am pleased to finish out the 2009 editorial year by moving from avid reader to guest editor.

Bacterial and parasitic diseases are encountered on a daily basis in exotic animal practice, and there has been a flood of new information in the literature in recent years. It is daunting pairing two diverse topics for a platform such as this, but I think this issue provides an excellent review of important and emerging bacterial and parasitic diseases likely to be encountered when treating special species. As each previous issue before it, this will be a great resource for busy practitioners, veterinary students, and those studying for the American Board of Veterinary Practitioners.

This issue brings together a diverse group of authors from three continents and includes varied discipline specialists from university, zoological, research, and private practice settings. Unexpectedly, the rodent section was unable to be covered, creating an unfortunate gap in this issue. There is, however, a unique section on bacterial and parasitic zoonoses. Aside from excellent updates on rabbits and reptiles, this issue also reports on five avian families and some groups infrequently covered in many other exotic animal references (primates, amphibians, fish, and invertebrates). Additionally, this issue includes perhaps the most comprehensive review of bacterial and parasitic diseases of ferrets I have encountered to date. Several authors have provided a number of pictures and summary tables that highlight important aspects of the organisms and diseases they cause.

One of the advantages of writing an article or editing other's manuscripts is the opportunity to learn about the subject more thoroughly than merely reading the

Vet Clin Exot Anim 12 (2009) xi–xii
doi:10.1016/j.cvex.2009.07.003
1094-9194/09/$ – see front matter © 2009 Elsevier Inc. All rights reserved.

finished product. Another advantage of working on a project like this with a group of respected experts in the field is the opportunity to expand the network of colleagues. I had the pleasure of working with Roger Harlin on the columbiform section. Dr. Harlin is from the pigeon capital of the United States (Oklahoma City, Oklahoma) and brings a practical perspective from his many years of pigeon practice. I enjoyed providing supplemental material and literature updates for this section.

I thank Agnes Rupley for considering me for my first editing experience. It has been both a pleasure and a challenge working on this issue. Each of the authors and I have busy practices and many other writing, speaking, and life commitments. I thank all of the authors for their expansive donation of time and effort for their article contributions. My extreme thanks goes to editor John Vassallo, for his patience and perseverance with the many delays this issue experienced along the way.

Laura Wade, DVM, DABVP–Avian
Specialized Care for Avian and Exotic Pets
Broadway Veterinary Clinic, PC
5915 Broadway Street
Lancaster, NY 14086, USA

E-mail address:
buffalobirdnerd@gmail.com (L. Wade)

# Bacterial and Parasitic Zoonoses of Exotic Pets

Marcy J. Souza, DVM, MPH, DABVP–Avian

**KEYWORDS**

- Zoonoses • Exotic pets • Nontraditional pets
- Disease prevention

Zoonoses are estimated to make up approximately 75% of today's emerging infectious diseases.[1] Many of these zoonoses are associated with wildlife or exotic pets. Human cases, including tularemia from a hamster[2] and salmonellosis from a hedgehog,[3] reinforce the notion that veterinarians must not only be aware of zoonoses but also be ready to educate pet owners about the risks associated with exotic pet ownership. This article provides an overview of selected bacterial and parasitic zoonoses associated with common exotic pets (**Tables 1** and **2**).

## BACTERIAL ZOONOSES
### Salmonellosis

Salmonellosis in humans can be caused by many different serotypes of *Salmonella* (most cases are due to *S enterica* but recent outbreaks of *S bongori* have also been reported).[4–6] *Salmonella* classification has been revised to consist of two species, *S enterica* and *S bongori*, and thousands of serotypes. Serotypes are characterized by their heat-stable somatic antigens (O), heat-labile capsular antigens (Vi), and flagellar antigens (H).[7] *Salmonella* can be a normal intestinal inhabitant of humans and many animals with no clinical signs present; exposure occurs from ingestion of contaminated food or water, or feces. Approximately 1.4 million human *Salmonella* infections occur in the United States annually; most of these infections are food borne, but some are acquired from contact with animals.[8] Many people do not develop disease when exposed to *Salmonella*; however, others may develop diarrhea, abdominal cramps, and fever within 12 to 72 hours of exposure. Most recover within a week without treatment, but the disease can progress to sepsis leading to organ damage and possibly death. Diagnosis of non-typhoid salmonellosis in humans is made with a positive fecal culture and treatment entails primarily fluid replacement. Antibiotics are typically only given in severe cases. A few individuals who recover from salmonellosis may develop Reiter syndrome, a condition that involves inflammation of the conjunctiva, joints, and urogenital system.[4]

Department of Comparative Medicine, University of Tennessee College of Veterinary Medicine, Knoxville, TN 37996
E-mail address: msouza@utk.edu

Vet Clin Exot Anim 12 (2009) 401–415
doi:10.1016/j.cvex.2009.06.003
1094-9194/09/$ – see front matter © 2009 Elsevier Inc. All rights reserved.

**Table 1**
Selected bacterial zoonotic pathogens of exotic pets

| Pathogen | Exotic Pets Involved in Transmission | Route of Transmission | Clinical Signs in Animals | Clinical Signs in Humans | References |
|---|---|---|---|---|---|
| *Salmonella enterica*, numerous serotypes | Reptiles, amphibians, rodents, hedgehogs, sugar gliders | Ingestion | Often asymptomatic; GI disease; osteomyelitis, sepsis, dermatitis | Diarrhea (possibly bloody), abdominal cramps, fever, sepsis | 3–17,19 |
| *Mycobacterium* spp | Fish, reptiles, birds, nonhuman primates | Entry into skin wound; ingestion; inhalation | GI disease; respiratory disease; cutaneous lesions | Respiratory disease; cutaneous lesions | 4,22–34 |
| *Chlamydophila psittaci* | Birds, especially psittaciformes & columbiformes | Inhalation; possibly ingestion | Asymptomatic; respiratory disease; lethargy | Flulike symptoms; pneumonia; endocarditis | 4,35–39 |
| *Leptospira* spp | Rodents | Ingestion (often of soil, food, or water contaminated with infected urine); contact with infected tissues | Asymptomatic | Flu-like symptoms; liver & kidney failure | 4,67 |
| *Francisella tularensis* | Rabbits, rodents | Ticks; contact with tissue of infected animal | Asymptomatic; diarrhea; neurologic signs; death | Ulceroglandular form; septicemia; oropharyngeal form; pneumonic form | 2,4,68 |

| Organism | Host | Route of transmission | Signs in animals | Signs in humans | References |
| --- | --- | --- | --- | --- | --- |
| *Yersinia pestis* | Rodents | Flea bite; inhalation or ingestion of organism from infected carcass | Asymptomatic; lymphadenomegaly & subcutaneous hemorrhages; peracute death | Bubonic, pneumonic, septicemic forms | 4,69,70 |
| *Bartonella* spp | Rodents, felids | Flea or tick bite; scratch from infected animal | Typically asymptomatic | Fever, lymphadenopathy, lethargy, endocarditis, bacillary angiomatosis | 4,71,72 |
| *Pasteurella multocida* | Rabbits, rodents, felids | Animal bite; wound contamination | Asymptomatic; respiratory disease; abscesses; neurologic disease | Bite wound infection; bacterial contamination to cuts and abrasions | 4,73 |
| *Streptobacillus moniliformis* and *Spirillum minus* | Rodents, possibly others (felids) | Animal bite; ingestion of food or water contaminated with feces or urine; direct contact with ocular or nasal discharge of rat | Typically asymptomatic | "Rat bite fever"; flulike symptoms; complications including endocarditis, pericarditis, pneumonia, meningitis may result if not treated | 4,74,75 |
| *Aeromonas* spp | Fish, amphibians | Ingestion; wound contamination | Skin ulcers; raised scales; coelomic distention; erythema | Wound infection; gastroenteritis | 23,76 |

**Table 2**
Selected parasitic zoonotic pathogens of exotic pets

| Pathogen | Exotic Pets Involved in Transmission | Route of Transmission | Clinical Signs in Animals | Clinical Signs in Humans | References |
|---|---|---|---|---|---|
| Giardia intestinalis | Potentially any mammal (rodents, ferrets) | Ingestion of cyst | Diarrhea, typically no blood in feces or fever | Diarrhea, typically no blood in feces or fever | 4,41–46 |
| Cryptosporidium parvum | Potentially all mammals (rabbits) | Ingestion of oocysts | Watery diarrhea; reduced appetite; straining to defecate; weight loss | Watery diarrhea; nausea; vomiting; abdominal cramps; mild fever; headache | 4,42,47–54 |
| Toxoplasma gondii | Felids (fecal shedding); other vertebrates (bradyzoites in tissue) | Ingestion of sporulated oocysts from felid feces; ingestion of bradyzoites in raw or undercooked tissue | Felids typically asymptomatic; neurologic and ophthalmic lesions; pneumonia; peracute death; marsupials particularly susceptible | Most asymptomatic; flulike symptoms; severe neurologic disease in congenital infections; abortion | 4,54–58 |
| Baylisascaris procyonis | Raccoons | Ingestion of infective eggs from environment | Raccoons: gastrointestinal signs with heavy infections; neurologic, ocular and visceral larval migrans in others | Most asymptomatic; neurologic, ocular & visceral larval migrans | 59–63 |
| Sarcoptes scabiei | Most animals have their own subspecies | Direct contact with infected animal | Pruritus; scales; crusts; erythema, alopecia | Tiny, red bumps; pruritus; infection typically limited with S scabiei subspecies other than hominis | 4,77 |
| Encephalitozoon cuniculi | Rabbits, rodents | Possibly exposure to infected urine; organism is environmentally resistant | Neurologic disease; renal disease | Variable presentation; respiratory, neurologic, GI, renal, ocular | 78,79 |

### Reptiles and amphibians

There is no shortage of literature demonstrating the link between certain species of reptiles and human salmonellosis.[9-14] One study suggested that approximately 74,000 cases of human salmonellosis associated with reptile and amphibian exposure occur annually in the United States.[15] Most infected reptiles are asymptomatic and because shedding of *Salmonella* organisms can be intermittent, all reptiles should be assumed positive and managed and handled accordingly regardless of fecal culture results. In 1975, the US Food and Drug Administration (FDA) ruled it illegal to sell viable turtle eggs or turtles with a carapace length less than 4 inches. Exceptions were made for legitimate educational and scientific institutions. This law led to a drastic reduction in the number of cases of salmonellosis associated with turtle ownership. Despite the ban on the sale of turtles, outbreaks do still occur because of the distribution of pet turtles. In 2007, members of congress from Louisiana introduced bills and amendments that would end the FDA's ban on the sale of turtles. In 2007 to 2008, a multistate outbreak of human salmonellosis associated with exposure to turtles occurred; 103 cases from 33 states were reported.[10] Removing the ban could lead to a significant increase in the number of reptile-associated cases of human salmonellosis.[16] Clients must also be educated about the risks associated with ownership of other reptiles, such as lizards and snakes.[13,14]

### Rodents

Cases of rodent-associated human salmonellosis have been reported.[8,17] The most recent outbreak involved 28 patients and pet hamsters distributed throughout 10 states from a common source; *Salmonella enterica* serotype Typhimurium was isolated from both hamsters and humans.[8] Some animals showed clinical signs, including diarrhea, lethargy, and rough hair coat; these clinical signs are similar to "wet tail" which frequently affects hamsters and is caused by *Lawsonia intracellularis*.[18] Wet tail is often used to describe diarrhea in young hamsters and disease often occurs shortly after transport to a pet store or new home. Hamsters or other rodents that have diarrhea should have fecal cultures performed to determine if *Salmonella* species are present.

### Hedgehogs

*Salmonella* serotype Tilene has been isolated from African pygmy hedgehogs and associated with clinical disease in a 10-year-old child.[3] *Salmonella* serotype Typhimurium was isolated from wild hedgehogs in Norway and isolates were identical to those identified in human cases of salmonellosis.[19] The prevalence of *Salmonella* carriage in pet hedgehogs is unknown.

Recommendations for prevention of zoonotic salmonellosis:
> Prevention of salmonellosis is best accomplished by reducing exposure to feces from infected animals.
> Gloves should be worn when cleaning enclosures and caging should not be cleaned in kitchens or bathrooms.
> Reptiles should not be allowed to soak in bathtubs or showers used by humans.
> Thorough hand washing should be performed after handling any animal, especially those potentially infected with *Salmonella*.

### Mycobacteriosis

Various *Mycobacterium* species and subspecies are responsible for disease in humans and animals, and clinical signs vary depending on which species or subspecies is present. Transmission of *Mycobacterium* sp can occur through aerosolization and inhalation of the organisms, direct contact with infected animals or environments, or ingestion of the organism. Incubation and development of disease are variable. Tuberculosis, a severe respiratory disease caused by *M tuberculosis*, is the most common bacterial cause of human deaths worldwide.[4] Tuberculosis can be difficult to treat and many multidrug–resistant strains of *M tuberculosis* have evolved. Historically, transmission of *M bovis* in unpasteurized dairy products commonly led to disease in humans, but with improvements in food safety regulations, cases are now rarely reported in North America.[4] Recent studies have suggested a link between *M avium paratuberculosis*, the causative agent of Johne disease in cattle, and Crohn's disease in humans.[20,21] Numerous *Mycobacterium* spp have been associated with exotic pets, including fish, reptiles, birds, and various mammals.

### Fish

Mycobacteriosis is a common disease of fish and is usually caused by *M marinum*, *M fortuitum*, or less commonly *M chelonei*.[22,23] Fish can be long-time carriers of *Mycobacterium* spp before showing clinical signs When clinical signs do appear, they include skin ulcerations, loss of scales, poor body condition, distention of the coelomic cavity, and exophthalmia.[24] Granulomas can also affect the liver, kidneys, and spleen.[25] Regardless of whether clinical signs are present, infected animals shed the organism into the environment through feces, infected tissues (including dead animals), and skin ulcerations.[24] In the United States, the approximate incidence rate of confirmed *M marinum* infections in humans is 0.27 cases per 100,000 inhabitants.[26] Humans are typically exposed when placing forelimbs into fish tanks, and the bacterium can enter the subcutaneous tissue through small cuts or abrasions in the skin. Infections in humans typically occur on the extremities and result in either ulcerative or raised granulomas.[27] Other names for this disease are fish tank granuloma and swimming pool granuloma. Although most infections are limited to the forearms, some can lead to systemic disease, especially in immune-compromised individuals. All individuals who have clinical disease should seek medical advice. Definitive diagnosis in humans is made with culture, histopathology, or PCR, and treatment should include long-term antibiotics, such as doxycycline, clarithromycin, and rifampicin.[27,28]

Recommendations for prevention of zoonotic mycobacteriosis from fish:

People should wear gloves that extend to the elbows to reduce potential exposure to *Mycobacterium* spp while cleaning filled fish tanks.

Water should not be disposed of where cutaneous inoculation or ingestion of *Mycobacterium* organisms could occur (sinks, bathtubs).

### Birds

Mycobacterial infections in birds are most commonly caused by *M avium avium* or *M genavense*, and disease typically affects the gastrointestinal tract and liver leading to a wasting syndrome.[29,30] These organisms are ubiquitous in the environment and can lead to exposure of both humans and animals.[31] A recent report detailed the isolation of *M avium hominissuis* (a proposed but not officially recognized subspecies name) in an Amazon parrot; *M avium hominissuis* is not a typical pathogen of birds but has been shown to infect humans, especially those who are immunocompromised.[29] Owners should be advised that there is potential for a pet bird to contract mycobacteriosis from an infected owner. Mycobacterial infections in humans typically result in either dermatologic or respiratory disease.[31] Although the exact risk for acquiring a mycobacterial infection from a pet bird is unknown, the morbidity and mortality associated with infection in humans warrants steps to avoid exposure.[30]

Recommendations for prevention of zoonotic mycobacteriosis from birds:

Euthanasia should be recommended for birds that have confirmed cases of mycobacteriosis, regardless of which species of *Mycobacterium* is present.

If owners will not euthanize an infected animal, the bird must be placed in permanent, strict quarantine. Multidrug treatment protocols are published.

Potentially exposed animals should be monitored every 6 to 12 weeks for infection. Monitoring may include acid-fast staining of fecal samples, complete blood counts, and histopathology of liver or spleen biopsies.

Cages should be designed for easy disinfection; numerous compounds, including alcohol and aldehydes, have been shown to have antimycobacterial activity.

Humans should take precautions, such as wearing gloves, masks, and gowns, when cleaning cages of infected or potentially infected animals.

### Nonhuman primates

Humans are the typical reservoir of *M tuberculosis*, but nonhuman primates can harbor the organism and develop disease. Clinical signs in nonhuman primates include weight loss, lethargy, coughing, and pneumonia.[32] The prevalence of *M tuberculosis* in nonhuman primates is low, and infection is typically due to exposure to an infected human.[33] Although documented cases of transmission from a nonhuman primate to a human are rare, the severity of infection in humans warrants preventive measures.[32]

Recommendations for prevention of zoonotic mycobacteriosis from non-human primates:

All nonhuman primates should be screened regularly for mycobacteriosis.

Initial screening should include a series of three intradermal injections (usually in the eyelid) of an appropriate strength of old tuberculin. Positive reactions can result from infection with *M tuberculosis* or other non-tuberculosis *Mycobacterium* species.

Suspect animals should have further testing performed, including chest radiographs, gastric and tracheal washes for mycobacterial culture, and complete blood counts.

Animals established in a collection should be tested annually with an intradermal injection of old tuberculin at the time of physical examinations.

Human caretakers should be screened for infection and precautions, such as gloves, masks, and gowns, worn to reduce exposure.

### Hedgehogs

One case of *Mycobacterium marinum* has been reported in a pet European hedgehog.[34] Although no reports of mycobacteriosis have been reported in African pygmy hedgehogs, which are more commonly kept as pets in the United States, care should be taken when handling these animals.

Recommendations for prevention of zoonotic mycobacteriosis from hedgehogs:

Gardening gloves should be worn to prevent injuries from the spines, which could introduce pathogens subcutaneously.

### Psittacosis

*Chlamydophila psittaci*, an intracellular bacterium, can cause disease in birds and humans. The National Association of State Public Health Veterinarians has published a document detailing the disease, diagnosis, treatment and prevention of *C psittaci* infections in humans and birds.[35] The disease in humans has numerous names, including chlamydophilosis, ornithosis, and parrot fever. Between 2002 and 2007, 91 cases of psittacosis were reported to the Centers for Disease Control (CDC); however, this is likely an underrepresentation of the true number of cases.[36] Clinical signs in humans include flulike symptoms, pneumonia, and even death if left untreated.[35,37] C psittaci is most commonly associated with parrots, but has also been isolated from many other birds, including columbiformes.[38] Most infected birds are asymptomatic but may show respiratory illness, lethargy, diarrhea, and biliverdinuria.[35] Birds shed the organism in respiratory secretions and feces. Despite a longstanding awareness of this disease, C psittaci still presents a public health risk.[39] In December 2007, a large chain pet store suspended all bird sales in more than 700 stores in 46 states after C psittaci caused illness in at least 22 birds. All birds were treated with medicated feed and employees were instructed to wear protective masks, gloves, and gowns when entering quarantined areas.[40] Numerous steps can be taken to reduce the risk for psittacosis.[35]

Recommendations for prevention of zoonotic chlamydiosis from birds:
Do not purchase birds that appear to be sick (fluffed, lethargic, anorexic).
Reduce stress in newly acquired birds by providing a quiet environment (reducing exposure to other pets, such as barking dogs and stalking cats), appropriate amounts of time for sleep, and appropriate food sources that the bird recognizes as food. Some birds that have been raised on seed diets may not recognize pelleted diets as food and therefore can lose significant amounts of weight.
All new birds should be examined immediately by a veterinarian and then placed in strict quarantine for a minimum of 30 days. Appropriate diagnostic testing should be performed (serology, antigen detection, complete blood count).
Caretakers should take precautions to reduce risk for exposure, including wearing protective gloves, masks, and gowns.
Appropriate disinfectants, such as quaternary ammonium compounds and dilute bleach, should be used when cleaning cages and environments. Use these disinfectants in well-ventilated areas because they can be respiratory irritants for humans and animals.
In an outbreak, affected birds should be kept separate from healthy birds. Healthy birds should be cared for first, and then sick birds can be treated.

## PARASITIC ZOONOSES
### Giardiasis

*Giardia intestinalis* (also known as *G lamblia* or *G duodenalis*) is most commonly associated with disease in humans and has been reported in ferrets and rodents.[41–43] Approximately 20,000 cases of human giardiasis were reported to the CDC annually from 2003 to 2005.[44] The classification of *Giardia* species is evolving and the zoonotic potential of some species, including *Giardia psittaci*, is unknown.[42] *G psittaci* is most commonly found in cockatiels and budgerigars.[45] Cysts are intermittently passed in the feces of an infected animal and are immediately infective; only a small number of cysts must be ingested to cause disease.[46] Clinical signs in humans and animals are similar and include severe diarrhea, cramps, gas, and fatigue. There is not typically blood in the stool or a fever.[4] Diagnosis of infection is typically made with light microscopy; PCR and indirect immunofluorescence are available but infrequently used because of cost.[42] Additionally, a SNAP Giardia test (IDEXX Laboratories, Inc.) is available for use in dogs and cats but has not been validated for use in exotic pets. Furazolidone is the only approved treatment of human giardiasis in the United States;

however, metronidazole is frequently used to treat infections. Numerous medications have been used to treat infections in animals, including metronidazole, fenbendazole, and albendazole.[42]

### Cryptosporidiosis

*Cryptosporidium parvum* is most commonly associated with clinical disease in humans, and approximately 6000 cases of human cryptosporidiosis were reported to the CDC in 2006.[47] Human cases are typically associated with recreational water use, but can also occur after exposure to infected animals. Infective oocysts are passed in the feces of an infected person or animal; infection occurs after ingestion of a very small number of oocysts that have contaminated the environment, food, or water. Some humans and animals can be asymptomatic but others may have watery diarrhea, decreased appetite, weight loss, and vomiting.[4] Numerous reviews are available detailing human cryptosporidiosis associated with animal exposure, and most commonly the humans have been exposed to ruminants.[48–50] *C parvum* can potentially be carried and spread by any mammal and infections in pet rabbits[51] and hedgehogs[52] have been reported. Cryptosporidiosis was also reported in ferrets, but the species of *Cryptosporidium* was not stated.[53] Numerous other species of *Cryptosporium* have been identified, including *C muris* (rodents), *C wrairi* (guinea pigs), *C serpentensis* (reptiles), and *C molnari* (fish); however, none have been shown to be zoonotic at this point.[42] Diagnosis of infection is typically made with light microscopy sometimes with the use of various stains and concentrating protocols; ELISA, immunofluorescence, and PCR are also available but are cost prohibitive and not clinically practical.[42] Disease in humans is typically self-limiting, but nitazoxanide is now approved for treatment in the United States. Currently, there is no reliable, definitive treatment of animals infected with *Cryptosporidium*.[42]

### Toxoplasmosis

Felids are the definitive host for *Toxoplasma gondii* and only felids shed oocysts in their feces. Non-felids can become infected by ingesting sporulated oocysts from the environment or by ingesting bradyzoites contained in raw or undercooked tissue from an infected animal. Additionally, if a human or animal becomes infected while pregnant, the organism can cross the placenta, infect the fetus, and cause abortion or significant disease in the fetus. Virtually all vertebrate species are susceptible to infection with *T gondii*, but marsupials are particularly prone to developing severe disease and infections are often fatal.[54,55] Felids are typically asymptomatic but can develop pneumonia, hepatitis, or neurologic signs. Approximately 60 million people in the United States are estimated to be infected with *T gondii* and most never have clinical signs related to infection.[4] Toxoplasmosis that is acquired after birth in a healthy person may lead to mild clinical signs, including flulike symptoms. Infections in immunocompromised individuals can be more severe and include central neurologic and ophthalmic lesions. Approximately 3000 cases of human congenital toxoplasmosis occur annually in the United States; congenital cases are the most severe and can lead to mental retardation, hydrocephalus, convulsions, deafness, blindness, or cerebral palsy.[4] Some studies have suggested a link between *T gondii* infection and schizophrenia; however, the validity of such studies has been questioned.[56–58] Fecal examinations can be performed on felids to determine if oocysts are being shed; however, felids typically only shed oocysts for approximately 1 to 3 weeks after initial infection.[54] Serology or histopathology can be used for diagnosis in non-felid species. Treatment of symptomatic animals that have toxoplasmosis may include clindamycin, pyrimethamine, and sulfonamides.[54]

## Baylisascaris

The raccoon (*Procyon lotor*) is the definitive host of the nematode *Baylisascaris procyonis*. Although raccoons are not commonly kept as pets, the severity of this zoonotic disease in humans warrants discussion. Most raccoons do not have clinical signs associated with infection unless they have a high intestinal parasite burden; younger raccoons are more commonly infected and shed more eggs into the environment than older animals.[59] Large numbers of environmentally resistant eggs are shed in feces and become infective to humans and other animals after 2 to 4 weeks.[60] Historically, prevalence levels in raccoons have been highest in the northeast, midwest, and west coast of the United States, but recent studies suggest that *B procyonis* may be an emerging disease in the southeastern United States.[61,62] Human infection occurs after ingestion of infective eggs from the environment and risk factors for developing disease include (1) contact with raccoons, their feces, or a contaminated environment; and (2) geophagia.[60] Human cases of *B procyonis* infection most commonly affect children and developmentally delayed individuals and have occurred in regions where prevalence is highest in raccoons. Most cases of *B procyonis* in humans are likely asymptomatic, but clinical signs are associated with migration of the larva through various tissues, including the central nervous system, visceral organs, and eyes. Two human cases were recently reported in New York; one case involved ocular larval migrans in a young adult and the other involved neural larval migrans in an infant.[63] Infections in raccoons can be easily diagnosed through fecal examination and then treated with most anthelmintics. Diagnosing *B procyonis* infections in humans is challenging and a combination of serology, brain biopsies, and neuroimaging are typically used.[60] Because of the difficulty of diagnosis, the actual prevalence of infection in humans is unknown. Treatment of humans with clinical signs includes anthelmintics, such as albendazole, and corticosteroids. Regardless of treatment, patients who have neural larval migrans have a grave prognosis for recovery.[60] Owners of pet raccoons should be strongly cautioned of the zoonotic risks associated with *B procyonis*.

Recommendations for prevention of zoonotic baylisascariasis from raccoons:

  Prevention of infection with many zoonotic parasites can be accomplished by eliminating exposure to feces of potentially infected animals and washing hands thoroughly after cleaning or handling animals.

  Owners should be made aware of potential parasites acquired through fecal exposure.

  Do not eat or drink potentially contaminated food or water. Any water collected while hiking or camping should be treated appropriately (filtration, UV light pens) to kill pathogenic parasites.

  Children should not clean up after potentially infected animals and gloves should be worn by adults while cleaning.

  Do not clean caging or litter boxes in the kitchen or bathroom. Feces should be placed into a plastic bag that is then closed and disposed of in the garbage. Flushing potentially contaminated feces is not recommended because standard water treatment procedures may not kill some parasites, such as *Cryptosporidium parvum*.

  Raccoons should be dewormed initially and then according to potential exposure to *B procyonis* (going outside).

### RISKS AND PREVENTION

Undoubtedly, risks associated with pet ownership exist, and studies have been published describing zoonoses and the risks associated with animal contact and the ownership of pets.[64–66] Unfortunately, these studies are based on literature searches and often do not differentiate risks associated with the different types of nontraditional pets. Livestock, such as cattle and goats, along with rabbits and hamsters, are considered nontraditional pets in one recent article.[65] Without differentiating the various types of nontraditional pets, it is unreasonable to make broad statements regarding risk for zoonoses. Finally, few prospective studies have been published evaluating the risk associated with a specific zoonosis in a specific species of animal. Recommendations are often made solely on the basis of case reports and literature searches. Prospective research needs to be performed to develop accurate, justified recommendations regarding the ownership of exotic pets. Until specific, prospective research is available, numerous steps, as outlined in this article, can be taken to reduce the risk for contracting a zoonotic disease from an exotic pet.

## ACKNOWLEDGMENT

The author thanks Drs. David Bemis, John New, and Sharon Patton for review of this manuscript.

## REFERENCES

1. Taylor LH, Latham SM, Woolhouse ME. Risk factors for human disease emergence. Philos Trans R Soc Lond B Biol Sci 2001;356:983–9.
2. Centers for Disease Control and Prevention (CDC). Brief report. Tularemia associated with a hamster bite – Colorado, 2004. MMWR Morb Mortal Wkly Rep 2005; 53:1202–3.
3. Centers for Disease Control and Prevention (CDC). African pygmy hedgehog-associated salmonellosis – Washington, 1994. MMWR Morb Mortal Wkly Rep 1995;44:462–3.
4. Colville JL, Berryhill DL. Handbook of zoonoses, identification and prevention. St. Louis (MO): Mosby Elsevier; 2007.
5. Giammanco GM, Pignato S, Mammina C, et al. Persistant endemicity of *Salmonella bongori* 48:$z_{35}$:- in Southern Italy: molecular characterization of human, animal, and environmental isolates. J Clin Microbiol 2002;40:3502–5.
6. Foti M, Daidone A, Aleo A, et al. *Salmonella bongori* 48:$z_{35}$:- in migratory birds, Italy. Emerg Infect Dis 2009;15:502–3.
7. Mitchell MA. Salmonella: diagnostic methods for reptiles. In: Mader DR, editor. Reptile medicine and surgery. St. Louis (MO): Saunders Elsevier; 2006. p. 900–5.
8. Swanson SJ, Snider C, Braden CR, et al. Multidrug-resistant *Salmonella enterica* serotype Typhimurium associated with pet rodents. N Engl J Med 2007;356:21–8.
9. Johnson-Delaney CA. Reptile zoonoses and threats to public health. In: Mader DR, editor. Reptile medicine and surgery. St. Louis (MO): Saunders Elsevier; 2006. p. 1017–30.
10. Centers for Disease Control and Prevention (CDC). Multistate outbreak of human Salmonella infections associated with exposure to turtles – United States, 2007–2008. MMWR Morb Mortal Wkly Rep 2008;57:69–72.
11. Centers for Disease Control and Prevention (CDC). Reptile-associated Salmonellosis – selected states, 1998–2002. MMWR Morb Mortal Wkly Rep 2003;52: 1206–9.
12. Centers for Disease Control and Prevention (CDC). Turtle-associated Salmonellosis in humans – United States, 2006–2007. MMWR Morb Mortal Wkly Rep 2007;56:649–52.

13. Burnham BR, Atchley DH, DeFusco RP, et al. Prevalence of fecal shedding of *Salmonella* organisms among captive green iguanas and potential public health implications. J Am Vet Med Assoc 1998;213:28–50.

14. Woodward DL, Khakhria R, Johnson WM. Human salmonellosis associated with exotic pets. J Clin Microbiol 1997;35:2786–90.

15. Mermin J, Hutwagner L, Vugia D, et al. Reptiles, amphibians, and human *Salmonella* infection: a population-based, case-controlled study. Clin Infect Dis 2004; 38(Suppl 3):S253–61.

16. Cima G. Turtle producers fighting in the courts and Capitol to sell hatchlings. J Am Vet Med Assoc 2008;233:1378–9.

17. Fish NA, Fletch AL, Butler WE. Family outbreak of salmonellosis due to contact with guinea pigs. Can Med Assoc J 1968;99:418–20.

18. Donnelly TM. Disease problems of small rodents. In: Quesenberry KE, Carpenter JW, editors. Ferrets, rabbits, and rodents clinical medicine and surgery. St. Louis (MO): Saunders; 2004. p. 299–315.

19. Handeland K, Refsum T, Johansen BS, et al. Prevalence of *Salmonella* Typhimurium infection in Norwegian hedgehog populations associated with two human disease outbreaks. Epidemiol Infect 2002;128:523–7.

20. Uzoigwe JC, Khaitsa ML, Gibbs PS. Epidemiological evidence for *Mycobacterium avium* subspecies *paratuberculosis* as a cause of Crohn's disease. Epidemiol Infect 2007;135:1057–68.

21. Sechi LA, Scanu AM, Molicotti P, et al. Detection and isolation of *Mycobacterium avium* subspecies *paratuberculosis* from intestinal mucosal biopsies of patients with and without Crohn's disease in Sardinia. Am J Gastroenterol 2005;100: 1529–36.

22. Noga EJ. Fish disease, diagnosis and treatment. Ames (IA): Iowa State University Press; 2000.

23. Lowry T, Smith SA. Aquatic zoonoses associated with food, bait, ornamental, and tropical fish. J Am Vet Med Assoc 2007;231:876–80.

24. Smith SA. Mycobacterial infections in pet fish. Semin Avian Exotic Pet Med 1997; 6:40–5.

25. Stamm LM, Brown EJ. *Mycobacterium marinum*: the generalization and specialization of a pathogenic mycobacterium. Microbes Infect 2004;6:1418–28.

26. Sciacca-Kirby J, Kim E, Jaffer S. *Mycobacterium marinum* infection of the skin 2002. Available at: http://emedicine.medscape.com/article/1105126-overview. Accessed May 28, 2009.

27. Petrini B. *Mycobacterium marinum*: ubiquitous agent of waterborne granulomatous skin infections. Eur J Clin Microbiol Infect Dis 2006;25:609–13.

28. Fabroni C, Buggiani G, Lotti T. Therapy of environmental mycobacterial infections. Dermatol Ther 2008;21:162–6.

29. Shitaye EJ, Grymova V, Grym M, et al. *Mycobacterium avium* subsp. *hominissuis* infection in a pet parrot. Emerg Infect Dis 2009;4:617–9.

30. Pollack CG. Implications of mycobacteria in clinical disorders. In: Harrison GJ, Lightfoot TL, editors. Clinical avian medicine, vol. II. Palm Beach (FL): Spix Publishing Inc.; 2006. p. 681–90.

31. Jorn KS, Thompson KM, Larson JM, et al. Polly can make you sick: pet bird-associated diseases. Cleve Clin J Med 2009;76:235–43.

32. Joslin JO. Other primates excluding great apes. In: Fowler ME, Miller RE, editors. Zoo and wild animal medicine. St Louis (MO): Saunders; 2003. p. 346–81.

33. Montali RJ, Mikota SK, Cheng LI. Mycobacterium tuberculosis in zoo and wildlife species. Rev Sci Tech 2001;20:291–303.

34. Tappe JP, Weitzman I, Liu S, et al. Systemic *Mycobacterium marinum* infection in a European hedgehog. J Am Vet Med Assoc 1983;183:1280–1.
35. National Association of State Public Health Veterinarians. Compendium of measures to control *Chlamydophila psittaci* infection among humans (psittacosis) and pet birds (avian chlamydiosis) 2009. Available at: http://www.nasphv.org/Documents/Psittacosis.pdf. Accessed April 15, 2009.
36. Centers for Disease Control and Prevention (CDC). Notice to readers: final 2007 reports of nationally notifiable infectious diseases. MMWR Morb Mortal Wkly Rep 2008;57:901, 903–13.
37. Petrovay F, Balla E. Two fatal cases of psittacosis caused by *Chlamydophila psittaci*. J Med Microbiol 2008;57:1296–8.
38. Magnino S, Haag-Wackernagel D, Geigenfeind I, et al. Chlamydial infections in feral pigeons in Europe: review of data and focus on public health implications. Vet Microbiol 2009;135:54–67.
39. Harkinezhad T, Geens T, Vanrompay D. *Chlamydophila psittaci* infections in birds: a review with emphasis on zoonotic consequences. Vet Microbiol 2009; 135:68–77.
40. Gordon R. Psittacosis concerns suspend bird sales at Petsmart stores. Veterinary Practice News 2008. Available at: http://www.veterinarypracticenews.com/vet-breaking-news/psittacosis-concerns-suspend-bird-sales-at-petsmart-stores.aspx. Accessed April 15, 2009.
41. Abe N, Read C, Thompson RCA, et al. Zoonotic genotype of *Giardia intestinalis* detected in a ferret. J Parasitol 2005;91:179–82.
42. Thompson RCA, Palmer CS, O'Handley R. The public health and clinical significance of *Giardia* and *Cryptosporidium* in domestic animals. Vet J 2008;177: 18–25.
43. Donnelly TM. Disease problems in chinchillas. In: Quesenberry KE, Carpenter JW, editors. Ferrets, rabbits, and rodents clinical medicine and surgery. St. Louis (MO): Saunders; 2004. p. 255–65.
44. Yoder JS, Beach MJ. Giardiasis surveillance – United States, 2003–2005. MMWR Morb Mortal Wkly Rep 2007;56(SS07):11–8.
45. Greiner EC, Ritchie BW. Parasites. In: Ritchie BW, Harrison GJ, Harrison LR, editors. Avian medicine: principles and application. Lake Worth (FL): Wingers Publishing, Inc.; 1994. p. 1007–29.
46. Bowman DD, Lynn RC. Georgis' parasitology for veterinarians. 7th edition. Phildelphia: WB Saunders Co.; 1999. p. 83–85.
47. Centers for Disease Control and Prevention (CDC). Summary of notifiable diseases – United States, 2006. MMWR Morb Mortal Wkly Rep 2008;55:1–94.
48. LeJeune JT, Davis MA. Outbreaks of zoonotic enteric disease associated with animal exhibits. J Am Vet Med Assoc 2004;224:1440–5.
49. Steinmuller N, Demma L, Bender JB, et al. Outbreaks of enteric disease associated with animal contact: not just a foodborne problem anymore. Clin Infect Dis 2006;43:1596–602.
50. Bender JB, Shulman SA. Reports of zoonotic disease outbreaks associated with animal exhibits and availability of recommendations for preventing zoonotic disease transmission from animals to people in such settings. J Am Vet Med Assoc 2004;224:1105–9.
51. Shibashi T, Imai T, Sato Y, et al. *Cryptosporidium* infection in juvenile pet rabbits. J Vet Med Sci 2006;68:281–2.
52. Graczyk TK, Cranfield MR, Dunning C, et al. Fatal cryptosporidiosis in a juvenile captive African hedgehog *(Ateletrix albiventris)*. J Parasitol 1998;84:178–80.

53. Rehg JE, Gigliotti F, Stoke DC. Cryptosporidiosis in ferrets. Lab Anim Sci 1988;38: 155–8.
54. Wolfe BA. Toxoplasmosis. In: Fowler ME, Miller RE, editors. Zoo and wild animal medicine. 5th edition. St. Louis (MO): Saunders; 2003. p. 745–9.
55. Holz P. Marsupialia (marsupials). In: Fowler ME, Miller RE, editors. Zoo and wild animal medicine. 5th edition. St. Louis (MO): Saunders; 2003. p. 288–303.
56. Niebuhr DW, Millikan AM, Cowan DN, et al. Selected infectious agents and risk of schizophrenia among U.S. military personnel. Am J Psychiatry 2008;165:99–106.
57. Mortensen PB, Norgaard-Pedersen B, Waltoft BL, et al. Early infections of *Toxoplasma gondii* and the later development of schizophrenia. Schizophr Bull 2007;33:741–4.
58. Hinze-Selch D, Daubener W, Egger L, et al. A controlled prospective study of *Toxoplasma gondii* infection in individuals with schizophrenia: beyond seroprevalence. Schizophr Bull 2007;33:782–8.
59. Snyder DE, Fitzgerald PR. The relationship of Baylisascaris procyonis to Illinois raccoons (*Procyon lotor*). J Parasitol 1985;71:596–8.
60. Gavin PJ, Kazacos KR, Shulman ST. Baylisascaris. Clin Microbiol Rev 2005;18: 703–18.
61. Eberhard ML, Nace EK, Won KY, et al. *Baylisascaris procyonis* in the metropolitan Atlanta area. Emerg Infect Dis 2003;9:1636–7.
62. Souza MJ, Ramsay EC, Patton S, et al. Baylisascaris procyonis in raccoons (Procyon lotor) in eastern Tennessee. J Wild Dis, in press.
63. International Society for Infectious Diseases (ISID). Baylisascaris – USA: New York (Archive No.20090410.1380). Available at: http://www.promedmail.org. Accessed April 10, 2009.
64. Hemsworth S, Pizer B. Pet ownership in immunocompromised children – a review of the literature and survey of existing guidelines. Eur J Oncol Nurs 2006;10:117–27.
65. Pickering LK, Marano N, Bocchini JA, et al. Exposure to nontraditional pets at home and to animals in public settings: risks to children. Pediatrics 2008;122: 876–86.
66. Stirling J, Griffith M, Dooley JSG, et al. Zoonoses associated with petting farms and open zoos. Vector Borne Zoonotic Dis 2007;8:85–92.
67. Gaudie CM, Featherstone CA, Phillips WS, et al. Human *Leptospira interrogans* serogroup icterohaemorrhagiae infection (Weil's disease) acquired from pet rats. Vet Rec 2008;163:599–601.
68. Petersen JM, Schriefer ME, Carter LG, et al. Laboratory analysis of Tularemia in wild-trapped, commercially traded prairie dogs, Texas, 2002. Emerg Infect Dis 2004;10:419–25.
69. Sainsbury AW. Rodentia (rodents). In: Fowler ME, Miller RE, editors. Zoo and wild animal medicine. 5th edition. St. Louis (MO): Saunders; 2003. p. 420–42.
70. Williams ES. Plague. In: Fowler ME, Miller RE, editors. Zoo and wild animal medicine. 5th edition. St. Louis (MO): Saunders; 2003. p. 705–9.
71. Iralu J, Bai Y, Crook L, et al. Rodent-associated *Bartonella* febrile illness, Southwestern United States. Emerg Infect Dis 2006;12:1081–6.
72. Inoue K, Maruyama S, Kabeya H, et al. Exotic small mammals as potential reservoirs of zoonotic *Bartonella* spp. Emerg Infect Dis 2009;15:526–32.
73. Silberfein EJ, Lin PH, Bush RL, et al. Aortic endograft infection due to *Pasteurella multocida* following a rabbit bite. J Vasc Surg 2006;43:393–5.
74. Gaastra W, Boot R, Ho HTK, et al. Rat bite fever. Vet Microbiol 2009;133:211–28.
75. Elliot SP. Rat bite fever and *Streptobacillus moniliformis*. Clin Microbiol Rev 2007; 20:13–22.

76. Crawshaw G. Anurans (anura, salienta): frogs, toads. In: Fowler ME, Miller RE, editors. Zoo and wild animal medicine. 5th edition. St. Louis (MO): Saunders; 2003. p. 22–33.

77. Mitchell MA, Tully TN. Zoonotic diseases. In: Quesenberry KE, Carpenter JW, editors. Ferrets, rabbits, and rodents clinical medicine and surgery. St. Louis (MO): Saunders; 2004. p. 429–34.

78. Deplazes P, Mathis A, Baumgartner R, et al. Immunologic and molecular characteristics of *Encephalitozoon*-like microsporidia isolated from humans and rabbits indicate the *Encephalitozoon cuninculi* is a zoonotic parasite. Clin Infect Dis 1996;22:557–9.

79. Mathis A, Weber R, Deplazes P. Zoonotic potential of the microsporidia. Clin Microbiol Rev 2005;18:423–45.

# Bacterial and Parasitic Diseases of Parrots

Robert J.T. Doneley, BVSc, FACVSc (Avian Medicine)

**KEYWORDS**

- Psittacine • Parrot • Bacteria • Parasites • Infection • Flora

The relatively close confines of captivity mean an increased pathogen load in the environment in which companion and aviary parrots live. This increased pathogen load leads to greater exposure of these birds to bacteria and parasites, and consequently a greater risk of infection and disease. This article discusses bacterial and parasitic infections in companion and aviary parrots. It covers the origins, pathogens, diagnosis, treatment, and some of the associated risk factors.

## BACTERIAL INFECTIONS

*If I could live my life over again, I would devote it to proving that germs seek their natural habitat—diseased tissues—rather than causing disease. Rudolf Virchow, 1821–1902*

Rudolf Virchow, the German doctor, anthropologist, public health activist, pathologist, prehistorian, biologist, and politician, is often described as the "Father of Pathology" and the originator of the theory of biogenesis—the concept that living cells can arise only from pre-existing living cells. He argued that bacteria (germs) do not cause disease but, rather that they invade already diseased tissue. This went against the work of Louis Pasteur (1822–1895), who believed that bacteria were the primary cause of disease. Today, we acknowledge that both men were correct. While some bacteria are primary agents, capable of causing disease in their own right, many are secondary infections taking advantage of diseased tissue or a compromised immune system. Other bacteria sometimes found in birds are simply transient or even normal flora. Clinicians should not be content with diagnosing a bacterial infection in their patient based only on a culture or Gram stain. The patient's history, clinical signs, and other ancillary diagnostics such as hematology should be used to confirm that the isolate is, in fact, significant. They must also always ask themselves, "Why does this bird have an infection?"

West Toowoomba Veterinary Surgery, 194 West Street, Toowoomba, Queensland 4350, Australia
E-mail address: drbob@wtvs.com.au

Vet Clin Exot Anim 12 (2009) 417–432
doi:10.1016/j.cvex.2009.06.009
1094-9194/09/$ – see front matter © 2009 Elsevier Inc. All rights reserved.

vetexotic.theclinics.com

## Normal Bacterial Flora

It is a long-held belief in avian medicine that the normal bacterial flora of healthy parrots is predominantly gram-positive bacilli; conversely, gram-negative bacteria have been considered abnormal and potentially pathogenic.[1–4] Various surveys have been conducted of both healthy and diseased parrots to ascertain normal and abnormal bacterial flora[3,5–7]; all agree that gram-positive bacilli are the predominant flora, but there is some disagreement on the significance and normality of the presence of gram-negative bacteria.

Bangert and colleagues[5] reported that fecal isolates from healthy parrots included gram-positive bacilli (*Lactobacillus* spp, *Bacillus* spp, *Corynebacterium* spp, *Streptomyces* spp), gram-positive cocci, (*Staphylococcus epidermidis*, *Streptococcus* spp., *Aerococcus* spp., and *Micrococcus* spp) and, in a low number of birds, gram-negative bacteria (*Escherichia coli*). They further reported that the number of birds yielding *Corynebacterium* and gram-negative bacteria increased with age; whereas the number of birds yielding lactobacilli decreased with age. Flammer and Drewes[6] reported that 91% of 506 clinically normal parrots had gram-positive bacilli recovered from cloacal cultures. However, *E coli* was recovered from 31% of these birds, *Enterobacter* spp from 4%, *Klebsiella* from 0.6%, and *Pseudomonas* spp from 0.8%. Species differences were noted: *E coli* was recovered from 60% of the cockatoos (*Cacatua* spp) cultured (168 birds), but from only 18% of non-cockatoo species (338 birds). All birds were housed in the same facility with similar diets and husbandry, suggesting that these were species-related differences, rather than differences in diet and management. Jones and Nisbet[7] cultured *E coli* from the intestinal tract of 46% of 54 parrots necropsied for non- intestinal diseases. These birds were all specimens from a zoologic collection and could be expected to have had similar diets and husbandry.

On the other hand, Harrison and McDonald[3] state that the normal fecal flora of parrots is comprised of 100% gram-positive, non–spore-forming rods and cocci, and that gram-negative bacteria should not be present in the feces of parrots on a healthy diet. This belief is reinforced by the work of Stanford[8] that showed that gram-negative bacteria in the feces of Grey parrots (*Psittacus erithacus*) were reduced to almost zero after conversion from a typical seed-based diet to a nutritionally balanced one.

Respiratory tract flora appears to follow a somewhat different pattern. Fudge[4] states that tracheal washes are usually sterile, but that contamination from the oropharyngeal area during collection of samples can be misleading. Drewes and Flammer,[9] and Tully,[10] state that the bacterial flora from the upper respiratory tract is predominantly gram-positive bacilli. Jesus and Correia,[11] on the other hand, cultured the choana of nineteen healthy parrots. Of the 36 bacterial isolates recovered, 26% were gram-positive bacteria and 62% were gram-negative bacteria. Isolates recovered were α-hemolytic *Streptococcus* spp, non-hemolytic *Streptococcus* sp, *Gemella morbillorum*, *Leuconostoc* sp, *Staphylococcus* sp, *Staphylococcus hominis*, *Bacillus* sp, *Actinomyces* sp, *Alcaligenes* sp, *Acinetobacter baumannii*, *Enterobacter cloacae*, *Erwinia nigrifluens*, *Klebsiella pneumoniae*, *Klebsiella oxytoca*, *Moraxella lacunata*, *Pasteurella* spp, *Pseudomonas alcaligenes*, *Pseudomonas stutzeri*, and *Xanthomonas maltophilia*. Some of these bacteria are known as potential pathogens, suggesting that the resident flora of the upper respiratory tract of healthy parrots can, given the right opportunity, behave as opportunistic pathogens.

The findings discussed above suggest that the normal bacterial flora in healthy parrots, while predominantly gram-positive bacteria, may include some gram-negative bacteria as well. From a clinician's point of view, it must be remembered that most patients presented for veterinary examination are rarely on a nutritionally balanced diet, nor is their husbandry identical or even optimal. As such, it can be expected that the bacterial flora in these birds will possibly include low numbers of gram-negative bacteria. This does not constitute evidence of a bacterial infection, nor does it always warrant antimicrobial therapy.

### Predisposing Factors in Bacterial Infections

Bacteria can be primary disease-causing agents or secondary invaders. Birds may be exposed to them through environmental contact, or they may be resident flora. Their ability to cause disease is determined by the interaction of host factors and pathogen factors.

Host factors include the state of the bird's defense system, its general health, the presence of concurrent disease, and external stressors. The defense system consists of both nonspecific defenses (epithelial surfaces, normal flora, and leukocytes) and specific defenses (the humoral immune system and the cell-mediated immune system).

The skin and the mucosal linings of the intestinal, respiratory, urinary, and reproductive tracts are the first line of defense in preventing pathogen access to the body. In a healthy bird, this is achieved by providing both a physical barrier to pathogens and establishing a resident population of bacteria with a low pathogenicity (normal flora), thereby inhibiting the entry and growth of pathogenic microorganisms (**Figs. 1** and **2**). This normal flora takes up available space, occupies receptors and acts competitively against invaders by various mechanisms such as inhibitory metabolic products, bacteriocins, and production of a low-pH environment that inhibits the proliferation of gram-negative rods and yeast.[3,12] If pathogenic bacteria do succeed in colonizing and penetrating this first line of defense, leukocytes are the body's "first responders" in identifying and phagocytizing bacteria that do not belong.

While nonspecific defenses either deny pathogenic bacteria entry to the body or destroy them when they enter the body, specific defenses play a prophylactic role by defending the body against initial and recurrent infections. The specific defense mechanism relies mainly on B and T lymphocytes to recognize antigens and to produce microorganism-specific antibodies (humoral immune system), or to provoke cell-mediated reactions (cell-mediated immune system).[12]

These defense mechanisms function best in a healthy bird. Birds that are malnourished (protein-, vitamin-, and mineral-deficient diets; ie, predominantly seed-based

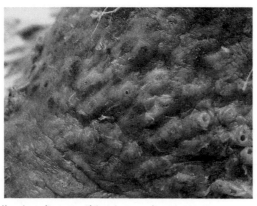

**Fig. 1.** Dermatitis following dog mouthing in a cockatoo.

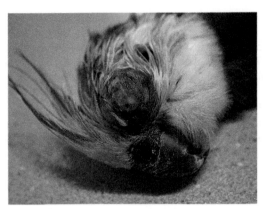

**Fig. 2.** Sinusitis in a cockatiel (*Nymphicus hollandicus*).

diets), suffering from concurrent disease (eg, psittacine beak and feather disease herpes virus infection, chlamydiosis, and mycotoxicosis), or are subjected to repeated external stressors (overcrowding, noise, abnormal diurnal rhythms, etc) are less able to mount an effective defense against real or potential pathogens.

Pathogen factors include the virulence of the microorganism in question and the concentration of bacteria to which the bird is exposed. Bacterial pathogens, once they have entered the body, have to survive the natural host defenses and compete with the established nonpathogenic flora to become established. This requires the ability to colonize the site of infection, determined by the physical characteristics of the microorganism (eg, the presence or absence of flagella), adherence factors, and enzymes. Pathogenic bacteria also possess virulence factors that enable them to cause primary damage to targeted organs, such as invasion, secretion of cytotoxins or enterotoxins, and resistance to phagocytosis.[13]

Exposure to relatively low numbers of even virulent bacteria usually presents little challenge to a healthy bird with a well-functioning immune system. Those same bacteria, allowed to concentrate in the bird's environment or food, can present the bird's natural defenses and immune system with an overwhelming challenge, leading to infection. Good hygiene and appropriate storage of food is essential to reduce the concentration of potential pathogens the bird may be exposed.

The interaction of these host and pathogen factors is the determinant of infection. Birds that are immunosuppressed or immunocompromised for any reason, when challenged by potential pathogens, may rapidly succumb to infection. Mildly virulent bacteria, when met with an ineffective response from the nonspecific and specific defense mechanisms, are able to colonize various entry portals and penetrate beyond them. On the other hand, well-nourished healthy birds, when challenged with a low to moderately virulent bacteria, are usually able to prevent this same colonization and penetration.

### Diagnosis of Bacterial Infections

When revisiting Virchow's belief that bacteria "*seek their natural habitat—diseased tissues—rather than causing disease*," it follows that simply identifying the presence of abnormal or potentially pathogenic bacteria in a bird does not mean that an infection or disease process is present. These bacteria may be resident flora or simply transitioning through the bird after being ingested or inhaled. Determining whether these bacteria are playing a role in the bird's current health status is the "art of avian practice."[14]

Traditionally veterinarians have employed antibiotics in the treatment of "sick birds," especially when the subjective finding that the bird is ill is supported by the presence of gram-negative bacteria in a fecal or choanal swab. This approach had some validity in the earlier days of avian medicine when birds were housed poorly, fed a suboptimal diet, and poor hygiene was the order of the day. The opportunities for pathogenic bacteria to become secondary or even primary disease agents were much greater. Now most birds are fed better diets, housed more appropriately, and the importance of good hygiene is well understood. The chances of birds coming into contact with significant levels of pathogens are fewer, and the bird's defense mechanisms are better. Infectious microorganisms, both bacterial and viral, play a smaller role in disease than these organisms did 15 years ago.[14]

In making an assessment of the significance of gram-negative bacteria identified in a bird by Gram stain or culture, the clinician must look beyond the laboratory report.[4] The patient's history, physical findings, hemogram, clinical biochemistries and other diagnostic aids must be employed in making the final determination of the significance of microbiological findings.[4,14] If we accept Virchow's belief that bacteria are most commonly (always?) secondary invaders, the clinician's role—in a diagnostic sense—is to determine the primary problem that allowed these bacteria to colonize and penetrate the patient's body. A diagnosis of a primary bacterial infection in an adult parrot is usually a disease of exclusion. If all other disease processes are ruled out, a primary bacterial infection may then be considered.[14]

**Table 1** lists many of the more common bacterial organisms that affect psittacine birds. Not included are less common organisms, such as *Mycobacteria* sp, *Listeria monocytogenes, Coxiella* sp, *Clostridia piliforme*, and others.[17–20]


## PARASITIC DISEASES

The dictionary definition of the word parasite is, "a plant or animal that lives on or in an organism of another species from which it derives sustenance or protection without benefit to, and usually with harmful effects on, the host." The word "parasite" is derived from the Greek "parasitos"—one who eats at the table of another. Parasite life cycles can be either direct (transmission from host to host) or indirect (the parasite's life cycle includes a vector that carries it from one host to another). The author is fortunate to live in a country with a large free-living parrot population and can verify that wild parrots frequently carry moderate loads of parasites—but rarely as severe as those seen in captive parrots. Captivity—keeping an animal confined in a relatively small area—increases the exposure of parrots to both direct and indirect parasitic life cycles.

Some parasitic infections can result in illness and death; other parasites are more successful, rarely affecting their host. An interesting alternate view on successful parasitism was reported by Bize and colleagues.[21] "Parasite fitness"—the ability of a parasite to survive and reproduce—is a balance between the amount of nutritive resources extracted from the host body and the parasite's ability to deal with the host's immune response. As both nutritive resources and immunity increase with increasing host body condition, finding a balance between the two can become more difficult with well-nourished, healthy birds. Although parasites may avoid individuals in very good condition (with a strong immune response), they may also avoid those in poor condition (that do not provide adequate resources). This balancing act highlights the

**Table 1**
Common bacterial pathogens in parrots

| Genus | Species | Source | Common Sites of Infection | Comments |
|---|---|---|---|---|
| Aeromonas | A hydrophila | Water | Gastrointestinal (GI) and upper respiratory tract | Often presents as a septicemic condition. |
| Bordatella | B avium | Food, water and airborne | Upper respiratory tract | Cockatiel "lockjaw" syndrome |
| Campylobacter | C fetus C intestinalis C jejuni | Fecal or aerosol contact, contaminated fomites, infected vectors | GI tract | Potentially zoonotic |
| Clostridia | C perfringens | Contaminated food or fomites | GI tract | Often associated with dietary change or prolonged use of antibiotics |
| Enterobacter | E cloacae | Resident flora in GI tract | Septicemia | Only in immunocompromised patients |
| Enterococcus | E faecalis | Resident flora in GI tract | Wound infections following fecal contamination | Highly resistant to most antibiotics |
| Escherichia | E coli | Contaminated food, water and fomites—often associated with poor hygiene | All organ systems | Often difficult to distinguish between pathogenic strains and resident or transient strains |
| Klebsiella | K pneumoniae K ozaenae K oxytoca | Water | Initial GI colonization with hematogenous spread to the lungs and air sacs | Often associated with artificially incubated chicks, where the water in the incubator has become contaminated |

| Pasteurella | P multocida | Cat bites | Rapid septicemic spread | Death can occur in 6-12 hours after the bite is inflicted—urgent antibiotic therapy must be instituted |
|---|---|---|---|---|
| Pseudomonas | P aeruginosa | Water | Upper respiratory tract, eyes | Can survive in many disinfectants and in polyvinyl chloride water pipes—resistant to many antibiotics |
| Salmonella | S typhimurium S arizonae | Ingestion or inhalation of contaminated food or fecal dust—birds that survive infection can become carriers | GI tract, with rapid, septicemic spread | Can be a primary pathogen, capable of penetrating intact intestinal mucosa |
| Staphylococcus | S aureus | Resident flora on the skin of many birds | Skin and feet—can also become a septicemic infection and may localize in internal organs | — |
| Spirochetaceae (Helicobacter)[15,16] | — | May be resident flora in the oropharynx, but has been associated with pharyngitis in cockatiels, lovebirds | Oropharynx (palatine salivary gland)[15] | Unable to culture to date—usually diagnosed by cytology |
| Yersinia | Y enterocolitica Y pseudotuberculosis | Contamination of food and water by rodent urine and feces | GI tract, liver, respiratory tract | Replicates in the environment at low temperatures, making infections more common in winter months |

complex interactions between host and parasite and may help our understanding of parasitic infections in parrots.

Parasites of parrots include helminths (nematodes, cestodes, and trematodes), protozoa, and arthropods. Most, if not all, organ systems can be affected—the skin, respiratory tract, gastrointestinal tract, kidneys, muscles, and blood. Parasites may be successful (causing little damage) or unsuccessful (causing illness or death), and may be either primary or opportunistic pathogens. None has a symbiotic relationship with parrots, where both host and parasite gain from the relationship.

As the husbandry and nutrition of captive parrots has improved, the incidence of parasitic infections has decreased. However, parasitic infections can be a serious health and management issue in some parrot collections and individuals, and the clinician should always be alert to their presence.

The parasites described below are the more common species found in parrots. This is not a complete list, as there is a wide geographic variation in the type and occurrence of parasites—to describe them all is beyond the scope of this article.

### Protozoal Parasites

#### Coccidia

Coccidia (*Eimeria* spp and *Isospora* spp) are very host specific, nonmotile protozoa found in the intestinal mucosa of most parrot species around the world. Infected birds may not show clinical signs until stressed or until overwhelmingly large numbers of coccidial schizonts are present. Affected birds are lethargic with weight loss and diarrhea (sometimes hemorrhagic); severely affected birds often die. This parasite requires 6 to 8 days to complete its direct life cycle. As the oocysts undergo schizogony in intestine, the intestinal mucosa is damaged, causing enteritis. Clinical signs are seen 4 to 6 days after infection. Nonsporulated oocysts are shed in the feces and sporulate in a warm, moist environment to become infective. It is important to note that clinical signs may become apparent before oocysts are detectable in the feces. Treatment with amprolium, toltrazuril, and other anticoccidial drugs is usually effective. Two treatments must be given, 5 days apart, for the best effect (Garry Cross, personal communication). Prevention and control revolves around preventing access to infected fecal material (eg, by placing food and water dishes above the ground) and strategic treatments in collections where infection has become a problem.

#### Cryptosporidia

Cryptosporidium is a coccidian parasite (its oocysts are the smallest of any coccidia) that can infect any epithelial surface, including the gastrointestinal, respiratory, and urinary tracts, the conjunctival sac, and the bursa. It is not host specific (although it does not appear to move from birds to mammals), and often acts as a secondary pathogen. Although some infected birds can be asymptomatic, immunosuppressed birds often develop clinical disease. Signs include depression, dehydration, pyrexia, anorexia, persistent diarrhea, bulky droppings (associated with malabsorption), abdominal pain, vomiting, coughing, sneezing, and nasal discharge. It has a direct life cycle with fully sporulated infective oocysts passed in the droppings to be ingested or inhaled by another (or the same) bird. Diagnosis is made through the detection of oocysts in the droppings or by histopathology of necropsy specimens. The recommended treatment is paromomycin sulfate but this is expensive and difficult to obtain. It is poorly absorbed and excreted by way of the gastrointestinal tract. In this environment, the oocysts are resistant to many disinfectants.

### Microsporidiosis

Microsporidiosis (Encephalitozoonosis) is caused by *Encephalitozoon hellum*, an obligate intracellular protozoan parasite that can infect multiple tissues. It has been associated with enteritis, hepatitis, nephritis, keratoconjunctivitis, sinusitis, and lower respiratory tract infections.[22,23] Infection is often associated with some element of immunosuppression such as stress, overcrowding, or concurrent disease. It has a direct life cycle, with transmission by ingestion and possibly inhalation. Diagnosis is made by polymerase chain reaction or histopathology. Although not proven, it should be considered a potentially zoonotic disease. Treatment with albendazole may be of benefit.

### Sarcocystis falcatula

*Sarcocystis falcatula* is a coccidian parasite that has an obligatory two-host life cycle; it undergoes sexual multiplication in the intestine of the definitive host (the opossum, *Didelphis virginiana*). Oocysts sporulate internally and are infectious when passed in the feces. Sporocysts are ingested by cowbirds and grackles (the normal intermediate host) either directly or after ingestion by an insect. They then invade various tissues where they undergo schizogony or merogony and then form sarcocysts in the cardiac or striated muscles. The cycle is completed when the definitive host eats the intermediate host and ingests the cysts in its muscle tissue.[24] Parrots become infected when they eat insects (especially flies and cockroaches) that have ingested the infective sporocysts. Infection is rapidly fatal in cockatoos, cockatiels, and Grey parrots. The disease presents in parrots in three different clinical forms: an acute pulmonary disease, muscular disease, and neurologic disease.[25] It has also been reported to cause myocarditis in parrots.[26] The diagnosis of sarcocystosis is usually made on necropsy; antemortem testing includes muscle biopsy and indirect immunofluorescent assay.[25] This can give a false-negative result in acute cases, as clinical disease is present before detectable antibodies are present. Recommended treatments include pyrimethamine in combination with trimethoprim-sulfadiazine or trimethoprim-sulfamethoxazole. Control involves keeping both possums and insects away from susceptible birds.

### Toxoplasma gondii

*Toxoplasma gondii* is another coccidian parasite, but rarely reported in parrots. Cats are definitive hosts, shedding the infective oocysts in their droppings. Parrots become infected when they ingest these oocysts. Clinical signs are rare, and include weight loss, anorexia, general debility, ataxia, blindness, conjunctivitis, and death. Diagnosis is usually made by finding *Toxoplasma* tissue stages on histopathology. Serology has also been used for antemortem diagnosis. Treatment is similar to that for sarcocystosis, although clindamycin has been used also.

### Giardia psittaci

*Giardia psittaci* is a motile protozoan parasite found in the intestinal tract of parrots throughout the world. Infective cysts are passed intermittently in the feces of infected birds and are then ingested by another parrot.[27] Clinical signs reflect enteritis and a possible malabsorption syndrome. They include weight loss, depression, ruffled feathers, chronic diarrhea, neonatal mortality, and persistent feather picking and pruritis in cockatiels. Diagnosis is by direct examination of fresh feces to identify the motile trophozoites or infective cysts. Note that the trophozoites are only shed intermittently and they are unstable outside the host. Fecal samples should be examined within 10 minutes of elimination, using warmed saline rather than tap water. The trophozoites are destroyed in salt or sugar flotation solutions. Treatment with metronidazole and other nitroimidazoles is effective. Good hygiene is essential in preventing further infections. Giardia cysts may survive chlorinated water, but are inactivated by quaternary ammonium compounds.

### Trichomonas gallinae

*Trichomonas gallinae* is a motile protozoan parasite characterized by a clear, narrow, longitudinal axial rod (axostyle), an undulating membrane and four anterior flagella. In Australia, it is a common infection of budgerigars and occasionally other psittacine species; in the United States, it is considered uncommon. The life cycle is direct; contaminated food and water, and mutual feeding, are the routes of infection. It lives in the crop of affected birds where it causes ingluvitis, often with caseous diphtheritic membranes extending from the oropharynx to the thoracic esophagus. Clinical signs include weight loss, ptyalism, vomiting, and diarrhea. Death through starvation is common in advanced cases. Diagnosis is usually straight forward, achieved by microscopic examination of a fresh crop wash suspended in saline. Treatment with the nitroimidazoles (ronidazole, carnidazole, etc) is usually effective, although some patients with severe ulceration and diphtheritic membranes will die despite treatment.

### Cochlosoma spp

*Cochlosoma* spp are flagellated protozoa with a sucking disc similar to *Giardia*. However, other physical structures have led to its classification as a *Trichomonas*-like organism. It has a direct life cycle through the ingestion of contaminated fecal material, food, and water. In Australia it is found in the intestinal tract of cockatiels quite commonly; it causes enteritis with diarrhea, weight loss, and death. In some birds, it is associated with pruritis and feather picking behavior. Treatment can be frustrating; resistance to the nitroimidazoles (ronidazole, carnidazole, etc) is common.

### Spironucleus meleagridis

*Spironucleus meleagridis* (formerly *Hexamita* spp) has been reported in Australian King Parrots, cockatiels, and Splendid Grass parakeets.[28] It is a motile protozoan with eight flagella (six anterior and two trailing) found in the intestinal tract. It causes chronic, often intractable, diarrhea, weight loss, and death. Infective cysts are passed in the droppings; then they contaminate the food and water or are ingested. Diagnosis is made through the identification of the protozoa swimming in a smooth linear fashion in a very fresh fecal sample. Treatment with the nitroimidazoles (ronidazole, carnidazole, etc) is usually successful, although severely emaciated birds may not recover.

### Haemoproteus

*Haemoproteus* is a hemoprotozoa found only in birds. It has a worldwide distribution; in the United States, it is reported as common in imported cockatoos. Once infected, a bird remains a carrier for life. This parasite is transmitted by blood sucking insects such as the hippoboscids or louse flies. It is rarely pathogenic in parrots. It can be found in the endothelial cells of the blood vessels in various tissues (especially the lung, liver, and spleen) as numerous multinucleated bodies within an enlarged endothelial cell. It can also be found in erythrocytes, partially encircling the nucleus without displacing it. Chloroquine and primaquine have been reported to be effective, but treatment is rarely required. Control requires the elimination of biting insects within the bird's environment.

### Plasmodium

*Plasmodium* (avian malaria) also has worldwide distribution. Birds, especially small passerines, are the definitive (and reservoir) host. It is transmitted by *Culex* and *Aedes* mosquitoes. Many birds, once infected, become lifelong carriers. Others, when faced with an overwhelming infection, show clinical signs consistent with anemia and tissue destruction: depression, anorexia, vomiting, dyspnea, hemoglobinuria, pale mucus membranes, and death. The organism can be identified within erythrocytes (where it may displace the nucleus) in thrombocytes, leucocytes, and endothelial cells. Treatment is often too late by the time the bird is showing clinical signs, but in-contact birds should be treated with chloroquine and primaquine. Prophylactic weekly dosing with these drugs before, during, and after known biting insect seasons may be appropriate.

### Leucocytozoon
*Leucocytozoon* is a protozoan parasite of both erythrocytes and leucocytes, transmitted by biting flies. It is an uncommon parasite of parrots, although relatively common in waterfowl, turkeys, young raptors and some passerines. It causes gross distortion of the parasitized cell and the tissue phase of its life cycle can cause disruption of skeletal, cardiac, and gizzard muscles. Clinical signs include anorexia, depression, dehydration, and hemoglobinuria (due to hemolytic anemia). The recommended treatment is chloroquine and primaquine.

### Nematode Parasites

### Ascarids
Ascarids (roundworms) are a common parasite of birds with access to the ground. It is particularly common in Australian parrots, especially budgerigars, cockatiels, and Princess Parrots (**Fig. 3**). Several species have been identified in parrots: *Ascaridia hermaphrodita* (identified in a Hyacinth macaw), *A columbae* (shared between pigeons and parrots), *A galli* (shared between gallinaceous birds and parrots), and *A platycerci* (restricted to parrots). The life cycle is direct; ingestion of contaminated food, water, and feces is the route of transmission. Clinical signs include lethargy, poor condition, diarrhea, and death. Necropsy reveals large numbers of roundworms in the small intestine, particularly in the duodenal loop. Diagnosis is usually straightforward, with the thick-shelled eggs readily detected in the feces. Most anthelminthics are effective against roundworm. Control is achieved by preventing access to contaminated feces, food, and water. If this is not feasible, regular worming (every 2–3 months), may be necessary.

### Capillaria
*Capillaria* (hairworm and threadworm) is a small nematode that infects the crop, esophagus, and oral cavity; burrowing into the mucosa to create tracts that fill with

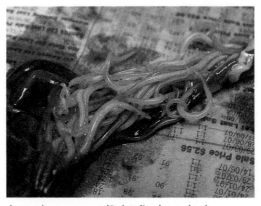

**Fig. 3.** Roundworms in a princess parrot (*Polytelis alexandrae*).

blood to produce hyperemic streaks and some diphtheritic lesions. Clinical signs include anorexia, dysphagia, diarrhea, and weight loss. Species reported in parrots include *C annulata* and *C obsignata*. Eggs are passed in the droppings and become infective in 2 weeks; they may remain infectious in the environment for several months. Transmission may be direct or indirect (insects and earthworms are the intermediate hosts). Diagnosis is made by detecting the characteristic double-operculated egg in the feces. Treatment can be difficult, as anthelminthics resistance is common. Response to therapy needs to be monitored. Environmental control to prevent access to insects and contaminated feces is essential.

## Cestode Parasites

There are many species of tapeworms infecting parrots, but the more common species include *Raillietaenia*, *Choanataenia*, *Gastronemia*, *Idiogenes*, and *Amoebataenia*. Their life cycle requires an intermediate host (such as grasshoppers, beetles, ants, and horse flies) and may be complete in as little as 3 to 4 weeks. Typical clinical signs include anorexia, weight loss, and diarrhea. Tapeworm segments may be seen in affected bird's droppings or even hanging from the vent. Fecal examination may reveal the characteristic eggs with oncosphere hooks. Treatment with praziquantel and fenbendazole is usually effective. Prevention lies with insect control.

## Arthropod Parasites

### Knemidocoptes pilae

*Knemidocoptes pilae* (scaly face or leg mite) is commonly seen in budgerigars (**Fig. 4**), Kakarikis, *Neophema*, and *Polytelis* parrots, producing the characteristic proliferative crusty lesions on not only the beak, cere, face, and legs—but also on the margins of the vent and the wing tips. Its entire life cycle is spent on the host, although it may be transmitted by way of dead skin and scales. Immunosuppression and genetic factors may play a role in producing clinical signs. Diagnosis is usually straightforward because the appearance of the lesions is classical. If doubt exists, a skin scraping can be used to identify the mite in the lesions. Treatment with ivermectin or moxidectin topically, orally, or parenterally—repeated every two weeks until the lesions

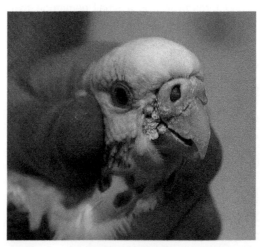

**Fig. 4.** *Knemidocoptes pilae* in a budgerigar (*Melopsittacus undulatus*).

resolve—is usually effective. The use of topical creams and liquids are rarely as effective, as the whole bird must be treated.

### Dermanyssus gallinae
*Dermanyssus gallinae* (red or roost mites) are common in aviaries, especially those that allow access by wild birds. These bloodsucking mites feed on the birds at night and leave them during the day. They can live in the environment, surviving long periods without feeding. They cause skin irritation and anemia (especially in juveniles or small birds) and may bite humans. Treatment with carbaryl dusting powder, or oral ivermectin or moxidectin, is usually effective. It is essential to treat the bird's environment at the same time with safe residual insecticides.

### Quill mites
Quill mites, such as *Syringophilus* spp, *Dermoglyphus* spp, *Pterolichus* spp, *Analges* spp, or *Harporhynchus* spp (**Fig. 5**), are an uncommon cause of feather loss in parrots. They spend their entire life cycle on the host, and can be found by examining the pulp material within a developing or damaged feather. Treatment with ivermectin or moxidectin is usually effective.

### Air sac mites
Air sac mites (*Cytodites nudus* and *Sternostoma tracheacolum*) are more common in canaries and Gouldian finches than in parrots, but have been reported in budgerigars and cockatiels as a rare parasite. Little is known of its life cycle, although it is assumed direct. Chicks may be infected in the nest by their parents. The irritation caused by the mites causes a sucking or clicking noise, loss or change of voice, dyspnea, and generalized debilitation. Diagnosis can be difficult at times. Sometimes, the mites can be visualized within the trachea by transillumination with a focal intense light or eggs may be noted in feces or tracheal wash. Treatment with ivermectin or moxidectin can reduce the mite population, and concurrent antibiotics may be necessary for the airway disease caused by the mites' presence.

### Biting lice
Biting lice (*Neopsittaconirmus* spp, *Psittaconirmus* spp, *Eomenopon* spp, and *Pacifimenopon* spp) are reasonably common in aviary birds but their significance as a cause of feather damaging behavior in pet birds is vastly exaggerated. Their eggs (nits) are

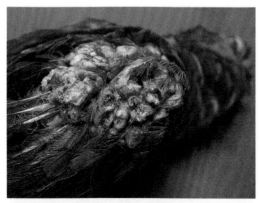

**Fig. 5.** Harporhynchus mites in a wild Scaly-breasted Lorikeet (*Trichoglossus chlorolepidotus*).

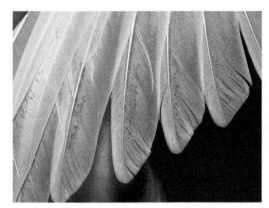

**Fig. 6.** Feather lice in a budgerigar (*Melopsittacus undulatus*).

glued to feather shafts (**Figs. 6** and **7**); they hatch out in 4 to 7 days into nymphs, which undergo three molts before maturity. Adult lice feed on skin scales and feather debris, resulting in pruritis and poor feather quality. The entire life cycle is usually spent on the one host. Treatment with carbaryl dusting powder or pyrethrin sprays is usually effective.

### Hippoboscid fly
The hippoboscid fly (louse fly, parrot fly) is more common in wild parrots than aviary or companion birds. It seldom leaves its host but it is not host specific. A bloodsucking parasite, it major significance is a vector of *Hemoproteus*. It lays it eggs off the host in a secluded spot. It can be treated with pyrethrin sprays or carbaryl dusting powder.

### Stickfast flea
The stickfast flea, *Echidnophaga gallinacea,* although a poultry parasite, can occasionally affect parrots housed in close proximity to chickens. The adult fleas are bloodsucking parasites, often attached to the skin of the head. They cause irritation and blood loss, sometimes resulting in depression, anemia, and pruritis. Treatment with pyrethrin sprays is usually effective.

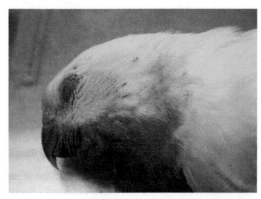

**Fig. 7.** Feather lice in a Princess parrot (*Polytelis alexandrae*), lutino mutation.

## SUMMARY

In the earlier days of avian medicine, when many birds were wild-caught and highly stressed, bacterial and parasitic infections were considered common problems. Diagnostic tests were developed and treatment regimes devised to overcome these infections. Even today, it is common to see antibiotics and ivermectin used to treat nearly every "sick" bird.

As wild-caught birds become increasingly rare in aviculture, there is a corresponding decline in the incidence of bacterial and parasitic problems and an increase in the recognition of the importance of maintaining health through better nutrition and husbandry. If such an infection is detected today, the clinician's first thought should be, "Why?"

## REFERENCES

1. Fiennes RNT-W. Report of the society's pathologist for the year 1957. Proc Zool Soc Lond 1959;132:129–46.
2. Fiennes RNT-W. Diseases of bacterial origin. In: Petrak ML, editor. Diseases of cage and aviary birds. Philadelphia: Lea and Febiger; 1969. p. 357–72.
3. Harrison GJ, McDonald D. Nutritional considerations—section II: nutritional disorders. In: Harrison GJ, Lightfoot TL, editors, Clinical avian medicine, vol. 1. Palm Beach (FL): Spix Publishing; 1996. p. 108–40.
4. Fudge AM. Diagnosis and treatment of avian bacterial infections. Seminars in Avian and Exotic Pet Practice 2001;10(1):3–11.
5. Bangert RL, Cho BR, Widders PR, et al. A survey of aerobic bacteria and fungi in the feces of healthy psittacine birds. Avian Dis 1988;32(1):46–52.
6. Flammer K, Drewes LA. Species-related differences in the incidence of gram negative bacteria isolated from the cloaca of clinically normal psittacine birds. Avian Dis 1988;32:79–83.
7. Jones DM, Nisbet DL. The gram negative bacterial flora of the avian gut. Avian Pathol 1980;9:33–8.
8. Stanford M. Effects of dietary change on fecal Gram's stains in the African grey parrot. Exotic DVM 2003;4(6):12–3.
9. Drewes LA, Flammer K. Clinical microbiology. In: Harrison GL, Harrison LR, editors. Clinical avian medicine and surgery. Philadelphia: W.B. Saunders Co.; 1986. p. 157–71.
10. Tully TN. Avian respiratory diseases: clinical overview. J Avian Med Surg 1995;9: 162–74.
11. Jesus SO, Correia JHD. Potential pathogens recovered from the upper respiratory tract of psittacine birds. Proceedings of International Virtual Conference in veterinary medicine: diseases of Psittacine birds. University of Georgia College of Veterinary Medicine, 1998.
12. Batt RM. Bacterial enteropathogens in dogs. Proc WSAVA Congress 2002. Available at: http://www.vin.com/Members/proceedings/Proceedings.plx?CID=WSAVA2002&Category=&PID=2581&O=VIN. Accessed May 2009.
13. Gerlach H. Defense mechanisms of the avian host. In: Ritchie BW, Harrison GJ, Harrison LR, editors. Avian medicine: principles and application. Lake Worth (FL): Wingers Publishing; 1994. p. 109–20.
14. Rosenthal KL. Microbiology: revisiting the Gram stain and culture. Proc Annu Conf Assoc Avian Vet Australian Committee 2006:183–6.
15. Wade LL, Bartick T. Pathology of spiral bacteria (Helicobacter species) in cockatiels (Nymphicus hollandicus). Proc Annu Conf Assoc Avian Vet 2004;345–8.

16. Wade LL, et al. Identification of oral spiral bacteria in cockatiels (Nymphicus hollandicus). Proc Annu Conf Assoc Avian Vet 2003;23–5.
17. Lennox A. Mycobacteriosis in companion psittacine birds: a review. J Avian Med Surg 2007;21(3):181–7.
18. Shivaprasad HL, Kokka R, Walker RL. Listeriosis in a cockatiel (Nymphicus hollandicus). Avian Dis 2007;51(3):800–4.
19. Soc-Colburn AM, Garner MM, Bradway D, et al. Fatal coxiellosis in Swainson's Blue Mountain rainbow lorikeets (Trichoglossus haematodus moluccanus). Vet Pathol 2008;45:247–54.
20. Raymond JT, Topham K, Shirota T, et al. Tyzzer's disease in a neonatal rainbow lorikeet (Trichoglossuz haematodus). Vet Pathol 2001;38:326–7.
21. Bize P, Jeanneret C, Klopfenstein A, et al. What makes a host profitable? Parasites balance host nutritive resources against immunity. Am Nat 2008;171(1): 107–18.
22. Black SS, Steinhort LA, Bertucci DC, et al. Encephalitozoon hellum in budgerigars (Melopsittacus undulates). Vet Pathol 1997;34:189–98.
23. Suter C, Mathis A, Hoop R, et al. Encephalitozoon hellem infection in a yellow-streaked lorry (Chalcopsitta scintillata) imported from Indonesia. Vet Rec 1998; 143:694–5.
24. Helmer P. Psittacine sarcocystis. Presented at the Proceedings of the Western Veterinary Conference. Las Vegas, Nevada, February 15–19, 2004.
25. Villar D, Kramer M, Howard L, et al. Clinical presentation and pathology of sarcocystosis in psittaciform birds: 11 cases. Avian Dis 2008;52(1):187–94.
26. Oglesbee B. Overview of avian cardiology. Proc Western Veterinary Conference 2003. Available at: http://www.vin.com/Members/Proceedings/Proceedings.plx?CID=WVC2003&Category=&PID=3384&O=VIN. Accessed May 2009.
27. Erlandsen SL, Bemrich WJ. SEM evidence for a new species of Giardia psittaci. J Parasitol 1987;73(3):623–9.
28. Philbey AQ, Andrew PL, Gestier AW, et al. Spironucleosis in Australian king parrots (Alisterus scapularis). Aust Vet J 2002;80(3):154–60.

# Bacterial and Parasitic Diseases of Passerines

Gerry M. Dorrestein, DVM, PhD, DRDCVP

**KEYWORDS**

• Bacterial diseases • Parasitic diseases • Passeriformes

Many veterinarians are relatively unfamiliar with the passerines. The aviculture, diagnostic procedures, and common diseases, and their treatment are discussed in several recent publications.[1–4]

Owners of passerines (songbirds) are using veterinary care in increasing numbers as aviculturists recognize the advances in avian medical and surgical treatment of these patients.

Diseases in these avian species are often influenced by nutrition, housing, and stress. For a complete understanding of diseases associated with problems of passerines, including diagnosis and treatment, clinicians must become familiar with the aviculture, housing, and husbandry of their patients. Supportive care and measures to minimize stress are often needed to maintain the host's defense mechanisms.

Many infectious diseases are species-specific, although salmonellosis and pseudotuberculosis are exceptions. Coccidiosis is often diagnosed in finches and these coccidia are often said to belong to the *Isospora lacazei* group. However, most species appear to have their own coccidian species.

## BACTERIAL INFECTIONS

Bacterial infections, mostly in the intestines, are a common finding in canaries and finches. The evaluation of the fecal smear (**Fig. 1**), or any other site where bacterial problems are suspected, using a quick stain helps to get an impression of the bacterial organisms present. It is also useful because most bacteria do not grow in a standard culture. The same quick staining can be used to evaluate the results of a treatment.

The most commonly encountered bacterial infections in passerines are *Escherichia coli* (and other Enterobacteriaceae), *Yersinia pseudotuberculosis, Salmonella typhimurium, Campylobacter fetus,* different species of cocci, *Pseudomonas* and *Aeromonas* sp, several *Mycobacterium* spp, *Chlamydophila* sp, and Mycoplasmata.

### Escherichia coli (and Other Enterobacteriaceae)

In normal healthy passerines, *E coli* (and other Enterobacteriaceae) are absent in the intestines. However, these bacteria are very often demonstrated (by cytology) and

Diagnostic Pathology Laboratory, Dutch Research Institute for Avian and Exotic Animals (NOIVBD), Wintelresedijk 51, NL-5507 PP Veldhoven, The Netherlands
*E-mail address:* dorresteingm@noivbd.nl

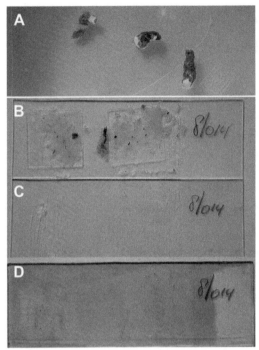

**Fig. 1.** Fecal exam canary (*Serinus canaria*). (*A*) Macroscopy, (*B*) wet mount (with saline), (*C*) thin smear air dried, (*D*) thin smear (*C*) stained with a quick stain.

isolated from the feces or intestinal contents of diseased passerine birds both with and without diarrhea.

*E coli* septicemia is suspected to be a major cause of epizootic mortality in newly arrived shipments of finches. *Citrobacter* spp infection has also been reported as a cause of mortality in finches, and gross necropsy can, as with *E coli*, be unrewarding. The Enterobacteriaceae present a secondary problem in finches more frequently than in canaries. The clinical signs and gross necropsy are not specific and include depression, conjunctivitis, and rhinitis, and may be fatal in some birds. These are secondary pathogens, however, and should be considered as a sign of poor health or management conditions. Other primary diseases may be present (eg, atoxoplasmosis or coccidiosis). Cultures are necessary for diagnosis, and a sensitivity test is essential for treatment. At the same time, clinicians must search for the primary underlying cause to prevent recurrence.

Enterobacteriaceae are regularly cultured from passerine nestlings with diarrhea ("sweating disease"). The antibiotics of choice are neomycin or spectinomycin, because they are effective and not resorbed from the gut. The selected drug is administered via the soft food, whereas fledglings require extra water, chopped greens, and vegetables to prevent dehydration. As always, the clinician should remember that a specific culture and sensitivity is recommended to select the most effective antibiotic.

### Yersiniosis (Pseudotuberculosis)

Infection with *Yersinia pseudotuberculosis* is regularly seen in canaries and wild finches in the wintertime in Europe. The clinical signs are nonspecific: ruffling of the feathers, debilitation, and high mortality. At necropsy, a dark, swollen, congested liver and spleen with small, yellow, focal bacterial granulomata are often found, with an associated acute catarrhal pneumonia and typhilitis. Many rod-shaped bacteria are seen in impression smears from all the organs, and diagnosis is confirmed after culturing the microorganisms. The treatment of choice is amoxicillin via drinking water and soft food. Once sensitivity test results have been obtained, the antibiotic might need to be changed. Cleaning and disinfection are essential to prevent a relapse after therapy has been completed.

Mynahs are very susceptible to yersiniosis, and mortality can be high owing to peracute pneumonia. Postmortem examination of affected birds demonstrates hepatomegaly, sometimes with small white foci, splenomegaly, and an acute to peracute pneumonia.

### Salmonellosis (Paratyphoid)

Infection with *Salmonella typhimurium* in small passerines appears similarly to pseudo-tuberculosis, both clinically and at necropsy (**Fig. 2**), although salmonellosis more often has a chronic course. Carriers are unknown in canaries. The diagnosis is confirmed after culturing the microorganism. Fatal septicemias are also reported in mynahs.

Antibiotics that are most effective are trimethoprim (with or without sulfa), amoxicillin, or enrofloxacin, and must be combined with proper hygiene measures. A bacteriological examination of a pooled fecal sample in an enrichment medium should be performed 3 to 6 weeks after therapy to evaluate its success. The therapy and hygiene measures can be repeated until the bacteriological control remains negative.

### Campylobacter Fetus

*Campylobacter fetus* subsp *jejuni* is often found in tropical finches, especially in juvenile Estrildidae. Society finches are commonly identified as carriers without conspicuous clinical symptoms. Clinical signs include apathy, retarded moulting, yellow droppings, and a high mortality, especially among fledglings. The yellow droppings are caused by large amounts of undigested starch (amylum) (**Fig. 3**) and occasionally parts of or whole seeds are found in the droppings. At necropsy the intestine is filled with a yellow amylum or whole seeds, resembling the beads of a rosary. Other necropsy findings are cachexia and a congested gastrointestinal tract. The diagnosis is confirmed by demonstrating the curved rods in stained smears from the droppings or gut contents, and cultivating the bacteria on special microaerophilic media. *Campylobacter* spp have also been isolated from recently imported mynahs.

Treatment can be attempted with several antibiotics, but hygienic measurements are most important. Although campylobacteriosis is considered a potential zoonosis, there are no published reports of *Campylobacter* spp transmission from passerines to humans.

### Cocci Infections

*Streptococcus* spp and *Staphylococcus* spp are often demonstrated in passerines. The clinical signs include abscesses, dermatitis, "bumble foot," conjunctivitis, sinusitis, arthritis, pneumonia, and death. In patients suffering from these infections, cocci will be seen in the impression smears. The treatment of choice for cocci infections is local and systemic treatment with ampicillin or amoxicillin.

*Enterococcus faecalis* has been associated with chronic tracheitis, pneumonia, and air sac infections in canaries. Clinically affected birds have harsh respiratory sounds, voice changes, and dyspnea.

### Pseudomonas spp and Aeromonas spp Infections

Improperly prepared sprouted or germinated seeds, dirty drinking vessels or baths, and water are often the source of *Pseudomonas* spp or *Aeromonas* spp bacteria. A polluted

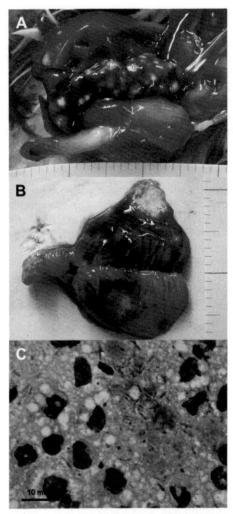

**Fig. 2.** Canary (*Serinus canaria*) with salmonellosis. Necropsy showing enlarged spleen with miliary necrosis (*A*), necrosis in the lungs (*B*), and rod-shaped bacteria in the air sacs (*C*) (Hemacolor).

flower-spraying mister, used for spraying the birds, can cause a severe necropurulent pneumonia and aerosacculitis. *Pseudomonas* spp are often found as the result of an improper antibiotic treatment. Proper treatment includes locating the source of the trouble and administration of an antibiotic (after performing a sensitivity test). Until the results are available, the first choice antibiotic in these infections is enrofloxacin. Painstaking hygiene is essential, because many strains are resistant to antibiotic treatment.

### Avian Tuberculosis

The classic tuberculosis with tubercles in the organs is seldom seen in small passerines. Tuberculosis (so-called atypical *Mycobacterium avium* or *Mycobacterium-avium-intracellulare* complex) is most commonly found accidentally at necropsy in canaries and finches (Estrildidae). *Mycobacterium genavense* is also associated

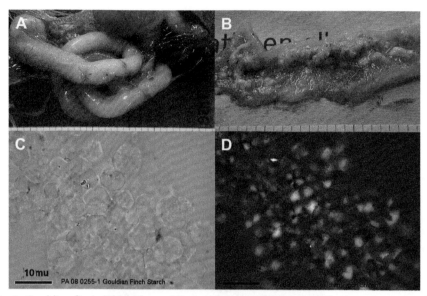

**Fig. 3.** Gouldian finch (*Chloebia gouldiae*) with Campylobacteriose. The intestines are pale and edematous (*A* and *B*). In a stained smear of the intestinal contents undigested starch can be recognized (*C*) that will show "crosses" in polarized light (*D*).

with avian tuberculosis, and is commonly isolated from patients with AIDS.[5,6] So far there is only one report of a canary with a tuberculous nodule in the lung caused by *Mycobacterium tuberculosis*; it is the first description of *M tuberculosis* in a non-psittacine bird species.[7] Other mycobacteria from the *Mycobacterium fortuitum* group are also documented in Gouldian finches infected with the so-called atypical form by *Mycobacterium peregrinum*.[8]

Incidental infections with acid-fast bacilli are diagnosed relatively often. On histological examination, macrophages loaded with acid-fast bacilli can be found in many organs, especially in the liver or intestines. No signs are apparent at necropsy, except perhaps a dark, slightly swollen liver. In a flock of zebra finches with signs of a central nervous system disease, acid-fast bacteria were demonstrated in impression smears of brain, liver, and intestines, and the bacterium was identified as *M genavense* by using polymerase chain reaction (PCR).[9]

Infections with *Mycobacterium* spp have also been reported in mynahs as a catarrhal enteritis, as well as classical tuberculosis.[10]

The diagnosis is confirmed by demonstrating nonstaining rod-shaped bacteria (ghost cells) in a stained impression smear (**Fig. 4**). With a Ziehl Neelson stain, the bacteria stain red (acid-fast) in tissue smears, whereas differentiation is possible using PCR techniques.

Treatment is not often practiced. There is a zoonosis aspect, mostly for people with an immunocompromised physiological status. The enclosures need to be cleaned and disinfected. In infected soil, *Mycobacterium* spp can survive for 2 years.

### Avian Chlamydiosis

This is a relatively uncommon problem in passerines and softbills. The annual incidence of avian chlamydiosis in canaries at necropsy in the Netherlands is between

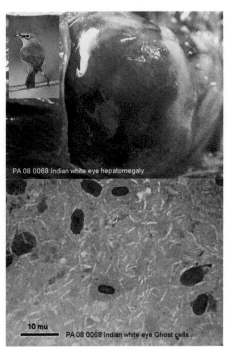

PA 08 0068 Indian white eye hepatomegaly

10 mu

PA 08 0068 Indian white eye Ghost cells

**Fig. 4.** Indian white eye (*Zosterops palpebrosus*) with atypical avian tuberculosis: an enlarged liver without tubercles. In the stained impression smear ghost cells can be seen as non stained rods (Hemacolor).

0.0% and 1.4%. *Chlamydophila psittaci* spp have been isolated from the droppings of clinically normal finches in households in which clinical cases of chlamydiosis (psittacosis) occurred in psittacines.[11] In a study in Israel, 26% of the Passeriformes tested by immunofluorescence test were positive, ranging from 10% in zoo collections up to 41% in pet birds.[12] Of these, 12% were found in the winter (December to February) and 41% in the summer (June to August). In a study of wild birds in Austria using an enzyme-linked immunosorbent assay (ELISA) test, 5 of 29 passerines were positive for the antigen and 15 of 17 showed antibodies.[13] Based on reviews, geographical areas and different test systems give large differences.

The clinical signs associated with this disease are nonspecific, and can include apathy, diarrhea, debilitation, nasal exudates, and conjunctivitis. The mortality is generally less then 10%. Avian chlamydiosis should be expected in passerines with recurrent respiratory disease, especially if they are exposed to psittacines.

The diagnosis is made at necropsy by the presence of the chlamydial organism in impression smears from the altered air sacs and organs, using special staining techniques, or a PCR test from swabs.

In mynahs, shedding has been demonstrated in clinically healthy birds.[10]

Treatment with chlortetracycline (30 days) or doxycycline (30 days) via drinking water and soft food is clinically effective, but only when the birds continue to eat and drink the normal amount of food and water.

### Mycoplasma spp

*Mycoplasma* spp have been isolated from canaries, and many cases of conjunctivitis and upper respiratory disease in canaries respond to tylosin; however, there has been no conclusive work proving that *Mycoplasma* spp are associated with this syndrome. An epizootic of conjunctivitis in house finches (*Carpodacus mexicanus*) associated with *Mycoplasma gallisepticum* (MG) infection was reported in 1994 and 1995 from the United States and has been spreading from east to west in 10 years.[14,15] Ever since *M gallisepticum* emerged among house finches in North America, it has been suggested that bird aggregations at feeders are an important cause of the epidemic of mycoplasmal conjunctivitis because diseased birds could deposit droplets of pathogen onto the feeders and thereby promote indirect transmission by fomites. House finches infected via this route, however, developed only mild disease and recovered much more rapidly than birds infected from the same source birds but directly into the conjunctiva. Although it is certainly probable that house finch aggregations at artificial feeders enhance pathogen transmission, to some degree transmission of *M gallisepticum* by fomites may serve to immunize birds against developing more severe infections. Some such birds develop *M gallisepticum* antibodies, providing indication of an immune response, although no direct evidence of protection.[16] The clinical signs ranged from mildly swollen eyelids with clear ocular discharge to severe conjunctivitis and apparent blindness.

Tetracyclines and enrofloxacin are believed to be effective against many *Mycoplasma* spp. Clinical signs of conjunctivitis associated with MG infection in house finches resolved following oral tylosin (1 mg/mL drinking water for at least 21 days) as the sole source of drinking water, in conjunction with topical ciprofloxacin HCl ophthalmic solution for 5 to 7 days.[17]

### Other Bacterial Infections

Gram-negative oviduct infections, which if untreated can cause high mortality among canary hens sitting on their second round of eggs, are seen in epidemic proportions in canary breeding establishments in some years.[11]

*Erysipelothrix rhusiopathia*, *Listeria monocytogenes,* and *Pasteurella multocida* (catbite) are occasionally isolated from dead passerine and softbill birds.

Megabacteria were recently classified as yeast-like organisms (*Macrorhabdus ornithogaster*).

### PARASITIC INFECTIONS
### Protozoal Infections

The most important protozoal infections in canaries are atoxoplasmosis, coccidiosis, toxoplasmosis, and trichomoniasis. Atoxoplasma-like infections and cryptosporidiosis are found only occasionally in finches, starlings, and mynahs, and are mostly restricted to individual birds; in those species of birds the infection is never seen as a flock problem. Coccidiosis, cochlosomosis, and trichomoniasis are common in finches. In softbills, *Giardia* spp and coccidiosis are occasionally noted in fecal examination or postmortem examination. There is one report of microsporidiosis in a flock of tricolor parrot finches (*Erythrura tricolor*). These birds showed a pale thickening of the serosal surfaces of the gastrointestinal tract, pancreas, and air sacs.[18] Unknown protozoa can be found in cytology smear in all parts of the digestive tract, eg, the proventriculus (**Fig. 5**).

### Atoxoplasmosis

Atoxoplasmosis (formerly *Lankesterella*) in canaries is caused by *Isospora serini*, a coccidium with an asexual life cycle in the organs and a sexual cycle in the intestinal mucosa. Atoxoplasmosis is a disease of young canaries ranging in age from 2 to 9 months. The clinical signs include huddling and ruffling of the feathers, debilitation,

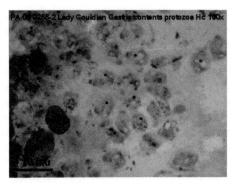

**Fig. 5.** Gouldian finch (*Chloebia gouldiae*). Incidental finding of protozoa (*) in a scraping of the proventriculus (Hemacolor).

diarrhea, neurological signs (20%), and death. Mortality can be as high as 80%. An enlarged liver may be observed as a blue spot on the right side of the abdomen caudal to the sternum, referred to by fanciers as "thick liver disease." At necropsy, an enlarged and sometimes spotted liver (with necrosis in the acute phase) is noted, along with a huge, dark-red colored spleen and, often, an edematous duodenum with vascularization. In the imprints of the liver, spleen, and lungs, parasites are found in the cytoplasm of the monocytes (**Fig. 6**). The nucleus of the host cell is crescent-

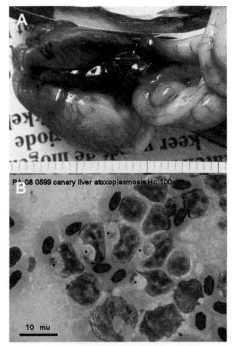

**Fig. 6.** Canary (*Serinus* canaria) acute atoxoplasmosis. At necropsy a typical enlarged spleen can be seen (*A*). In a stained impression smear the parasites (*) can be recognized as indents in the nuclei of the monocytes (*B*) (Hemacolor).

shaped. Coccidia are seldom found in the feces or intestinal contents because, after the acute phase is passed, only a few coccidia (100–200/24 hours) are excreted. The therapeutic agent of choice is sulphachlorpyrazine (150 mg/L drinking water) until after moulting for 5 days a week. This treatment affects the production of oocysts, but does not influence the intracellular stages. Other coccidiostats are used, like toltrazuril and diclazuril, but real controlled studies are not yet available.[19]

Other measures to improve health of young birds include feeding one part egg food and one part seed mixture until after moulting, prevention of crowding (eg, stress reduction), and better hygiene (ie, cleaning and changing the floor coating). These measures alone can prevent clinical outbreaks in infected canaries. This infection is also a common problem in other European finches kept in captivity (eg, goldfinches, siskins, greenfinches, bullfinches).

### Atoxoplasma-like infections

Atoxoplasma-like infections are seen in tropical finches, mynahs, and other Sturnidae. Atoxoplasmosis and hemochromatosis are the primary medical problems in captive Bali mynahs. Atoxoplasma oocysts have been found in the feces of wild Bali mynahs; however, it is unknown whether this disease is contributing to the birds' decline.[19]

### Coccidiosis

*Isospora* spp have been described in more than 50 species of passerines throughout the world. Although this species was formerly named *Isospora lacazei*, the author is convinced that there are many different species. A recent experimental infection supports this assumption. *Isospora michaelbakeri* is one of the *Isospora* species most commonly found in the wild, which can cause severe infection and mortality in young sparrows. This *Isospora* was orally inoculated to russet sparrows (*Passer rutilans*), spotted munia (*Lonchura punctulata*), canaries (*Serinus canaria*), Java sparrows (*Padda oryzivora*), chickens (*Gallus domesticus*), ducks (*Anas platyrhynchos*), and BALB/c mice. The results indicated that *I michaelbakeri* infected only russet sparrows and not any other species experimentally inoculated with *I michaelbakeri* in that study.[20]

In canaries, *Isospora canaria* is identified as a specific intestinal coccidiosis, and can be a problem in canaries older than 2 months of age. The primary clinical signs observed in *I canaria*–infected patients are diarrhea and emaciation. At necropsy the duodenum is edematous, often with extensive hemorrhages in the gut wall. Trophozoites and/or gamonts of the parasite can be found in scrapings of the duodenal mucosa, and large amounts of oocysts are seen in wet preparations from the droppings (**Fig. 7**). Therapy consists of strict hygiene measures and treatment with coccidiostatic drugs. Amprolium solution has been recommended for the treatment of coccidiosis at a dosage of 50 to 100 mg/L for 5 days, or sulphachlorpyrazine 300 mg/L drinking water, 5 days a week for 2 to 3 weeks.

*Eimeria* spp are not common in passerines, but single cases are being reported, based on the morphology of sporulated oocysts (*Eimeria* spp four sporocysts with two sporozoites, 4:2; *Isospora* spp 2:4). In hill mynahs, *Eimeria* spp are associated with hemorrhagic enteritis.[10]

Other coccidia, eg, *Dorisiella* spp (2:8) and *Wendyonella* spp (4:4), have also been identified in passerines.

*Sarcocystis* has been identified in skeletal muscle of many Passeriformes, especially in North America. Cowbirds, grackles, and other Passeriformes have been shown to be intermediate hosts for *Sarcocystis falculata*, for which opossums are

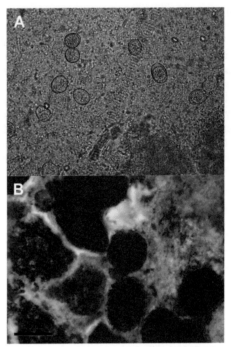

**Fig. 7.** Yellow grosbeak (*Pheucticus chrysopeplus*) showing coccidia in the wet mount of the feces (*A*) and gamonts in the mucosal scraping of the duodenum (*B*) (Hemacolor).

the definitive hosts. *Sarcocystis* is usually found incidentally when necropsy examinations are performed.

### Toxoplasmosis

In the acute phase of toxoplasmosis, the birds (canaries and mynahs) may show severe respiratory signs. In canaries this phase is often not diagnosed, and the owner is alarmed only when several birds become blind many weeks after becoming infected. In a flock, many birds were affected with blindness, which developed over a 3-month span, and two birds developed torticollis. The route of infection is not known, but it is likely that oocysts excreted in cat feces get into the aviary. In the acute phase, hepatomegaly and splenomegaly, and mostly a severe catarrhal pneumonia and a myositis of the pectoral muscle, are found in canaries and mynahs at necropsy. The trophozoites are easily identified in impression smears. Microscopic alterations within the eye consisted of a nonsuppurative chorioretinitis with large numbers of macrophages that contained the tachyzoite form of *Toxoplasma gondii* in the subretinal space, and aggregates of tachyzoites were found in the nerve fiber layer of the retina with and without necrosis. Tissue cysts with bradyzoites were scattered throughout the meninges and neuropil of the cerebrum and cerebellum.[21] In histological slides from the brains, (pseudo)cysts are relatively easy to find. Serology, immunofluorescence on brain tissue slides, or a PCR confirms the diagnosis. The Sabin–Feldman dye test will not detect *T gondii* antibodies in the serum of birds.[22] No effective treatment is known, although some effect is claimed using trimethoprim 0.08 g/mL $H_2O$ and sulfadiazine 0.04 g/mL in water for 2 weeks. A second treatment regime was given for 3 weeks.[21]

### Cryptosporidiosis

Cryptosporidiosis has been associated with acute onset, severe diarrhea and death in a diamond firetail finch, but is not common in passerines. The case in the firetail finch showed focal cuboidal metaplasia of the glandular epithelium of the proventriculus and amyloid deposits in the proventriculus and kidneys. In another case, canaries were infected with cryptosporidia in the proventriculus and *Salmonella* spp was concurrently isolated.[11] Although they are generally opportunistic and secondary invaders, they have been reported as primary pathogens producing respiratory and/or intestinal disease in birds.[23]

### Trichomoniasis

Trichomoniasis is commonly seen in many avian species. The protozoa are not very host-specific. In canaries, infections with *Trichomonas* spp are seen sporadically, and birds of all ages can be affected. Common clinical signs include respiratory symptoms, regurgitation, nasal discharge, and emaciation. The diagnosis can be made in a live bird, using a crop swab. At necropsy, trichomoniasis infections present as a thickened, opaque crop wall. The flagellates can be identified, even when the bird is not very fresh, in crop smears stained with Hemacolor or another "quick stain." The treatment is the same as for cochlosomosis.

In mynahs, the lesions look like trichomoniasis in pigeons with typical lesions in the oral cavity.

Another flagellate is seen in the crop of canaries, causing the same clinical signs in full-grown birds and mortality in nestlings. The diagnosis can be made with a wet mount, but the flagellates are difficult to recognize. The parasite does not move about in the preparation, but "waves" with its flagella.[24] The same flagellate is held responsible for pruritus, feather loss, and increased moulting time in individual kept canaries.[25] Using electron microscopy and PCR this flagellate was classified as an imperfect *Trichomonas* sp.

### Cochlosomosis

The flagellate *Cochlosoma* spp, living in the intestinal tract of society finches, can cause many deaths among Australian finches fostered by these carriers.[26] It is a problem in young birds from 10 days until 6 weeks of age. Typical signs are debilitation, shivering because of dehydration, and difficulties with moulting.

The diagnosis of cochlosomosis is based on demonstrating the flagellates in fresh feces. Treatment consists of ronidazole at 400 mg/kg egg food and 400 mg/L drinking water for 5 days. After a pause of 2 days, the regimen is repeated. This drug is relatively safe and no toxic signs have been seen. If dimetridazole is used, the concentration should not exceed 100 mg active drug per liter for 5 days. A sign of intoxication with dimetridazole is torticollis, and this will disappear after the medication is stopped. Metronidazole has also been reported to cause toxicity in finches.

Management should include disinfecting water containers, and the aviary should be kept clean and dry.

### Giardia spp

*Giardia* spp have been reported to be associated with gastrointestinal tract infections in finches (**Fig. 8**). Treatment for *Giardia* spp is the same as for trichomonads.

## Blood Parasites

Blood parasites may be detected on routine screening of apparently healthy passerines, but they are rarely implicated as the primary cause of disease or death. The most

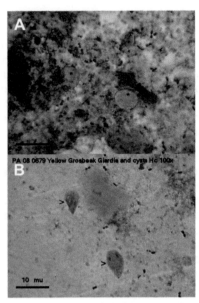

**Fig. 8.** Yellow grosbeak (*Pheucticus chrysopeplus*) showing in the intestines Giardia cyst (*A\**) and Giardia organisms (*B* >) (Hemacolor).

commonly encountered blood parasites include *Hemoproteus* spp, *Leukocytozoon* spp, *Trypanosoma* spp, *Plasmodium* spp (malaria), and microfilaria.

*Plasmodium* spp, the cause of avian malaria, are mosquito-borne protozoa that occur worldwide. Sporogony occurs in the invertebrate host, schizogony occurs in the erythrocytes, and golden or black refractile pigment granules are formed from the host cell hemoglobin. *Plasmodium* spp have been described in free-ranging passerines, including tits, finches, thrushes, starlings, and sparrows. They are occasionally found in captive-bred birds such as canaries and other finches. The diagnosis is based on the demonstration of the parasite in erythrocytes, and is differentiated from *Hemoproteus* spp by the demonstration of the schizont in malaria. Clinical and postmortem signs include anemia and splenomegaly. Molecular techniques (PCR) have also been developed and results of avian population surveys conducted with PCR assays suggest that prevalences of malarial infection are higher than previously documented, and that studies based on microscopic examination of blood smears may substantially underestimate the extent of parasitism by these apicomplexans. Nonetheless, because the published primers miss small numbers of infections detected by other methods, including inspection of smears, no assay now available for avian malaria is universally reliable.[27]

Treatment with chloroquine (250 mg/120 mL drinking water for 1–2 weeks) or pyrimethamine is successful in some cases, but a lasting immunity does not occur. Controlling of mosquito vectors is necessary to prevent infection.

*Hemoproteus* spp are also found worldwide, but cause only mild or nonapparent clinical symptoms. For most species of *Hemoproteus,* the intermediate hosts are hippoboscid flies, biting midges, or tabanids. Diagnosis is based on identification of typical pigment-containing gametocytes in erythrocytes; but schizonts are not found in blood and tissue cells. Treatment is seldom indicated, and will be identical to the treatment for avian malaria.

*Leukocytozoon* spp occur worldwide, and can infect either erythrocytes or leucocytes. Parasitized cells are so distorted by the parasite that it may be difficult to determine their origin. Pigment is not produced by *Leukocytozoon*, and schizonts cannot be found in peripheral blood. Megaloschizonts can be found in brain, liver, lung, kidney, intestinal, heart, muscle, and lymphoid tissue. Most infections are subclinical, although vague signs and death are reported.

*Trypanosoma* spp are also found worldwide, but their incidence is low and they are found only during summer months in temperate climates. Vectors are thought to include hippoboscid flies, red mites, simuliids, and mosquitoes; treatment is not warranted.

Microfilariasis is mostly an incidental finding in cytology smears. There is no obvious pathology connected to this finding. The adult filaria are even more rarely found, mostly in the air sacs (**Fig. 9**).

### Helminth Parasitism

Helminth parasites are usually of no significance in small passerines. Acanthocephalans, cestodes, and nematodes have mostly been reported in free-ranging and captive large passerines (eg, thrushes, grackles, and starlings). Insect-eating species in particular show more parasitic infections.

### Nematodes

Two main types of roundworms affect passerines: *Ascaridia* spp, which have a direct life cycle, and *Porrocaecum* spp, which have an indirect life cycle, with invertebrates such as earthworms as the intermediate host. Both types of roundworms may be associated with weight loss, diarrhea, general debility, and, sometimes, neurological signs. *Ascaridia* spp are uncommon in small passerines. *Porrocaecum* spp have been found in a variety of free-ranging passerines (eg, pipits, thrush, blackbirds, and corvids). Fenbendazole, piperazine, levamisole, and ivermectin, all orally applied, are useful in treating ascarid infections.

*Capillaria* spp are cosmopolitan in their distribution and affect a range of passerines, including mynahs. The life cycle is direct, or may involve earthworms as paratenic hosts. Susceptibility does not depend on dietary preferences, and the parasite has been found to cause disease in a variety of seed-eaters, insect-eaters, omnivorous species, and honey-eaters.

High parasite loads may lead to weight loss, diarrhea, general ill health, and death. These worms may localize to a variety of sites in the gastrointestinal tract. They may be associated with white or creamy-colored plaques in the buccal cavity or pharynx, and

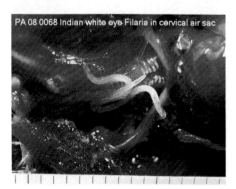

PA 08 0068 Indian white eye Filaria in cervical air sac

**Fig. 9.** Indian white eye (*Zosterops palpebrosus*) with filaria in the air sac as an incidental finding.

swelling of the crop, proventriculus, intestines, or bowel. The typical *Capillaria* spp egg has bipolar plugs and may be found by direct swabbing of lesions or feces, or by fecal flotation.

Treatment may be more difficult than for ascarids. Aviary hygiene and removal of earthworms are important control measures. Anthelmintics may be effective in some cases. In a cleaned, dry environment, the eggs will lose their infectious capacity within 3 weeks without further disinfection.[10]

*Syngamus trachea* (gapeworm) are found in outdoor aviaries and are a serious problem in mynahs, corvids, and starlings. Earthworms may act as a transport host. The signs include gasping for breath, and the small passerines often die from occlusion of the trachea by the worms and the mucus produced (**Fig. 10**). The diagnosis

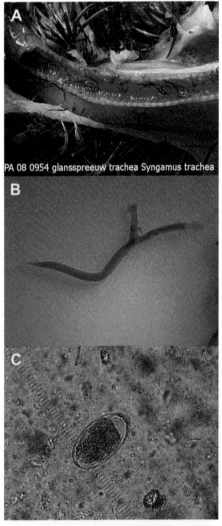

**Fig.10.** Superb starling (*Lamprotornis superbus*). Trachea blocked *Syngamus trachea* (*A*). The worms live in pairs attached (*B*) and the eggs are easily recognized in the feces (*C*).

is confirmed by demonstrating the worms in the trachea by using backlighting, or by finding the typical eggs in the droppings. The worms are easily identified in the trachea at necropsy. Ivermectin (injection 200 µg/kg) and levamisole or fenbendazole are effective in treating this parasite, but caution should be exercised when treating birds with heavy infections, because the dead worms can obstruct the trachea. In such a case with a heavy worm burden, treatment with a low dose of an anthelmintic (especially fenbendazole) over several days provides effective treatment.

### Spiruroids

*Geopetitia aspiculata* is a parasite that lives in the proventriculus and has been reported in tropical birds housed at zoological gardens in Europe and North America.[28,29] Insects (eg, cockroaches, crickets) serve as intermediate hosts. *G aspiculata* are pathogenic, leading to perforation of the wall of the proventriculus, often resulting in death. The parasite is not host-specific and is demonstrated in six avian orders, including Passeriformes (eg, Emberizidae, Estrildidae, Fringillidae, Icteridae, and Sturnidae, including a hill mynah). The diagnosis is confirmed by finding the embryonated spiruroid eggs in the feces (although this might not always be effective), followed by endoscopic demonstration of the proventricular lesions. At necropsy an enlarged abdomen is found, caused by a mass of tightly coiled parasites attached to the serosa of the proventriculus, and worms are sometimes found in the liver. Infected birds can be successfully treated with ivermectin (300–400 µg/kg body weight subcutaneously) or fenbendazole (25 mg/kg body weight orally for 3 days). To interrupt the development cycle of the parasite, emphasis should be laid on eradication of the intermediate host.

*Acuaria skrjabini* infections of the gizzard, with mucosal necrosis, have been reported in adult finches in Australia. The mortality rate was 4% to 5%, and oral treatment with 80 mg levamisole or 50 mg fenbendazole/L drinking water for 3 days was effective.

Feeding live food (such as maggots, mealworms, or termites) or providing a compost heap in the aviary to attract insects for the birds to eat are both common management practices in Australia. These practices increase the likelihood of infection, as insects are the intermediate hosts for gizzardworms and tapeworms.

Tapeworm (*Cestoda*) infestations in softbills and insectivorous finches are common. They are not normally seen in canaries or exclusively seed-eating birds, except in situations where parents feed insects to their offspring or insects are accidentally consumed with the seeds.[11] Some necropsies show small intestines literally packed with the tiny tapeworms. The typical hexacanth embryos are usually identified on fecal flotation. Effective treatment for passerines diagnosed with tapeworms include praziquantel and oxfenbendazole.

*Trematodes* have complicated life cycles that typically involve snails as initial intermediate hosts and other invertebrates as secondary intermediate hosts. Trematodes are seen occasionally in wild-caught passerines. *Schistozoma* spp are trematodes that live in blood vessels and have been reported in North American goldfinches and cardinals. *Prosthogonimus* spp are trematodes affecting the intestinal tract, cloaca, bursa of Fabricius, or oviduct. These parasites been found worldwide in passerines, and are not particularly pathogenic. Dragonflies and snails are intermediate hosts. Praziquantel (10 mg/kg) may be useful in treating trematodes.

### Arthropods

Ectoparasites, including blood-sucking mites (*Dermanyssus gallinae* and *Ornithonyssus sylviarum*), skin mites (eg, *Backericheyla* spp and *Neocheyletiella media*) and feather mites (eg, Epidermotidae, *Dermation* spp), are found in the calamus of the feathers. Meal-mites (*Tyroglyphus farinae*) are not parasites, but their large number on a bird can cause unrest and irritation.

The red mite (*Dermanyssus gallinae*) is a blood-sucking mite that can cause serious mortality among fledglings as well as adult birds. The common clinical sign in affected patients is anemia. A bird with respiratory symptoms and a PCV of less than 30% should be suspected of having serious problems with blood-sucking mites (**Fig. 11**). The main complaint from the owner is general depression; the mites are often not detected or their presence is even denied. The red mite spends the day in the nest or bird-room crevices, and ventures out at night to attack the birds. Treatment should be prompt, and consists of dusting or spraying the victims with an insecticide and vacating the cage or room during the day and thoroughly cleaning it.

The white or northern mite (*Ornithonyssus sylviarum*) is increasingly found to cause problems in aviaries. This blood-sucking mite spends its entire life on the host. Dusting with insecticides can be hazardous, especially to nestlings. A relatively safe method of treatment is to put one drop of 0.1% ivermectin in propylene glycol on the bare skin; however, the mites are killed only after sucking blood.

Other ectoparasites may cause some irritation or feather damage. They are considered a sign of inadequate hygiene and management.

Quill mites have been described in passerines, and infested birds show clinical signs of irritation, pruritus, feather-picking, and feather-loss. These signs are rarely severe. The mites seem to feed on the quill tissue, and not on blood or sebaceous fluid. Many different species of quill mites are described, including *Syringophylus* spp, *Harpyrhynchus* spp, *Dermatoglyphus* spp, and *Picobia* spp. Regularly new quill mites are being described in all bird species.[30] The diagnosis is made by inspection (usually with magnification) of quill material. Treatment with ivermectin (spot-on 0.1% ivermectin in propylene glycol) is very effective.[21]

*Kemidocoptes pilae* infections, or scaly mites, are occasionally seen on the beak base of finches. In general, they tend to cause hyperkeratotic lesions on the feet in Passeriformes. These mites are easily found and recognized in scrapings from the altered areas. Treatment with any oil or 0.1% ivermectin applied locally will cure the birds. This infestation should not be confused with the so-called "tassel foot" found in the European goldfinch (*Carduelis carduelis*), which is caused by a papillomavirus.

Lice are fairly common in Passeriformes. Some biting lice are not specialized for life on particular feathers, and are able to move quickly. Chewing lice are often more

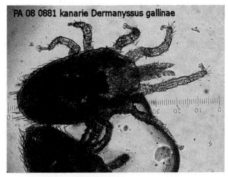

**Fig. 11.** *Dermanyssus gallinae* found in the package of a dead Canary (*Serinus canaria*) sent for necropsy.

adapted to a particular part of the body, and are more sluggish. Signs of the presence of lice include restlessness and biting, excessive preening, and damage to the plumage. Some cases of baldness in canaries are caused by lice. Lice undergo a complete life cycle on the bird, and a weekly dusting with pyrethrins is an effective method of control.[11] Some species of Estrildidae are hypersensitive to pyrethrin, and care must be taken in its use.

### Endoparasites

Air sac mites (*Sternostoma tracheacolum*) are occasionally found in canaries, but they are seen mostly commonly in Australian finches. They are not reported in softbills. This problem is also seen in wild Gouldian finches in Australia, and may have been introduced with domestic canaries. The mites' life cycle is unknown, but it is theorized that nestlings become infected by parents regurgitating nutrients with mites. Adults may be exposed via contamination of water and food, and by coughing or sneezing.

Clinical signs include a decline in physical condition, respiratory distress, wheezing, squeaking, coughing, sneezing, nasal discharge, loss of voice, head shaking, and gasping. The mortality is low. Diagnosis of air sac mites can sometimes be made by transillumination of the trachea in live birds, with the mites visible as tiny black points in the trachea. The throat of the bird must be wetted (eg, with alcohol) and the feathers parted. Postmortem examination, however, is more reliable, and the condition is diagnosed by finding in the mites in the air sacs, the lungs, and/or the trachea. Air sacculitis, tracheitis, and focal pneumonia may be evident.

Several therapeutic regimens have been described for air sac mite infestations. Pest strips make a reasonably good air sac mite preventative, provided the bird does not come into direct contact, and only if the bird is not held within a small enclosure. Ivermectin can be used for individual treatment by a spot-on method of 0.1% ivermectin in propylene glycol, one drop on the bare skin dorsolateral to the thorax inlet or on the chest. A small amount of alcohol to wet the skin is helpful to view the site of application.

*Cytodites nudus* is another mite that has occasionally been associated with respiratory disease in free-ranging passerines. It may be found in the abdominal cavity as well as the respiratory system.

### REFERENCES

1. Dorrestein Gerry M. Passerines. In: Tully TN, Dorrestein GM, editors. Handbook of avian medicine. 2nd edition. Edinburgh: Saunders Elsevier; 2009. p. 169–208.
2. Dorrestein GM. Passerines. In: Altman RB, Clubb SL, Dorrestein GM, editors. Avian medicine and surgery. Philadelphia: WB Saunders; 1997. p. 867–85.
3. Hawkins M. Passerine birds. Seminars in avian and exotic pet medicine 2003;12: 1–36.
4. Sandmeier P, Coutteel P. Management of canaries, finches and mynahs. In: Harrison G, Lightfoot T, editors, Clinical avian medicine, vol. II. Palm Beach (FL): Spix Publishing; 2006. p. 879–913.
5. Hoop RK, Ossen P, Pfyffer G. Mycobacterium genavense: a new cause of mycobacteriosis in pet birds? In: Proceedings of the 3rd European conference of the Association of Avian Veterinarians. Israel; 1995. p. 1–3.
6. Hoop RK, Bottger EC, Pfyffer G. Etiological agents of mycobacteriosis in pet birds between 1986 and 1995. J Clin Microbiol 1996;34:991–2.
7. Hoop RK. *Mycobacterium tuberculosis* infection in a canary (*Serinus canaria* L.) and a blue-fronted Amazon parrot (*Amazona amazona aestiva*). Avian Dis 2002;46:502–4.

8. Vitali SD, Eden PA, Payne KL, et al. An outbreak of mycobacteriosis in Gouldian finches caused by *Mycobacterium peregrinum*. Vet Clin North Am Exot Anim Pract 2006;9:519–22.

9. Sandmeier P, Hoop RK, Bosshart G. Cerebral mycobacteriosis in zebra finches (Taeniopygia guttata) caused by Mycobacterium genavense. In: Proceedings of the 4th conference of the European Association of Avian Veterinarians. London; 1997. p. 119–22.

10. Korbel R, Kösters J. Beos. In: Gabrisch K, Zwart P, editors. Krankheiten der Heimtiere. 4th edition. Hannover: Schlütersche; 1998. p. 397–428.

11. Macwhirter P. Passeriformes. In: Ritchie B, Harrison G, Harrison L, editors. Avian medicine: principles and application. Lake Worth (FL): Wingers; 1994. p. 1172–99.

12. Dublin A, Mechani S, Malkinson M, et al. A 4-year survey of the distribution of Chlamydia psittaci in 19 orders of birds in Israel with emphasis on seasonal variability. In: Proceedings of the 3rd European conference of the Association of Avian Veterinarians. Israel; 1995. p. 1.

13. Pohl U. Chlamydia psittaci in Austrian wild birds. In: Proceedings of the 3rd European conference of the Association of Avian Veterinarians. Israel; 1995. p. 15–17.

14. Fischer JR, Converse KA. Overview of conjunctivitis in house finches in the eastern United States, 1994–1995. In: Proceedings of the joint conferences AAZV, WDA, AAWV. American Association of Zoo Veterinarians. Pittsburgh (PA). Pittsburgh (PA); 1995. p. 508–9.

15. Ley DH, Shaeffer DS, Dhondt AA. Further western spread of *Mycoplasma gallisepticum* infection of house finches. J Wildl Dis 2006;42:429–31.

16. Dhondt AA, Dhondt KY, Hawley DM, et al. Experimental evidence for transmission of *Mycoplasma gallisepticum* in house finches by fomites. Avian Pathol 2007;36: 205–8.

17. Mashima TY, Ley DH, Stoskopf MK, et al. Evaluation of treatment of *Mycoplasma gallisepticum*-associated conjunctivitis in house finches (*Carpodacus mexicanus*). J Avian Med Surg 1997;11:20–4.

18. Gelis S, Raidal SR. Microsporidiosis in a flock of tricolor parrot finches (*Erythrura tricolor*). Vet Clin North Am Exot Anim Pract 2006;9:481–6.

19. Norton TM, Seibels RE, Greiner EC, et al. Bali mynah captive medical management and reintroduction program. In: proceedings of the main conference AAV; 1995. p. 125–36. Available at: http://www.riverbanks.org/subsite/aig/Atoxo-recommendations.htm. Accessed March 3, 2009.

20. Tung KC, Liu JS, Cheng FP, et al. Study on the species-specificity of *Isospora michaelbakeri* by experimental infection. Acta Vet Hung 2007;55:77–85.

21. Williams SM, Fulton RM, Render J, et al. Ocular and encephalic toxoplasmosis in canaries. Avian Dis 2001;45:262–7.

22. Patton S. Diagnosis of Toxoplasma gondii in birds. In: Proceedings of the Annual Conference Association of Avian Vetterinarians. Tampa (FL); 1996. p. 75–8.

23. Schmidt RE, Reavill DR, Phalen D. Pathology of pet and aviary birds. Ames (IA): Iowa State Press; 2003.

24. Van der Hage MH, Dorrestein GM. Flagellates in the crop of canary bird. In: Proceedings of the 1st European Association of Avian Veterinarians. Vienna; 1991. p. 303–7.

25. Cornelissen H, Dorrestein GM. A new dermatological disease in canaries (Serinus canarius) possibly caused by flagellates in the gastrointestinal tract. In: Proceedings of the 5th ECAMS scientific meeting. Tenerife; 2003. p. 17–8.

26. Poelma FG, Zwart P, Dorrestein GM, et al. Cochlosomose, a problem in raising Estrildidae in aviaries. Tijdschr Diergeneeskd 1978;103:589–93.
27. Fallon SM, Ricklefs RE, Swanson BL, et al. Detecting avian malaria: an improved polymerase chain reaction diagnostic. J Parasitol 2003;89:1044–7.
28. Kübber-Heiss A, Juncker M. Spiruridosis in birds at an Austrian Zoo. In: Proceedings of the 4th conference of the European Association of Avian Veterinarians. 1997. p. 102–6.
29. Tscherner W, Wittstatt U, Goltenboth R. *Geopetitia aspiculata* Webster, 1971— a pathogenic nematode in tropical birds in zoological gardens. Zool Garten NF 1997;67:108–20.
30. Bochkov V, Fain A, Skorackl M. New quill mites of the family Syringophilidae (Acari: cheyletoidea). Syst Parasitol 2004;57:135–50.

# Bacterial and Parasitic Diseases of Columbiformes

Roger Harlin, DVM[a],*, Laura Wade, DVM, ABVP–Avian[b]

KEYWORDS

- Bacterial • Parasitic • Diseases • Columbiformes
- Pigeons • Doves

Pigeons and doves have been associated with humans since 3000 to 5000 BC and make up an estimated 50% of all birds in captivity. Columbids are used for food, hobby, sport (racing homers), entertainment (rollers), display (exotic doves), shows and competitive exhibition (fancy breeds), research and communication (racing homers, tumblers and high fliers). All domestic pigeon breeds are derived from the common rock dove (*Columba livia*), and there are now more than 800 varieties. Common domesticated doves include the diamond dove (*Geopelia cuneata*) and European ringneck dove (*Streptopelia risoria*).

There are many excellent books, book chapters, journal articles, and conference proceedings manuscripts on the subject of pigeon medicine.[1–14] This article focuses on bacterial and parasitic diseases of domestic columbiform birds, with special mention of several important underlying viral infections.

## PREVENTIVE MEDICINE

One of the most important factors in preventing infectious disease in columbid flocks is to incorporate a sound preventative medicine program. Medications are thus rarely necessary if these guidelines are followed by the pigeon fancier:

Buy quality stock from quality breeders. Do not introduce new birds into an existing flock until they have been quarantined and physically examined. The optimal length of quarantine is the time for a pair to raise two or three sets of babies. When quarantine is over, introduce one pair at a time to the existing flock. Allow each pair to establish territory before adding the next pair. This method minimizes the stress of pairs finding a place in the loft.

Examine all new birds for ectoparasites, such as lice, mites, and pigeon flies. Perform fecal floatation and direct smears to check for helminths and *Coccidia*

[a] Southside Dog, Cat and Bird Hospital, 7020 South Shields Boulevard, Oklahoma City, OK 73149, USA
[b] Specialized Care for Avian and Exotic Pets, 5915 Broadway Street, Lancaster, NY 14086, USA
* Corresponding author.
*E-mail address:* rharlin@coxinet.net (R. Harlin).

Vet Clin Exot Anim 12 (2009) 453–473
doi:10.1016/j.cvex.2009.07.001
1094-9194/09/$ – see front matter © 2009 Elsevier Inc. All rights reserved.

sp. Examine throat aspirates for trichomonads and blood smears for *Hemoproteus* sp. If test results are negative, do not administer any medications, because evidence suggests that some drugs cause immunosuppression.

During quarantine, vaccinate all new acquisitions for paramyxovirus1 (PMV1). *Salmonella* vaccination is optional and is of questionable efficacy. Vaccination for pigeon pox is ideally done after other vaccines, because birds will have an active case of pox that can decrease the immune response to the other vaccines if these are given concurrently. Some practitioners administer all three vaccines at the same time, however, with no apparent ill effects.

Vaccinate all young birds at least 6 to 8 weeks before racing or show season. Do not add unvaccinated birds to the flock at this time because they could contract clinical poxvirus infection.

Keep pigeons in a clean, dry, well-ventilated loft. Do not overcrowd. Feed the birds according to their needs. If a problem arises, seek a diagnosis before administering medications.

## VIRAL DISEASES

Viral infection is often an underlying cause of illness of bacterial and parasitic disease and viral disease is probably much more common than actually diagnosed in pigeons. Most infections cause only mild illness, but subclinical infections can complicate the disease processes caused by other pathogens. Because the presence of viruses is usually confirmed on necropsy, other pathogens (eg, protozoa, gram-negative bacteria) are more likely to be implicated as the meteoric agents. A brief description of some important viral diseases is provided here.

Excluding PMV1 and pigeon pox virus, herpes virus and adenovirus are the most notable pathogens; however, circovirus, rotavirus, parvovirus, and influenza virus infections have been suggested as causes of immune system compromise.

### Pigeon Herpesvirus

Many pigeons are immune carriers of pigeon herpesvirus (PHV) and once infected are lifelong carriers, sometimes shedding without clinical signs. Young birds are most susceptible to clinical illness, but immunocompromised older birds can show symptoms.

A mild to necrotizing pharyngitis and esophagitis are the primary symptoms. Diphtheritic membranes and general signs of illness, including neurologic abnormalities, green droppings, and anorexia, can suggest PHV infection. Vomiting with no other symptoms and inclusion body hepatitis can occur.

### Adenovirus

Adenovirus infection had been shown to cause primary illness in pigeons. Young birds are most susceptible and the symptoms are as would be expected with hepatic necrosis of any cause. Basophilic intranuclear inclusion bodies are strongly suggestive of adenovirus infection.[15]

Treatment is supportive. Antibiotics are indicated for prevention of secondary bacterial infection. Protozoal and helminth parasites should be eliminated and adequate hydration and nutrition provided.

### Paramyxovirus-1

Although it has been a problem in Europe and many other parts of the world for a long time, PMV1 has been a problem in North America since 1984 and has spread over the whole continent since 1987 to 1989.

Fanciers with absolutely closed flocks are in the lowest risk. Those who race their pigeons frequently, or buy, sell, trade, or allow contact with feral pigeons are most likely to have infected flocks.

Primary signs of PMV-1 are polyuria (not diarrhea) and central nervous signs, ranging from incoordination, difficulty picking up grains, and mild head tilt, to severe ataxia and torticollis (**Fig. 1**). Surprisingly, affected pigeons do not seem to feel very ill and most eventually recover if given long-term supportive care. The most severely affected birds are unable to feed well enough to maintain body weight, and may need to be euthanized. Immune carriers are possible, and older and younger birds, especially, are most susceptible to infection. Viral shedding can precede clinical signs, and incubation has been suggested as lasting 1 week to as long as 6 weeks.

The author (R.H.) recommends expedient vaccination of all birds, including young birds, in the face of an outbreak. Devastation in outbreaks has been minimized by vaccination, suggesting that incubation is long (2–4 weeks) or that other factors cause a moderate to slow spread in a flock. Elimination of parasites, good nutrition, and loft cleanliness promote the strength of the pigeon's immune system.

Vaccination 1 to 2 months before breeding season and 6 to 8 weeks before racing or showing with oil emulsion vaccine SC has been recommended. The author (R.H.) vaccinates his young bird racing team on weaning and believes that lifelong immunity probably happens from that single immunization. The LaSota oral vaccine should not be depended on for adequate protection.

### Pox Virus

Pox virus is found in saliva and in nasal and lacrimal secretions. It enters the body through defects in the skin, especially on the wattle or cere. Direct contact, insect vectors, or airborne secretions can spread the disease. Birds develop scabs and proliferations of the cere, wattle, legs, feet, and commissures of the beak.

The first signs are usually conjunctivitis with excess lacrimation and swelling of the eye and cere. A diphtheroid form can occur, causing lesions on the mucosal surface

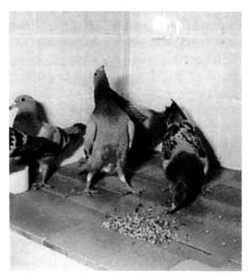

**Fig. 1.** Neurologic signs of paramyxovirus 1. Pigeons are exhibiting stargazing, torticollis, and polyuria.

inside the mouth. Secondary bacterial invasion can cause proliferative lesions, obstructing respiration and making eating difficult.

Treatment of infected birds is strictly supportive. Preventive measures (including practicing strict sanitation; providing proper nutrition; and using antibiotics, anthelminthics, and coccidiostats) should be taken in the event of an outbreak. Isolation of infected individual animals and insect control using screens or insecticides can slow the spread.

Birds develop immunity 3 to 4 weeks after administration of a commercially available vaccine. Feathers are pulled, and the vaccine is applied by a dropper or brush. The wing web is an acceptable site. An inflammatory reaction at the site suggests successful vaccination. Birds as young as 4 weeks of age can be vaccinated, and annual vaccination is recommended 4 weeks before mosquito season. Care should be taken not to introduce new birds into an already vaccinated loft. The incidence of pox varies greatly from year to year and by geographic area. Chances of outbreak increase in late summer and fall, especially in years when the first freeze comes late.

## Circovirus

Circovirus, a relative to psittacine beak and feather disease virus and chicken anemia agent, has been recognized since 1986 and has been reported in the United States since 1990. The victims are usually young birds 2 months to 1 year of age. Clinical signs are anorexia, lethargy, diarrhea, rapid weight loss, inability to fly, sneezing, respiratory distress, and death in 3 to 5 days.[16–21]

The incubation period is best estimated at about 2 weeks. Circovirus generally has an immunosuppressive effect, allowing concurrent infections to cause the demise of the bird. Among them are *Pasteurella* sp, herpes virus, *Chlamydophila psittaci*, *Trichomonas gallinae*, adenovirus, *Aspergillus* sp, and *Escherichia coli*.

It is the author's belief (R.H.) that the incidence of this viral illness is more common than reported. Often the concurrent agents previously mentioned are determined to be the cause of the illness, when they might have only been opportunistic. Recent research shows lesions and pathognomic botryoid inclusions in lymphoreticular tissues consistently in pigeons with "young bird sickness" (see later discussion). It is suggested that bursa be included with liver, spleen, and other tissue for histopathology in suspected viral illness.

### Young bird sickness

In Europe, young bird sickness is a condition affecting pigeons in their first year of life.[22] Birds exhibit slow crop emptying, regurgitation, diarrhea, weight loss, poor performance, and occasionally death. Lesions occur in the lymphoreticular system, alimentary tract, and respiratory system. Caused by underlying circovirus infection, birds exhibit protozoal, fungal, and mixed bacterial infections associated with ingluvitis and enteritis. Concurrent *C psittaci* pneumonitis is common.

### Viral Hepatitis

Since 1992, an acute hepatic disease in pigeons has occurred in Europe. The syndrome is much like Pacheco disease in parrots, except that there are no inclusions in the hepatocytes and the agent has yet to be identified. Old and young birds are affected.

The birds are sick for 24 to 48 hours and they either die or recover without treatment. Some birds develop yellow, slimy droppings and foul-smelling vomitus. The symptoms can continue for a course of 3 to 4 weeks. The mortality rate is about 30%.

Hepatomegaly with a pale-colored liver and complete destruction of all liver cells is found on postmortem examination and histopathology. Treatment is supportive only.

## BACTERIAL INFECTIONS
### Paratyphoid (Salmonellosis)

The most important bacterial disease in pigeons and doves is paratyphoid, caused most often by *Salmonella typhimurium* var *Copenhagen* (less often by *S arizonae*, *S pullorum*). The best-known signs are swollen wing and leg joints ("boils"), which should be considered almost pathognomonic by the practitioner when observed. Most pigeons with paratyphoid present with an array of other signs, however, including anorexia; weight loss; ruffled feathers; dropped wings; refusal to fly; diarrhea; green droppings; reproductive problems, such as embryonic or early squab death; or death of older birds (**Figs. 2** and **3**) Although not always present and not the most common sign, elbow swelling (also seen in the canalis triosseus) may occur months or years after infection due to antibodies to *Salmonella*. *Salmonella* is the second most common agent after PMV-1 causing neurologic signs and can cause severe hepatomegaly and bony lesions that mimic infection with *Mycobacterium* sp.[23]

Diagnosis is made by demonstration of the organism from the live bird or on necropsy. Selenite broth onto MacConkey or brilliant green agar is suitable for recovering the organism from intestinal or crop contents. Serology may also be useful.

Treatment should be determined by sensitivity testing, because many strains exist with variable drug susceptibility. Enrofloxacin has the most consistent efficacy record, although members of the penicillin, tetracycline, and aminoglycoside families sometimes can be suitable choices. Because *Salmonella* organisms are shed intermittently, pooling feces over 5 days may be useful. A recent study using 0.5 mg/mL florfenicol in

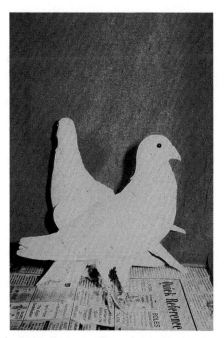

**Fig. 2.** Articular form of salmonellosis. Swelling of the tibiotarsal tarsometatarsal joint and wing, causing lameness and inability to fly (wing droop).

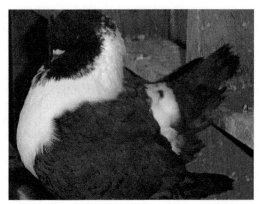

**Fig. 3.** Gazzi Modina breed pigeon with severe wing droop articular form of Salmonellosis.

drinking water reduced fecal excretion and clinical signs, but enhanced persistence of *Salmonella* in internal organs.[24] In most outbreaks, there may also be concurrent infections with *Klebsiella* sp and *E coli*, so it is beneficial to treat all isolates. Be sure to check for concurrent circovirus infection, which causes immune suppression, therefore increasing susceptibility.

Prevention is far superior to treatment. Before introducing new stock into a disease-free loft, birds should be quarantined in individual cages until they have raised a nest of healthy young. Cleanliness, acidification of floor litter, and strict control of stray pigeons are also helpful measures. Vaccination with killed bacterin may be beneficial. Vaccine does not protect against infection but stimulates immunity.

### Colibacillosis (Escherichia coli)

Colibacillosis is another important disease in pigeons. Disease syndromes previously attributed to paratyphoid recently have been shown to be caused by *E coli* when proper diagnostic tests were done. Excluding the swollen wing and limb joints, the symptoms of the two diseases are similar.

*E coli* is found in 97% of all pigeon intestinal tracts (part of normal flora) and is not usually a primary problem. It may be involved in septicemia as a facultative pathogen, especially with concurrent adenovirus infection. Disease can occur solely in nestlings or in pigeons of all ages.

Base antibiotic therapy on culture sensitivity. Quinolone resistance is common but enrofloxacin and trimethoprim sulfa are generally successful. Rule out circovirus and other concurrent viruses.

### Other Bacteria

Other bacteria, such as *Streptococcus*, *Staphylococcus*, *Pasteurella*, *Haemophilus*, and *Pseudomonas*, have been described as pathogens but are of lesser importance than *Salmonella* and *E coli* (**Table 1**).

Treatment of all bacterial diseases should involve culture and sensitivity testing. Often, fanciers and veterinarians "shotgun" flocks with antibiotics, resulting in many resistant strains of bacteria and many immunosuppressed pigeons. The author (R.H.) has noted several cases of peracute or at least acute death. Often they have full crops and no apparent lesions except what appear to be fluid-filled intestines. *Clostridium perfringens* is found on cultures. Possibly exotoxins damage the gut

**Table 1**
**Other bacterial diseases of columbiform birds**

| Genus | Species | Comments |
| --- | --- | --- |
| Pasteurella | P multocida | Unilateral (bilateral) epiphora, nasal discharge and swelling, otitis media/interna, arthritis, subcutaneous abscesses, septicemia |
| Mycoplasma | M columbinasale, M columborale, M columbinum | Persistent subclinical infections are common (resemble chlamydiosis and pasteurellosis). |
| Mycobacteria | M avium, M bovis | Pigeons and doves are susceptible to avian Mycobacteriosis. Host genetics (interspecies variations associated with color polymorphism) seem to play an important role in the susceptibility of doves to disease and immunity caused by this bacteria |
| Clostridium spp | C perfringens | Sometimes a cause of enteritis in individual birds |

Data from References.[25–32]

because of altered bacterial flora, much like hemorrhagic gastroenteritis syndrome in dogs.

### Limb deformities caused by enrofloxacin

Krautwald and colleagues[33] reported several problems with fluoroquinolone use in racing pigeons. Embryonic mortality was found with high parental doses and was due to streptococcal pneumonia, and secondary staphylococcal and candida infections. Young birds that survived often exhibited deformities, decreased food intake, delayed feather development, slow weight gain, and joint abnormalities, such as distal leg rotations, and intertarsal and stifle joint lesions. Thus far, the author (R.H.) has not appreciated these deformities.

### Streptococcus

An acute or even peracute death in pigeons has been attributed to Streptococcus gallolyticus (previously known as S bovis).[34] The primary sign in most birds is inability to fly (or deviant flying behavior) and dropped wings. Others have green, foamy droppings and sometimes loss of appetite, polyuria, polydipsia, and swollen abdomen. Birds that have acute disease presents with septicemia. Old and young birds are affected; young birds have pericarditis and old birds often have abnormal yellowing of the breast muscles. A chronic lameness has also been reported.

Nearly 40% of all pigeons carry streptococci in the gastrointestinal tract without clinical signs. It may be part of normal flora but can be a facultative pathogen. Clinical signs are usually not present if confined to the gastrointestinal tract. The disease can easily be mistaken for paramyxovirus and salmonellosis but is usually more acute. Amoxicillin is an effective treatment if instituted early enough. In the human literature, S gallolyticus is developing resistance to tetracyclines and erythromycin, so obtaining a culture before antibiotic administration is ideal.[35]

### Ornithosis Complex

The ornithosis complex (known as "eye colds" or "one-eyed croup") is common in domestic pigeons. *Chlamydophila psittaci* is the primary causal agent, but *Mycoplasma* spp and gram-negative bacteria are also involved. Many herpesvirus infections are also complicated with *C psittaci* so viral agents should be included in the complex. In addition, birds are often concurrently affected with *Trichomonas gallinae*. Frequently, the same eye of all the affected birds is in the windward side of wind currents (**Fig. 4**).

Treatment is usually successful with tylosin, but tetracyclines, lincomycin, or erythromycin are also effective. Intramuscular injection is irritating and should be avoided in racing birds. Oral administration and sinus flushing of antibiotics can be the best methods of treatment. Supportive therapy reduces stress and enhances immune response. Topical ophthalmic medications, such as tetracycline ointment, are also of benefit.

### Chlamydophila Psittaci

It is estimated that 30% to 90% of pigeons are infected (feral pigeons are the most common carriers of *C psittaci* in the United States) and doves are also susceptible.[36] Serotype B is most commonly isolated from pigeons. Usually considered part of the respiratory disease complex, *C psittaci* in columbiform birds exhibits low virulence and low zoonotic risk potential. Certain strains (ie, psittacine and turkey) are important causes of diarrhea and weight loss in young birds. Bacterial infections, especially salmonellosis, also complicate upper respiratory problems by pigeon strains leading to higher shedding and mortality. *C psittaci* may be accompanied by concurrent herpesvirus infections.

Polymerase chain reaction (PCR) testing can be performed and is best done by swabbing the superior conjunctiva and choana. If birds are PCR positive, this indicates active infection. Cloacal swabs are not recommended because a positive PCR means the bird has been exposed and the organism is passing through.[37] Treatment with 0.5 mg/mL doxycycline in the drinking water for 45 days is safe and efficacious for doves.[38]

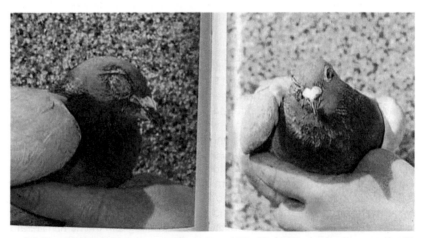

**Fig. 4.** Ornithosis complex (one-eye cold) conjunctivitis. Underlying organisms may be *Mycoplasma* sp, *Chlamydophila psittaci*, or bacteria.

## PARASITIC DISEASES
### Endoparasites

Gastrointestinal nematodes are the primary endoparasitic problem of pigeons (**Table 2**). Ascarids, *Capillaria*, *Ornithostrongylus*, and *Dispharynx* are of concern; geographic location determines the particular species that a clinician will encounter. Cestodes (*Raillietina* spp) are occasionally encountered, and trematodes (*Echinostoma* spp) are rarely, if ever, found in the United States. Although rare, ocular nematodes (*Ceratospira inglisi*) were found recently in a dove.[39]

Diagnosis is made by fecal flotation, direct smear, or intestinal or proventricular scrapings on necropsy. Cestode proglottids can be shed after food deprivation. Because cestodes and some nematodes (eg, *Tetrameres*) require intermediate hosts (eg, pill bugs), care should be taken to prevent pigeons from foraging where organisms are found. Raised lofts are the most common sites where pigeons are infected.

Deworm birds before the racing and breeding season (**Table 3**). Piperazine is effective only for ascarids. Fenbendazole and mebendazole are effective for ascarids, *Capillaria*, and probably other parasites that feed on blood or body tissue, but must be used for 3 days. Levamisole is effective against ascarids and has some value against *Capillaria* sp. Ivermectin is most effective against all nematodes, but other drugs, such as pyrantel pamoate, are better for ascarids. Praziquantel is the drug of choice for cestodes and trematodes.

### Benzimidazole toxicosis

Most reported cases of benzimidazole toxicosis in birds are Columbiformes. Fenbendazole and albendazole cause bone marrow suppression and direct intestinal tract cell damage.[41,42] Use of fenbendazole at reported literature dose of 50 mg/kg by mouth

| Table 2 Columbid helminths | | |
|---|---|---|
| **Name** | **Species** | **Comments** |
| Ascarids | *Ascaridia columbae* | Most common nematodes (common in feral pigeons, rare in racing pigeons); direct intestinal life cycle, larvae may encyst in lung and liver |
| *Capillaria* | *C caudinflata, C obsignata, C columbae* | Direct intestinal lifestyle; may cause vomiting, diarrhea, anemia |
| Roundworms | *Dispharynx* (previously *Acuaria*) *spiralis* (proventriculus) and *Ornithostrongylus* spp (intestine) | Most serious roundworms; cause severe hemorrhage. *Dispharynx* requires an intermediate host (pill bug). |
| Globular stomach worm | *Tetrameres* spp, *T columbicola* | Require an intermediate host (pill bug). Proventriculus has raspberry-like appearance on necropsy. Not as pathogenic, but causes poor condition |

| Table 3 Some common helminth treatment doses | | |
|---|---|---|
| **Drug** | **Effective** | **Dose** |
| Fenbendazole | Nematodes, including *Capillaria*, ascarids, strongyles, *Tetrameres* | 10–12 mg/kg po q 24 h × 3 d |
| Pyrantel pamoate | Nematodes, including ascarids | 20–25 mg/kg po |
| Ivermectin | Best for all nematodes, excellent for *Capillaria* and *Tetrameres* but less effective for *Ascaridia* spp | 0.2 mg/kg po >sq >im, repeat 10–14 d |
| Praziquantel | Cestodes, trematodes | 10–20 mg/kg po repeat in 10–14 d |

*Data from* Refs.[10,13,40]

every 24 hours for 5 days caused death in doves.[41] Avoid the use of fenbendazole in birds with developing primaries because it will cause weakness and breakage of growing remiges.

### Protozoa

#### Coccidia

The role of coccidian parasites as primary pathogens remains controversial because oocysts are commonly found in healthy birds. Often, pigeons are afflicted with other diseases or under stress shed large numbers of oocysts, particularly young birds. The physical examination should not end when a fecal flotation reveals oocysts but should be thorough in eliminating bacterial infections, trichomoniasis, nutritional deficiencies, husbandry errors, and helminths.

Infections in domestic pigeons are typically mixed and commonly include *Eimeria columbarum* and *Eimeria labbaena*. The estimated prevalence of infection is 5.1% to 71.9% and mortality in juvenile pigeons ranges from 5% to 70% worldwide. Most deaths occur in juveniles 3 to 4 months old.[43]

Evidence indicates that low-level exposure to mildly virulent strains of coccidia can help to produce immunity to more pathogenic strains. Immunity is species-specific and disappears if birds are not reinfected. Coccidiostatic drugs should be administered to poorly performing birds or when experiencing mortalities.

When a disease situation involving coccidia occurs and drugs must be used, sanitation and good husbandry to prevent fecal–oral contact should be the first therapy instituted. Heavily bred, heavily raced older birds, and young birds kept under less than optimal conditions are the most susceptible to disease.

Clazuril, amprolium, sulfachlorpyridazine, and other sulfas (eg, sulfadimethoxine and sulfamethazine) are effective coccidiostats (**Table 4**). There is evidence of growing resistance against sulfonamides and amprolium.[43] Because the sulfas reduce thiamine absorption, vitamin B supplementation after therapy is beneficial.

Nitrofurazone can help with secondary bacterial enteric infections but is not recommended for treatment of coccidiosis in pigeons. Three to 5 days are required for the oocyst to sporulate and become infective, so frequent cleaning is the best preventative measure.

**Table 4**
**Some common coccidiostats**

| Drug | Dose | Comments |
| --- | --- | --- |
| Amprolium | 0.2% solution (200 mg/L) for 5 d, 25 mg/kg/d po | — |
| Clazuril | 2.5 mg per pigeon once | Suppresses oocyst excretion for up to 2 wk |
| Toltrazuril | 20 mg/kg drinking water 2 d[42] | Effective for refractory coccidiosis |
| Sulfamethazine | 50–65 mg/pigeon orally × 5 d; 400 mg/L day 1 followed by 200–270 mg/L for 4 d | Supplement B vitamins for 5 d |
| Sulfadimethoxine | 25 mg/kg po q 12 h × 5 d; 330–400 mg/L day 1 followed by 200 mg/L for 4 d | Supplement B vitamins for 5 d |

*Data from* Refs.[10,13,40]

### Trichomoniasis

Primarily a columbid disease, most pigeons and doves carry *Trichomonas gallinae*. The parasite can be a primary pathogen or cause disease secondary to other illnesses or stressful conditions. The severity of trichomoniasis depends on the virulence of the strain and the magnitude of debility from concurrent diseases. The common name "canker" refers to the cheesy, white caseous deposits in the throats of birds that have advanced disease (**Fig. 5**). Mentioned by John Moore as far back as 1735, trichomoniasis is certainly not a new disease.

More often the condition is confused with respiratory diseases because the oculo-nasal and oral discharges are clear. The organism can easily be demonstrated by suctioning the mucus from the throat with a 1-mL needleless syringe and immediately observing the sample with immersion microscopy. There is no cyst stage, only the trophozoite, which moves in an undulate on wet mounts.

*Trichomonas* often accompanies the ornithosis complex, viral illnesses, parasitic diseases, and noninfectious stressful situations. Successful therapy involves resolving the other diseases and treatment of the trichomonads. The immune status of the bird is important to consider if recovery is to be expected. Exposure to strains of low

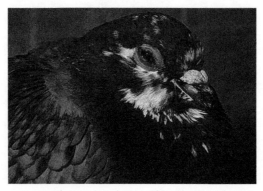

**Fig. 5.** Pigeon with caseous trichomoniasis lesion. This advanced form is canker complicated with secondary bacterial infection.

virulence in an immunocompetent bird can produce resistance against more pathogenic strains. Trichomoniasis causes caseous masses that are easily removed without bleeding, whereas poxvirus typically creates more voluminous masses localized to the front of the mouth, and the mucosa bleeds when removed.

Although trichomoniasis is primarily a disease of the upper alimentary tract, local lesions, including omphalitis, can occur, along with infection of the liver, lung, and other organs (**Figs. 6** and **7**) Erosion of the palatal flaps indicates previous or current infection. Tiny, pinpoint abscesses in the choanal region may be seen in chronic infections. Signs of infection depend on immunocompetency, previous exposure, and virulence of the infective strain. Most strains are low virulence and most affected pigeons do not show macroscopic lesions. Any debilitated, juvenile, or immunocompromised birds, especially squabs or circovirus-infected birds, are high-risk. A novel respiratory tract presentation has recently been reported.[44]

Trichomonas is transmitted via crop secretions from parent to squab or during courtship and through drinking water. Passive immunity is acquired from crop milk and resistance develops from previous exposure.

Effective treatment involves proper use of the 5-nitroimidazole derivatives, including ronidazole, carnidazole, dimetridazole, and metronidazole (**Table 5**). Carnidazole is the drug of choice. Dimetriazole is quite toxic and doses should be reduced in hot weather. Licensed for treatment of blackhead in turkeys, dimetriazole has been discontinued in US because the FDA found traces of the drug in pork. Prevention depends on reducing stress and controlling other diseases. Total eradication of the organism is not practical or desirable. Certain strains may have increased resistance and dosages may need to be adjusted.[45]

### Hexamita

Hexamitiasis occurs primarily in young pigeons. Host-specific, *Hexamita columbae* (previously *Spironucleus columbae*), can be primary or secondary (ie, complication

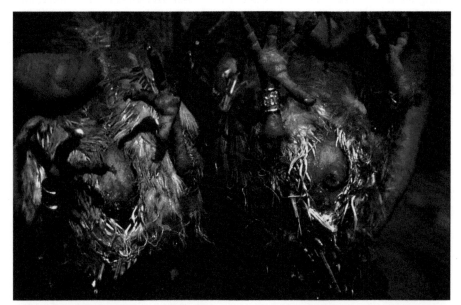

**Fig. 6.** Squab with omphalitis (right chick). This is an atypical presentation of trichomoniasis complicated with secondary bacteria. The squab on the left is normal for comparison.

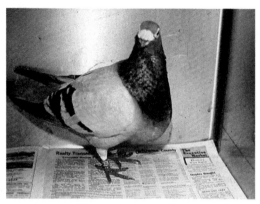

**Fig. 7.** Crop abscess secondary to trichomoniasis, readily corrected with surgery.

of adenovirus 1 infection). Carriers harbor organisms in cecal tonsils. Symptoms include weight loss, diarrhea, and general unthriftiness. Demonstration of the organism on fresh direct fecal smears is diagnostic.

Important differential diagnoses include: *Salmonella*, *E coli*, adenovirus, and PMV. Treat with ronidazole or metronidazole for 7 days. Use caution because pigeons that have polyuria may develop acute toxicosis. Severe infections may need secondary bacterial coverage; trimethoprim or enrofloxacin are good choices. Preventing fecal–oral contact is helpful in controlling hexamitiasis.

### Other enteric protozoa

Giardia is seldom a problem in captive columbids. Clinical toxoplasmosis and sarcocystosis are rarely reported in pigeons; however, there have been several reports in the last few years.[46–50] Enclosure contamination with cat (toxoplasma) and opossum (sarcocystis) feces should be considered. Intestinal cryptosporidiosis was reported in pigeons in that had diarrhea and weight loss.[51] Feral pigeons have recently been found to shed microsporidia (*Enterocytozoon* and *Encephalitozoon* spp), which could spread to domestic birds that come into contact with them.[52,53] There is little information on disease from microsporidia in pigeons at this time, however.

### Hemoprotozoa

"Pigeon malaria" is the name frequently given to hemoproteus infection (*H columbae*, *H sacharovi*, *H maccallumi*). Hemoproteus is usually nonpathogenic in domestic

| Table 5 | | |
|---------|---|---|
| **Some common antiprotozoal medications** | | |
| **Drug** | **Dose** | **Comments** |
| Carnidazole | 20 mg/kg once | Only drug labeled for use in pigeons in United States |
| Ronidazole | 2.5 mg/kg po × 6 d, 100–600 mg/L drinking water for 3–5 d | Flock treatment: lower end of dose range for preventative, higher dose range for treatment |
| Metronidazole | 25–50 mg/kg po q 12–24 h × 5 d; 1057 mg/L drinking water | Lower dose if twice daily |

*Data from* Refs.[10,13,40]

**Box 1**
**Possible pigeon diseases based on common clinical signs**

*Central nervous system*

Trauma

*Salmonella*

*Streptococcus gallolyticus*

Paramyxovirus

Herpesvirus

West Nile Virus

Eastern Equine Encephalities (EEE)

St. Louis Encephalitis

Rabies

*Toxoplasma*

Lead

Zinc

Sodium chloride

Pesticides (especially OP)

Mycotoxins

Benzimidazoles

Nitrofurazone

Ivermectin

Alphachloralose

Avitrol

*Clostridium botulinum* (exotoxin)

Neoplasia

*Diarrhea (with blood)*

*Salmonella* (B)

*Escherichia coli*

*S gallolyticus*

*Chlamydia psittaci*

Mycobacteria

Clostridia (B)

Herpesvirus

Adenovirus

Parvovirus

Reovirus

Rotavirus

Influenza A

EEE

Trichomoniasis (severe)

Hexamita (B)

Coccidia

Cestodes (B) (squabs)

Trematodes (B)

Asper (late)

Mycotoxins (B)

Insecticides

Rodenticides (cholecalciferol)

Lead

Zinc

Copper

Neoplasia

*Vomiting*

E coli

Adenovirus

Capillaria

Lead

Zinc

Copper

Rodenticides (cholecalciferol)

Levamisole

Foreign body

Neoplasia

*Respiratory*

Trauma

*Salmonella*

*C psittaci*

*E coli*

*Streptococcus intermedius*

*Pelistega europaea*

*Pasteurella*

*Mycoplasma*

Herpesvirus

Influenza A (acute)

Adenovirus (some)

Coronavirus

Aspergillus

Rodenticides (anticoagulants)

Pesticides

Neoplasia

(*continued on next page*)

---

**Box 1**
*(continued)*

*Polyuria (PU)/polydipsia (PD)*

*Salmonella (PU)*

*S gallolyticus (PU)*

Paramyxovirus

Herpes *(PD)*

Ethylene glycol *(PU)*

Rodenticides (cholecalciferol)

Sodium chloride

Avicides (2-chloro-4-acetotoliudine, 3-chloro-4-methybenzenamine)

*Lameness*

Trauma

*Salmonella*

*S gallolyticus*

*Mycobacteria*

*Staphylococci*

*Pasteurella*

Herpesvirus

Enrofloxacin

Neoplasia

*Data from Refs.*[1,6,56,57]

---

pigeons but disease is possible and is a sign of an overcrowded pigeon aviary. *Plasmodium* spp are rarely reported in pigeons, but can cause disease in young or debilitated birds. *Leukocytozoon* spp have caused deaths in some Columbids.

*Hemoproteus* is much more common in performing breeds than in fancy and utility pigeons, possibly because of stresses and exposure to insect vectors in racing situations that make the disease more apparent in racing pigeons then in sedentary exhibition pigeons. The disease is transmitted by the pigeon louse (hippoboscid) fly. Hemoproteus infection is diagnosed by demonstration of the organism in the red blood cell's cytoplasm without nuclear displacement (as apposed to *Plasmodium* sp), as shown on stained blood smears.

Control of insect vectors is the best prevention. Dusting or dipping with pyrethrin every 2 weeks can be effective in controlling pigeon flies in endemic areas. The disease has been effectively treated with quinacrine. Primaquine has been successfully used as a preventative.

### Ectoparasites

Pigeon flies (hippoboscids), lice, and mites are the most significant ectoparasites of pigeons. *Pseudolynchia canariensis*, the pigeon louse fly, seldom flies. It spends most of its time feeding on birds' blood, causing anemia and transmission of *Hemoproteus* (and also possibly pox, PMV-1). Louse flies cause considerable discomfort

**Box 2**
**Possible pigeon diseases associated with poor management, infectious/zoonotic risk, and circovirus infection**

*Poor management*

*Salmonella*

*Chlamydophila*

Paramyxovirus

Pox

*Aspergillus*

Ascarids

Coccidia

*Hemoproteus*

Hippoboscids

Lice

*Infectious/zoonotic (at-risk species)*

*Salmonella* (all)

*Chlamydophila* (humans, birds)

*E coli* (all)

*Clostridium* (all)

*Pasteurella* (birds)

Adenovirus (galliforms)

Herpes (psittacines, raptors?)

Influenza A (humans, birds)

Paramyxovirus (poultry, raptors, psittacines, passerines)

Hippoboscids (birds)

*Pigeon circovirus-associated*

*Salmonella*

*E coli*

*C psittaci*

*Pasteurella*

*Pseudomonas*

Paramyxovirus

Poxvirus

Adenovirus

Herpesvirus

*Candida*

*Aspergillus*

*Trichomonas*

*Hemoproteus*

*Tetrameres*

*Data from* Refs.[1,6,56]

to the bird and can be devastating to the general health of the flock. Louse flies have also been found to transport skin mites (*Myialges* sp) from one bird to another.[54]

*Columbicola columbae*, the slender pigeon louse, is the most common mallophagian parasite. It does not take blood but feeds on feathers, causing tiny pinpoint holes. When lice are found by the clinician, other diseases should be considered. Heavy louse infestations usually indicate a debilitated bird that might not feel well enough to groom properly. *Dermanyssus gallinae* and *Ornithonyssus sylviarum* cause skin irritation and feed on blood. They are called red mites or roost mites and are found on the bird at night. *Knemidokoptes mutans*, the scaly leg mite, causes considerable skin damage. *K laevis,* the depluming mite, is rare.

Ivermectin is effective for ectoparasites that feed on blood and body tissues and is recommended with dusting or preferably dipping with 0.15% pyrethrin or 5% carbaryl products. Ivermectin and pyrethrin are effective against lice when used properly. The author (L.W.) reports that fipronil (Frontline; Merial, Athens, Georgia) 0.29% spray has been used off-label successfully by wildlife rehabilitators on pigeons and raptor veterinarians to remove hippoboscids and also reduce black flies and mosquitoes. The suggested dose is two to three squirts under each wing and tail every 30 days. One of the metabolites of fipronil has higher toxicity to birds than the parent compound; use the product carefully because it shows variable toxicity in different avian families.[55]

## SUMMARY

Treatment of infectious diseases in columbiform birds typically involves consideration for both individual birds and the flock. An awareness of the pathogens involved, including underlying viruses and bacterial sensitivity patterns, greatly improves the successful treatment of ill pigeons and doves. Considering organ systems involved and possible differential diagnoses is also useful (**Boxes 1** and **2**).

## ACKNOWLEDGEMENT

The authors thank Jamie Gorman (Southside Dog, Cat and Bird Hospital, Oklahoma City, OK) for help with this manuscript.

## REFERENCES

1. Tudor DC. Pigeon health and disease. Ames (IA): Iowa State University Press; 1991.
2. Marx DA. Veterinary approach to pigeon health. Lake Charles (LA): Racing Pigeon Digest Co; 1997.
3. Hooimeijer J. Management of racing pigeons. In: Harrison GJ, Lightfoot TL, Flinchum GB, editors. Clinical avian medicine. Palm Beach (FL): Spix Pub; 2006. p. 849–60.
4. Rupiper DJ. Diseases that affect race performance of homing pigeons. Part I: husbandry, diagnostic strategies and viral diseases. J Avian Med Surg 1998; 12(2):70–7.
5. Rupiper DJ. Diseases that affect race performance of homing pigeons. Part II: bacterial, fungal and parasitic diseases. J Avian Med Surg 1998;12(3):138–48.
6. De Herdt P, Devriese L. Pigeons. In: Tully TN, Lawton MPC, Dorrestein GM, et al, editors. Avian medicine. Oxford: Butterworth Heinemann; 2000. p. 312–38.

7. Hooimeijer J, Dorrestein GM. Pigeons and doves. In: Altman RB, Clubb SL, Dorrestein GM, et al, editors. Avian medicine and surgery. Philadelphia: WB Saunders; 1997. p. 886–909.

8. Vogel C, Gerlach H, Loffler M. Columbiformes. In: Ritchie BW, Harrison GJ, Harrison LR, et al, editors. Avian medicine principles and application. Lake Worth (FL): Wingers Publishing; 1994. p. 1201–17.

9. Beynon PH, Forbes NA, Harcourt-Brown NH, editors. BSAVA manual of raptors, pigeons and waterfowl. Ames (IA): Iowa State University Press; 1996.

10. Harlin RW. Practical pigeon medicine. Proc Annu Conf Assoc Avian Vet 2006;249–62.

11. Powers LV. Veterinary care of columbiformes. Proc Annu Conf Assoc Avian Vet 2005;171–83.

12. Rupiper D, Ehrenberg M. Practical pigeon medicine. Proc Annu Conf Assoc Avian Vet 1997;479–97.

13. Harlin RW. Pigeon therapeutics. Veterinary Clin North Am Exot Anim Pract 2000; 3(1):19–34.

14. Ritchie BW. Avian viruses: function and control. Lake Worth (FL): Winger's Publishing; 1995.

15. Takase K, Yoshinaga N, Egashira T, et al. Avian adenovirus isolated from pigeons affected with inclusion body hepatitis. Nippon Juigaku Zasshi 1990; 52(2):207–15.

16. Schmidt V, Schlomer J, Luken C, et al. Experimental infection of domestic pigeons with pigeon circovirus. Avian Dis 2008;52(3):380–6.

17. Duchatel JP, Todd D, Smyth JA, et al. Observations on detection, excretion and transmission of pigeon circovirus in adult, young and embryonic pigeons. Avian Pathol 2006;35(1):30–4.

18. Abadie J, Nguyen F, Groizeleau C, et al. Pigeon circovirus infection: pathological observations and suggested pathogenesis. Avian Pathol 2001;30:149–58.

19. Lester VK, Wilson GH, Gregory CR, et al. Testing parameters for the control of pigeon circovirus. Proc Annu Conf Assoc Avian Vet 2003;11–2.

20. Woods LW, Latimer KS. Circovirus infection of nonpsittacine birds. J Avian Med Surg 2000;14(3):154–63.

21. Woods LW, Latimer KS, Niagro FD, et al. A retrospective study of circovirus infection in pigeons: 9 cases (1986–1993). J Vet Diagn Invest 1996;6:156–64. Available at: http://jvdi.org/cgi/reprint/6/2/156.pdf. Accessed June 24, 2009.

22. Scullion FT, Scullion MG. Pathologic findings in racing pigeons (Columba livia domestica) with "young bird sickness." J Avian Med Surg 2007;21(1):1–7.

23. Suedmeyer WK, Bermudez A, Shaiken L. Osteolysis and hepatomegaly caused by Salmonella typhimurium in a Temminck's fruit dove (Ptilinopus porphyrea). J Avian Med Surg 1998;12(3):184–9.

24. Martel A, Baert K, Lanckreit R, et al. The use of an oral formulation of florfenicol to control Salmonellosis in pigeons. Proc Annu Conf Assoc Avian Vet 2005;19–21.

25. Esposito JF. Respiratory medicine in pigeons. Veterinary Clin North Am Exot Anim Pract 2000;3(2):395–402.

26. Loria GR, Tamburello A, Liga F, et al. Isolation of mycoplasmas from pigeons suffering eye lesions and respiratory disease. Vet Rec 2005;157(21):664–5.

27. Nagatomo H, Kato H, Shimizu T, et al. Isolation of mycoplasmas from fantail pigeons. J Vet Med Sci 1997;59(6):461–2.

28. Saggese MD, Phalen DN. Serological and histological findings in doves with Mycobacteriosis. Proc Annu Conf Assoc Avian Vet 2005;71–3.

29. Bougiouklis P, Brellou G, Fragkiadaki E, et al. Outbreak of avian mycobacteriosis in a flock of 2 year old domestic pigeons (*Columba livia f domestica*). Avian Dis 2003;49(3):442–5.

30. Pond CL, Rush HC. Infection of white carneaux pigeons (*Columba livia*) with *Mycobacterium avium*. Lab Anim Sci 1981;31(2):196–9.

31. Fitzgerald SD, Zwick LS, Berry DE, et al. Experimental inoculation of pigeons (*Columba livia*) with Mycobacterium bovis. Avian Dis 2003;47(2):470–5.

32. Hejlicek K, Treml F. Epizoology and pathology of avian mycobacteriosis in domestic pigeons (*Columba livia f domestica*). Vet Med (Praha) 1994;39(10): 615–24.

33. Krautwald ME, Pieper K, Rullof R, et al. Further experience with the use of Baytril in pet birds. Proc Annu Conf Assoc Avian Vet 1990;226–36.

34. Chadfield MS, Christensen JP, Decastere A, et al. Geno-and phenotypic diversity of avian isolates of *Streptococcus gallolyticus* subsp. *gallolyticus* (*Streptococcus bovis*) and associated diagnostic problems. J Clin Microbiol 2007;54(3):822–7.

35. Leclercq R, Huet R, Picherot M, et al. Genetic basis of antibiotic resistance in clinical isolates of *Streptococcus gallolyticus* (*Streptococcus bovis*). Antimicrobial Agents Chemother 2005;49(4):1646–8.

36. Grimes JE, Small MF, French LL, et al. Chlamydiosis in captive white-winged doves (*Zenaida asiatica*). Avian Dis 1997;41(2):505–8.

37. Phalen DN, Hofle M, Dahlhausen B, et al. Diagnosis of *Chalmydia psittaci* infections in cockatiels and columbiformes. Proc Annu Conf Assoc Avian Vet 1999;13–7.

38. Padilla LR, Flammer K, Miller RE. Doxycycline-medicated drinking water for treatment of *Chlamydophila psittaci* in exotic doves. J Avian Med Surg 2005;19(2): 88–91.

39. Suedmeyer WK, Smith T, Moore C, et al. *Ceratospira inglisi* ocular infestation in a wompoo fruit-dove (*Ptilinopus magnificus*). J Avian Med Surg 1999;13(4): 261–4.

40. Carpenter JW. Exotic animal formulary. 3rd edition. St. Louis (MO): Elsevier Saunders. p. 135–344.

41. Howard LL, Papendick R, Stalis IH, et al. Fenbendazole and albendazole toxicity in pigeons and doves. J Avian Med Surg 2002;16(3):203–10.

42. Rivera SR, McClearen J, Reavill D. Suspected fenbendazole toxicity in pigeons (*Columba livia*). Proc Annu Conf Assoc Avian Vet 2000;207–9.

43. Krautwald-Junghanns ME, Zebisch R, Schmidt V. Relevance and treatment of coccidiosis in domestic pigeons (*Columba livia* forma domestica) with particular emphasis on toltrazuril. J Avian Med Surg 2009;23(1):1–5.

44. Stoute ST, Charlton BR, Bickford AA, et al. Respiratory tract trichomoniasis in breeder squab candidates in Northern California. Avian Dis 2009;53(1):139–42.

45. Franssen FF, Lumeij JT. In vitro nitroimidazole resistance of *Trichomonas gallinae* and successful therapy with an increased dosage of ronidazole in racing pigeons (*Columba livia domestica*). J Vet Pharmacol Ther 1992;15(4):409–15.

46. Mushi EZ, Binta MG, Chabo RG, et al. Seroprevalence of *T. gondii* and *C. psittaci* in domestic pigeons (*Columa livia domestica*) at Sebele, Gabarone, Botswana. Onderstepoort J Vet Res 2001;68(1):159–61.

47. Las RD, Shivaprasad HL. An outbreak of toxoplasmosis in an aviary collection of Nicobar pigeons (*Caloenus nicobara*). J S Afr Vet Assoc 2008;79(3):149–52.

48. Suedmeyer WK, Bermudez AJ, Barr BC, et al. Acute pulmonary Sarcocystis faculata-like infection in three Victoria crowned pigeons (Goura Victoria) housed indoors. J Zoo Wildl Med 2001;32(2):252–6.

49. Olias P, Gruber AD, Heydorn AO, et al. A novel sarcocystis-associated encephalitis and myositis in racing pigeons. Avian Pathol 2009;38(2):121–8.
50. Ecco R, Luppi MM, Malta MC, et al. An outbreak of sarcocystosis in psittacines and a pigeon in a zoological collection in Brazil. Avian Dis 2008;52(4): 706–10.
51. Rodriguez F, Oros J, Rodriguez JL, et al. Intestinal cryptosporidiosis in pigeons (*Columba livia*). Avian Dis 1997;41(3):748–50.
52. Haro M, Henriques-Gil N, Fennoy S, et al. Detection and genotyping of *Enterocytozoon bieneusi* in pigeons. J Eukaryot Microbiol 2006;53(1):S58–60.
53. Graczyk TK, Sunderland D, Rule AM, et al. Urban feral pigeons (*Columba livia*) as a source for air-and waterborne contamination with *Enterocytozoon bieneusi* spores. Appl Environ Microbiol 2007;73(13):4357–8.
54. Macchioni F, Magi M, Mancianti F, et al. Phoretic association of mites and mallophaga with the pigeon fly *Pseudolynchia canariensis*. Parasite 2005;12(3):277–9.
55. National pesticide telecommunications network fact sheet on fipronil. Available at: http://npic.orst.edu/factsheets/fipronil.pdf. Accessed June 24, 2009.
56. Wade L. Pigeon medicine. Proc Mid-Atlantic States Assoc Av Vet 2007;137–57.
57. Vandamme P, Segers P, Ryll M, et al. Pelistega europaea gen.nov., sp. nov., a bacterium associated with respiratory disease in pigeons:taxonomic structure and phylogenetic allocation. Int J Syst Bacteriol 2002;48(2):431–40.

# Bacterial and Parasitic Diseases of Anseriformes

Glenn H. Olsen, DVM, MS, PhD

**KEYWORDS**

- Anseriformes • Avian cholera • Bacteria • Ducks
- Geese • Parasites

Taxonomically, the order Anseriformes contains three families: (*i*) *Anhimidae*, the screamers, not common to North America but found in other parts of the world, (*ii*) *Anseranatidae,* which has only one species, the magpie goose (*Anseranas semipalmata*), and (*iii*) *Anatidae.* This last family consists of the ducks, geese, and swans found worldwide, and it is this family to which the diseases of this article are primarily directed. Waterfowl, in addition to being found in the wild throughout the world, are commonly raised in captivity for food and eggs and kept in zoologic and private collections.

The order Anseriformes is primarily associated with water and wetland habitats. *Anatidae* or true waterfowl, have dense, waterproof plumage, webbed feet, and shortened tarsometatarsal bones. They are strong swimmers and divers, but somewhat less gainly on land, walking with a waddling gait. Generally, waterfowl molt twice yearly. After breeding season they will undergo both a body molt and flight feather molt, becoming flightless for a short period of days or weeks. In the winter, just a body molt will result in birds coming into breeding plumage. From a disease standpoint, the tendency of waterfowl to aggregate in large numbers during postbreeding molt, fall migration, and winter and spring migration can lead to the ready transfer of disease-causing organisms.

## AVIAN CHOLERA

Avian cholera, caused by *Pasteurella multocida*, is a highly pathogenic bacterium found in many species, but often associated with large mortality events in waterfowl. Avian cholera is found worldwide. It is more common in the western United States where large die-offs have occurred: greater than 60,000 at Muleshoe Refuge, Texas in 1956 to 1957,[1] 70,000 birds in northern California in 1965 to 1966,[2] and 80,000 in the Rainwater Basin of Nebraska in 1980.[3] However, outbreaks have occurred in

United States Geologic Survey, Patuxent Wildlife Research Center, 12302 Beech Forest Road, Laurel, MD 20708, USA
*E-mail address:* golsen@usgs.gov

Vet Clin Exot Anim 12 (2009) 475–490
doi:10.1016/j.cvex.2009.07.004
1094-9194/09/$ – see front matter. Published by Elsevier Inc.

vetexotic.theclinics.com

the east on the Chesapeake Bay in 1970 and 1978,[4] and in Canada.[5] Avian cholera is less common in Europe but is present.[6]

## Etiology

*Pasteurella multocida* is a small pleomorphic, gram-negative coccobacillus. It is characterized as bipolar staining, nonhemolytic, aerobic but facultatively anaerobic. The bipolar-staining characteristic can be seen in tissues or body fluids stained with Wright's, Giemsa, or methylene blue stains.[7] *P. multocida* has variable pathogenicity and host predilection, depending upon the individual strain encountered. Three subspecies, *multocida*, *septica*, and *gallieida* are differentiated by culture and fermentation of sorbitol and dulcitol. Strains are identified by characteristics of the capsule and cell wall with five capsule antigens, identified as A, B, D, E, and F by indirect hemagglutination.[8] Sixteen somatic antigens have been identified. Strains are characterized by the letter of the capsule antigen and the numbers of the somatic antigens, as some strains can react to more than one somatic antigen. To confuse matters more, sometimes strains with identical antigenic identification will vary in pathogenicity and sometimes epizootics will involve more than one strain.

## Epizoology

Potential reservoirs for *P. multocida* include soil, water, and carrier birds.[9] However, soil and water are probably not year-round reservoirs.[9] In poultry, chronically infected carriers are important for transmission.[10] Poultry that recover from an infection may continue to harbor *P. multocida* in their nasal clefts and, through nasal discharges, serve as a future source of infection to other poultry. The role and carrier state in wild waterfowl is not as well documented. Among common eiders (*Somateria mollissima*), 1 of 236 apparently healthy birds had *P. multocida* in their tissues and 1 of 357 in the oropharynx.[11] Epizootics are associated with dense concentrations of waterfowl and, to some extent, the loss of wetland habitat across central North America has been a factor in concentrating waterfowl and potentiating these epizootics.[12] Again, because of loss of wetland habitat, waterfowl will use a wetland continually during the winter rather than moving among wetlands.[5] Other factors contributing to avian cholera outbreaks include overcrowding of ducks because of drought or poor management, and inclement weather.[13] The pathogenesis of avian cholera varies by species of ducks and temporally from year to year in the same location.

## Clinical Signs and Pathology

In poultry, avian cholera is seen as both an acute and chronic disease, but in ducks the disease is most often seen as a peracute septicemia with rapid mortality, sometimes in as little as 6 to 12 hours after exposure, but 24 to 48 hours is more common.[14] In fact, very few clinical signs appear, most ducks are simply found dead. Clinical signs that are seen may include diminished normal reflexes, lack of fear, and signs of nervous system involvement, such as abnormal flight and landings.[2] Captive waterfowl have developed a wasting disease associated with avian cholera characterized by dyspnea and diarrhea, and this is often seen in older birds.[6] Chronic bilateral caseous infraorbital sinusitis has been found in emaciated, weak lesser snow geese (*Chen hyperborea hyperborea*).[7]

When *P. multocida* gains entry into susceptible waterfowl, a rapid septicemia ensues, with the bacteria producing an endotoxin that produces fever, systemic hypertension, endotoxic shock, and rapid death.[15] Signs at necropsy can include petechial and ecchymotic hemorrhages, 1-mm to 3-mm pale necrotic foci in the liver, and scattered petechiae on the gizzard serosa, epicardium, myocardium, mesentery, and possibly other serous membranes. Intestines will be either empty or have catarrhal hemorrhagic enteritis,[6] while the upper gastrointestinal tract may contain food items because of the peracute onset and death of the duck or goose. Pulmonary hemorrhage or consolidation, fibrinopurulent pleurisy, pericarditis, and air sacculitis can be found in subacute or chronic cases.[6] Histopathology is nonspecific early inflammation of necrosis but with large numbers of bacteria present in the vascular system.[16] The definitive diagnosis is made by culture isolation and identification of *Pasteurella multocida*, usually in heart blood, liver, bone marrow, or exudate from the intestines. Serotyping and molecular identification should follow to identify the strain of *P. multocida*.

### Treatment and Control

In poultry, sanitation, vaccination, and chemotherapy are used to control *Pasteurella multocida*, but these techniques are not as effective in waterfowl collections or in wild waterfowl. When an outbreak of avian cholera occurs, lowering the density of waterfowl on a pond or wetland may help stop the outbreak, but this also risks spreading the infection if waterfowl move elsewhere. Control measures that have had some success include: (*i*) inspection of waterfowl areas on a regular basis to detect any mortality, (*ii*) retrieval of all dead birds and incineration of carcasses, (*iii*) draining and flushing water areas (ponds or small lakes) if possible, and (*iv*) discouraging scavengers from spreading disease by removing dead birds quickly.[7] Bacterin has been used to protect Canada geese (*Branta canadensis*) during an epizootic.[14] Furthermore, treatment of individual waterfowl with penicillin or tetracycline has been effective.[6] Tetracycline has been used in a flock of captive Canada geese with an initial intramuscular injection of 50-mg oxyteracyline followed by 30-day treatment with tetracycline in feed (500 g per ton).[14] Using poultry vaccines in waterfowl has not been effective and, in at least one case, a modified live poultry vaccine may have caused a disease outbreak when used in a nontarget species (pheasants).[6,17]

### AVIAN TUBERCULOSIS

Avian tuberculosis in waterfowl is caused by *Mycobacterium avium*. Over 50 serotypes of *M. avium* complex have been identified, only 3 of which are known to cause disease in birds.[18] Only serotypes 1 and 2 cause disease in North America; serotype 3 is common in Europe and Africa.[19] *M. avium* can cause disease in all waterfowl species; indeed, the organism can cause disease in all bird species, human beings, most domestic livestock, and other mammal species. Among birds kept in captivity, turkeys, quail, cranes, pheasants, and some species of raptors are more commonly infected than waterfowl,[18] but *M. avium* is still a common and often fatal disease of waterfowl. Among wild waterfowl, less then 1% of birds examined at necropsy in North America[20] and 0.7% to 2.4% in the Netherlands had avian tuberculosis.[21]

### Epizoology

Avian tuberculosis is found worldwide in wild, captive, and domestic waterfowl. The disease is often chronic and no seasonal trends have been identified.[18] However, exposure to the causative organism is probably highest in fall and winter for wild waterfowl when they tend to form larger flocks. Added to this is the tendency of wild waterfowl to use sewage lagoons or waste-water areas during these seasons because the areas are often free of hunters and the water is warmer and takes longer to freeze. Captive waterfowl fed inadequate diets or kept in wet, cold, crowded, or poorly ventilated areas are more likely to contract avian tuberculosis if exposed to the disease, and this possibly holds true for wild waterfowl as well.

### Clinical Signs and Pathology

There are no specific clinical signs of avian tuberculosis. The chronic nature of the disease results in signs, such as weight loss, emaciation, weakness, lethargy, plumage deterioration, or general debilitation, all signs similar to other chronic diseases.[6] Depending upon the location of lesions, gastrointestinal signs such as diarrhea, musculoskeletal signs such as lameness, or organ failure signs such as ascites, are possible. Acid-fast bacilli in the feces is suggestive of disease but not diagnostic, either negative or positive. Birds are intermittent shedders and will yield a false-negative result if not shedding bacteria when tested. Likewise, the presence of acid-fast bacilli in a fecal sample may indicate something the bird ingested that is passing through the gastrointestinal tract but not constitute an established infection, thus giving a false-positive result. Lesions can sometimes be detected and biopsied on endoscopic examination.[6]

Lesions at necropsy consist of pliable to solidified yellow, white, or gray caseous nodules that vary in size from less than 1 mm to several centimeters. The nodules are encased deeply in the infected organs, usually the intestines, lung, spleen, and most often the liver. Lesions on unfeathered portions of the skin can resemble avian pox.[22] The veterinarian can learn about the route of exposure by locating the site of the primary lesion. Gastrointestinal lesions point to ingestion as the route of exposure from contaminated feed or water, while lesions of the lungs can indicate an aerosol exposure. In Canada and Ross geese (*Chen rossi*) and mute swans (*Cygnus olor*) and Tundra swans (*Cyghus columbianus*), a form of the disease causes emaciation with ascites, diffuse liver enlargement, and hydropericardium as the most common necropsy findings.[23] No discrete nodules are present. The histologic picture resembles generalized amyloidosis. Acid-fast staining and mycobacterium cultures are required to differentiate this form of avian tuberculosis from generalized amyloidosis.[23]

Gross necropsy results are important for a preliminary diagnosis, and acid-fast staining of impression smears or histologic sections gives a presumptive diagnosis. A definitive diagnosis requires culture and identification of *M. avium* complex, including serotype. However, this bacterium is very slow growing and requires special culture techniques to prevent overgrowth by other common bacteria. In addition, the isolate of M. *avium* needs to be identified.

### Control and Treatment

Detection in wild or captive birds is difficult. Monitoring the health of a waterfowl population is of utmost importance and this should include necropsies. Culturing feces can be used to monitor waterfowl, especially captive waterfowl, for the disease. However, a negative test on a single bird is not always accurate, as various factors and the chronicity of the disease can lead to a negative test at any one point in time in a bird that actually has the disease.

*M. avium* can persist for long periods in the environment, up to 48 months in poultry litter, 28 months in poultry carcasses, and 24 months buried 5 cm in soil.[24] Treatment is ineffective and the general recommendation for captive waterfowl is to euthanize the flock and keep the area free of birds for 2 or more years. Removing vegetation and frequent tilling of the soil, to expose the soil to sunlight, will help destroy the organism. Tilling of topsoil or removal and replacement of topsoil has also been recommended.[6] When discovered in a flock of wild waterfowl, elimination of the flock is not usually possible. Management techniques should be examined to see if any factors have contributed to the outbreak, such as the use of waste water to fill refuse ponds. Draining ponds or wetlands, using clean water to flush ponds or wetlands, plus tilling the soil are helpful management tools in these situations.

*M. avium* is potentially zoonotic, but infections are most likely to occur in people with compromised immune systems, as seen with diseases such as AIDS.

## SALMONELLOSIS, *SALMONELLA TYPHIMURIUM*

Salmonellosis refers to a disease caused by one of the *Salmonellae* bacteria of which 2,500 different strains have been identified.[25] The strains are called "serovars" or "serotypes" and are based on antigen or antibody responses. The 2,500 serovars are considered as variants of two primary species, *Salmonella enterica* and *S. bongori*. In addition, *S. enterica* is divided into six subspecies. The most common *Salmonella* to infect waterfowl, the cause of paratyphoid disease, is thus named *Salmonella enterica enterica* (subspecies) typhimurium (serovar), sometimes just referred to as *Salmonella typhimurium*.

Salmonellosis is a cause of mortality in waterfowl and also in passerines; however, large-scale disease in wild birds appears rare, disease in individuals being more common. Species that have been documented as suffering mortality in epizootics include mute swans, tufted ducks (*Aythya fuligula*), scaup (*Aythya* sp), mergansers (*Mergus merganser*), and coots (*Fulica americana*).[26] Large-scale mortality events of noncolonial nesting birds appear to be rare.[25] The death of individual waterfowl in captive collections, though, is much more frequent.

### Clinical Signs and Pathology

In ducklings, the disease is seen as depression, lethargy, reluctance to move, drowsiness, wing droop, and loss of balance shortly before death.[23] Diarrhea and feces pasted around the vent are common signs at any age. Also present may be conjunctivitis and swollen or edematous eyelids, with discharge that may result in the eyelids being closed together.

Gross pathologic lesions can be highly variable. One needs to consider the virulence and source of infection. Acute infections can have few gross pathologic lesions. As the disease progresses from acute to chronic, lesions will include swollen, friable liver with darker red or pale foci, and tan to white and granular abscess-like lesions of the pectoral muscle and possibly other tissues.[25] Intestinal infections are characterized by a reddened mucosal lining of the posterior half of the small intestines, ceca, and colon. In more chronic situations, the mucosal lining is coated with pale-white or yellow-fibrinous material. The ceca may contain thickened friable, caseous, or necrotic centers. Rectal or cloacal impaction is common in ducklings.[25] The spleen may also be swollen.

Diagnosis requires microbiologic culture and identification of *Salmonella* sp, as gross lesions are similar to avian cholera and colibacillosis.[25] Isolation of *Salmonella* sp from the intestines without significant pathology or isolation of the bacteria from organs may only indicate the bird was a carrier. The disease can infect eggs, and when low hatchability is seen, eggs can be cultured.

### Control and Treatment

*Salmonella* spp have been isolated from a variety of waterfowl species and from differing habitats. However, the prevalence of *Salmonella* spp in wild waterfowl populations are generally low.[25] Ducks feeding in areas of sewage effluent or water seeping from landfills will have higher levels of *Salmonella* sp present. For captive waterfowl, using clean, safe water sources is required to prevent Samonellosis. In addition, cleaning feeding bowls occasionally with household bleach diluted 1:10 in water will help prevent disease. Salmonella carriers in waterfowl collections should be identified by frequent fecal cultures, and the carriers eliminated from the collection. Adult carriers should not be used for breeding, as vertical transmission to eggs and the next generation is possible. Rats and mice can bring *Salmonella* sp into a waterfowl collection by contaminating water or, more likely, food; therefore, a diligent rodent-control program is necessary. No control or treatment is usually done for wild waterfowl. Antibiotics are occasionally used for treatment of Salmonellosis on captive waterfowl, but may not totally eliminate the bacteria and can result in the creation of carrier ducks.

Salmonellosis is a potential human pathogen. The organism can reside in the tissue and feces of infected birds, so extra care with personal hygiene and protection (gloves, mask) when handling or being exposed to waterfowl is important.

## AVIAN CHLAMYDIOSIS

Chlamydiosis in waterfowl, formerly referred to as ornithosis (or psittacosis, parrot fever if the source was a psittacine bird), is caused by the bacterium *Chlamydophila psittaci* (formerly *Clamydia psittaci*). The disease was first reported in psittacine birds in the 1920s as psittacosis, and later in other species,[27] where it was thought to be a similar but different agent, hence the name ornithosis. The causative bacterium, *C. psittaci*, is the same for all the diseases; hence, the new preferred nomenclature, avian chlamydiosis.[28]

The disease is found worldwide and has been reported in 30 orders and 460 avian species.[29] Large-scale mortality events in waterfowl have been reported, including mallards (*Anas platyrhynchos*) in Montana in 1999,[30] domestic ducks in eastern Europe,[31] and Britain and Australia.[32]

### Clinical Signs and Pathology

The disease can be acute, subacute, or chronic, with signs being variable and nonspecific. Signs are dependent on the virulence of the strain and the bird species involved. Lethargy, anorexia, ruffled feathers, weight loss, conjunctivitis, serous or infraorbital sinusitis, mucopurulent nasal and ocular discharge, green to yellow feces frequently with diarrhea, emaciation, dehydration, and death are all possible.[30] Mortality up to 30% in ducks and 55% in goslings has been reported.[23] Clinical signs and resemble other diseases including *Mycoplasma* and *Riemerella anatipestifer*.

Gross pathologic lesions, like clinical signs, are nonspecific. The vascular endothelium is the primary target of the bacterium, resulting in exudation of fluid and fibrin, along with necrosis and inflammatory cell infiltration.[23] Muscular atrophy pericarditis, perihepatitis, and hepatomegoly, splenomegaly, focal necrosis of liver or spleen, peritonitis, air sacculitis, pulmonary edema, and hyperemia are all seen at various times.[23] Conjunctival scrapings, blood smears, and fecal and tracheal swabs are used for diagnosis, but special media is required. Diagnosis requires isolation of the organism or finding a fourfold rise in antibody titer that coincides with clinical disease or pathology.[33] Recent diagnostic tools being tested include enzyme-linked immunosorbent assay (ELISA) and polymerase chain reaction.[33]

The organism is excreted in nasal discharges and in feces and may remain viable for several months. Inhalation is the primary route of exposure. Dried bird feces that become airborne are an excellent source of infection. Infections can occur at any season because of carrier birds and latent infections in bird populations. Stressors, such as crowding, chilling, breeding, shipping, and other factors have triggered shedding of the organism and outbreaks of infection.[34]

### Control and Treatment

All birds with avian chlamydiosis should be collected and euthanized. Carcasses should be incinerated to reduce infected material in an area. Human beings working around infected birds or dried bird feces should wear a mask or respirator in addition to protective clothing and gloves. Dried bird droppings can be wetted with a 5% bleach solution or other disinfectant. Before the development of antibiotics, mortality among human beings developing avian chlamydiosis was as high as 20%.[34] Secondary spread of the disease between human beings is considered rare.[35] Pregnant women should avoid contact with potential cases or sources of avian chamydiosis, as the organism can cause miscarriage. Tetracyclines are still the recommended antibiotic of choice, but erythromycin is also often used, especially among children and pregnant women.[30]

Treatment of wild waterfowl is not possible but individual ducks or small groups in captivity can be treated. The ducks with avian chlamydiosis should be isolated. Doxycycline, given orally, in drinking water or as an injectable form have all been used in pet birds.[35] Chlortetracycline-treated feed (400 g per ton) is recommended for treating poultry.[28] Premises and cages should be cleaned and disinfected with 1% bleach solution, 1% Lysol, or 70% isopropyl alcohol.[35]

For wild waterfowl, removing and incinerating infected carcasses is recommended. Infected waterfowl should be disturbed as little as possible to avoid dispersal to other areas and spread of the disease. Field personnel should wear protective clothing as described above. The area should be closed to the public. In any outbreak, it may be required to notify public health officials.

### NEW DUCK DISEASE, DUCK SEPTICEMIA

The bacterium *Reimerella anatipestifer* is the causative organism of a disease called new duck disease, duck septicemia, infectious serositis, or goose influenza. The disease has been reported worldwide. The organism is a gram-negative, nonmotile, rod-shaped bacterium that can occur singly, in pairs, or in filaments. It may stain bipolar with Wright's or new methylene blue stains. The organism is very similar to *Pasteurella multocida*.

### Clinical Signs and Pathology

The disease in domestic ducks is found almost exclusively in 1- to 8-week-old ducklings. Ducklings younger than 5 weeks die within 24 to 48 hours.[36] Signs of the disease include greenish diarrhea, serous to more solid ocular discharges, weakness and lethargy, ataxia, head tremor or head bobbing, opisthotonus, swimming in circles, or inability to stand on land.[23] However, birds may die suddenly with no previous signs of illness. Ducks that survive may develop salpingitis and have depressed egg production.[37]

Fibrinous polyserositis is a common but not consistent finding at necropsy.[38,39] Usually the most prominent of these fibrinous coverings are on the surfaces of the liver, heart, and respiratory system. Meningitis is found on histologic examination.[38] Culture and identification of the bacterium is required for a diagnosis as *P. multocida*, *Staphylococcus aureus*, *Mycoplasma*, and *Escherichia coli* all cause similar disease. *R. anatipestifer* sometimes is difficult to culture, so samples from several organs should be submitted.

## Treatment, Prevention, and Control

Treatment with antibiotics is possible.[36] Sulfamethazine, 0.2% to 0.25% in drinking water or feed prevents onset of clinical sighs in ducks under experimental exposure to the bacterium.[40] Sulfaquinoxaline, 0.025% to 0.05% in feed has been used both experimentally and in field outbreaks to reduce mortality.[41] Novobiocin (0.030%–0.0368%) or lincomycin (0.011%–0.022%) as feed additives are effective in reducing mortality when given starting 3 days before experimental exposure.[41] Subcutaneous injections of lincomycin-spectonomycin, penicillin, or penicillin-dihydrodtreptomycin will also reduce mortality.[41] Bacterins and live-virus vaccines have also been developed and proved effective to prevent disease or reduce mortality after onset.[42,43]

In free-living or wild ducks, the disease is very sporadic and, in most cases, ducks are widely separated when ducklings are young. In captive situations, crowding or stress contribute to the severity of outbreaks, as do unsanitary conditions.

## AVIAN BOTULISM

Avian botulism, also called limberneck, western duck disease, and alkali poisoning, is a paralytic and fatal disease of waterfowl and other birds. Waterfowl are sickened and die after ingesting the toxin produced by *Clostridium botulinum*. There are seven distinct toxin types, given letter labels. Waterfowl are most affected by Type C.[44] *C. botulinum* is a gram-positive anaerobic bacterium that forms spores that can remain viable for years in mud or soil. The bacterium produces toxin, but only when infected by a virus that triggers the production of the toxin protein through an introduced gene into the bacterium.[44] Outbreaks are favored by warm weather above 25°C, thus outbreaks are more common in summer and fall. Decomposing animal carcasses (vertebrate or invertebrate) are good media for *C. botulinum* growth. Raw sewage or rotting vegetation can also promote bacterial growth. Waterfowl are usually stricken when ingesting invertebrates feeding in a contaminated area. The invertebrates are not affected by the toxin.

## Clinical Signs and Pathology

The toxin affects peripheral nerves by preventing impulse transmission by interference with the release of acetylcholine, resulting in muscle paralysis.[45] Waterfowl cannot fly or walk and may use wings to push themselves along. The third eyelid is often prominent and the bird may fail to hold its head erect. Death can be from drowning or respiratory arrest.[44]

No characteristic lesions are found at necropsy. Diagnosis is by mouse inoculation testing or by the newer ELISA test.[44]

## Treatment, Prevention, and Control

Recovery rates of 75% to 90% are possible if sickened waterfowl are given good supportive care (fluids or fresh water) and kept in a shaded, quiet environment. Antitoxin injections, when available, are also useful for treatment.

It is not feasible to eliminate botulism spores from the environment where waterfowl live normally. Avoid management actions that can result in large-scale plant or animal mortality in warmer months, such as flooding areas, thus killing vegetation, or draining areas, thus killing fish in the water column.[44] Removing dead animals quickly in areas where outbreaks occur is useful.

**Table 1**
Miscellaneous bacterial diseases of waterfowl

| Disease Common Name | Etiologic Agents | Signs | Pathology | Treatment or Control |
|---|---|---|---|---|
| Colibacillosis | Escherichia coli | Nonspecific, enteritis, lethargic, weight loss, fall and winter more common[46] | Pericarditis, perihepatitis, swollen liver | Control exposure to feces, antibiotics based on sensitivity testing as may resistant strains exist[46] |
| Bumblefoot | Staphylococcus aureus | Wounds and swelling on feet, lameness, death if septicemic | Acute to chronic granulomatous lesions on feet, culture and sensitivity testing, gram-positive cocci | Antibiotic, supply duck with soft surfaces for walking |
| Necrotic enteritis | Clostridium sp | Mortality 1%–40%,[23] sudden acute onset, sometimes related to stress or diet change | Hemorrhagic necrotizing enteritis | Avoid stress or sudden diet changes |
| Erysipelas | Erysipelothrix rhusiopathiae | Lethargy, death, acute disease | Small gram-positive rods, septicemia, lesions such as generalized congestion, petechial or ecchymotic hemorrhages in pericardial fat, pleura, skeletal muscle | Potential zoonotic but of low pathogenicity for humans. Susceptible to penicillin, cephalosporin, cefotaxime, clindamycin, fluoroquinolones. Remove and incinerate carcasses[47] |
| Mycoplasmosis | Mycoplasma anatis, M. anseris, M. imitavis[48] | Sinusitis, reduced hatching, infertile eggs, inflamed phallus in ganders[49] | Sinusitis, air sacculitis, salpingitis, peritonitis, pulmonary edema, meningitis[50] | Cleaning and disinfection of cages and feeders for captive waterfowl |

**Table 2**
Common parasitic diseases of waterfowl

| Disease Common Name | Etiologic Agent | Clinical Signs | Pathology | Treatment and Control |
|---|---|---|---|---|
| Tapeworms | Cestodes: 264 species in waterfowl[51] | Segments in feces, debilitation in severe cases | Indirect life cycle, require intermediate host, look for proglotids in droppings | Dibutyltin dilaurate as a food additive is used in chickens.[52] Praziquantel (Droncit) 10 mg/kg–20 mg/kg PO, repeat in 10–14 days[53] |
| Roundworms, gizzard worms, stomach worms | *Amidostomum* sp, *Epomidiostomum* sp | In heavy infestations may see poor growth, emaciation, weakness | Direct life cycle, inflamed hemorrhagic or sloughed gizzard lining, necrosis of gizzard muscle | Good sanitation, removing feces to break cycle. Ivermecin 0.2 mg/kg IM, PO once[53] |
| Thorny-headed worms | Acanthocephalans, 52 species[54] | Emaciation, enteritis | Granulomatous hemorrhagic enteritis, pentonitis with penetration of intestinal wall, parasite in intestine bright yellow orange 0.5 cm–1.0 cm long | Epizootic mortality during periods of stress, control by removing intermediate hosts, thiabendazole for treatment[55] |
| Flukes | Trematodes: 536 species in waterfowl,[56] only 10% of species pathogenic *Sphaeridiotrema globulus* most common | Bloody cloacal discharge, wing droop, death in 5 to 6 days, chronic enteritis possible, weight loss, lameness | *S. gobulus*: Fibreno hemorrhagic uncreative enteritis lower small intestine in Scaup, Canvasback Long-tailed Ducks, Swans, Mallards | Freshwater snails first and second intermediate hosts of *S. globulus*, prevent access to invertebrate intermediate hosts in captive setting |

| Leeches | Theromyzon sp, 14 species[57] | Attach in nasal respiratory passages and conjunctiva, ketato conjunctivitis shaking head, sneezing scratching head | Partial or complete occlusion of nasal passages by leeches, respiratory mucosal irritation, anemia, leeches may leave dead bird before necropsy | No preventative measures in wild, in captivity prevent birds from using water with heavy leech infestations, mechanical removal, submerging bill in 10%–20% NaCl solution for 10 seconds[58] |
|---|---|---|---|---|
| Lice | Mallophaga Trinoton anserinum vector for swan heartworm disease | Emaciation, poor feathers in severe cases | Usually no pathology other than finding lice on feathers | Pyrethrin or carbaryl powder on feathers |
| Hemosporidiosis, Avian malaria | Plasmodium Haemoproteus Leucocytozoa | Emaciation, appetite loss, listless, dyspnea lameness, death | Biting insects are vectors, 75% of waterfowl have one or more species,[59] enlarged liver and spleen, anemic, liver and spleen brown to black colored because of hemozoin pigment deposits, diagnose on blood smears | Reduce or control vectors |
| Intestinal Coccidiosis | Eimeria sp: 13 species reported in ducks[60] | Nonspecific lethargic, anemic, weight loss, watery diarrhea, tremors, convulsions, lameness,[61] up to 70% mortality[60] | Life-cycle completed in 1 to 2 weeks, hemorrhagic enteritis in upper intestinal tract seen in Scaup[61] | Change contaminated litter frequently to break life cycle, coccidiostatic medications in food or water (Amprolium 0.0125%–0.0175% or Sulfadimethoxine 0.0125% as feed additives[60] |

(continued on next page)

**Table 2**
*(continued)*

| Disease Common Name | Etiologic Agent | Clinical Signs | Pathology | Treatment and Control |
|---|---|---|---|---|
| Renal coccidiosis | *Eimeria* sp Ducks *E. boschadis E. somatarie* Geese *E. truncata* Swans *E. christiansani*[62] | Most common during breeding and wintering seasons, emaciation, weakness, nonspecific signs | Enlarged, pale kidneys, spots or mottled pattern on kidneys, chalky tenture because of urates[62] | Avoid crowding, good sanitation |
| Sarcocystis, Rice breast disease, Sarcosporidiosis | *Sarcocystis rileyi* | Most common in dabbling ducks, usually no signs, possibly loss of muscle mass, lameness in severe cases | Indirect life cycle requiring carnivore as primary host, duck is intermediate host, rice-grain size, white streaks in muscle tissues (Macrocysts) | No known treatment or control measures |
| Heartworm of swans and geese | Nematodes of subfamily *Filarioidea*, *Sarconema eurycera* most common[63] | No specific signs | Indirect life cycle requires biting louse for transmission, adult parasite found within myocardium, blood smears for filarial worms | In captivity, control biting lice with pyrethrin, carbaryl, ivermectin |

## MISCELLANEOUS BACTERIAL AND PARASITIC DISEASES

There are many other bacterial diseases that effect waterfowl and some of the more common, not previously covered, are described in **Table 1**.

Parasitic diseases of waterfowl are quite common but generally are not major mortality factors. However, parasites, if present during other disease outbreaks, can contribute to mortality. **Table 2** describes the major internal and eternal parasites encountered on waterfowl.

## SUMMARY

It is not possible in the short section of one article to completely cover the many bacterial and parasitic diseases of waterfowl. The author recommends several of the references as excellent sources of further information, in particular the books *Diseases of Wild Waterfowl* by G. Wobeser, *Field Manual of Wildlife Diseases* by M. Friend and J. C. Franson, editors, and *Infectious Diseases of Wild Birds* by N. J. Thomas, D. B. Hunter, and C. T. Atkinson, editors (these editors also recently published a second book, *Parasitic Diseases of Wild Birds*, available through Blackwell Publishing).

## REFERENCES

1. Jensen WI, Williams C. Botulism and fowl cholera. In: Linduska JP, editor. Waterfowl tomorrow. Washington, DC: U.S. Government Printing Office; 1964. p. 333–41.
2. Rosen MN. Avian cholera. In: Davis JW, Anderson RC, Karstad L, et al, editors. Infectious and parasitic diseases of wild birds. Ames (IA): Iowa State University Press; 1971. p. 59–74.
3. Smith GJ, Higgins KF, Gritzner CF. Land use relationships to avian cholera outbreaks in the Nebraska rainwater basin area. Prairie Nat 1989;21:125–36.
4. Montgomery RD, Stein G, Stotts VD, et al. The 1978 epornitic of avian cholera on the Chesapeake Bay. Avian Dis 1979;24:966–78.
5. Wobeser G. Avian cholera and waterfowl biology. J Wildl Dis 1992;28:674–82.
6. Routh A, Sanderson S. Waterfowl. In: Tully TN, Lawton MPC, Dorrestein GM, editors. Avian medicine. Oxford: Butterworth Heinemann; 2000. p. 234–65.
7. Wobeser GA. Avian cholera. In: Wobeser GA, editor. Diseases of Wild Waterfowl. 2nd edition. New York: Plenum Press; 1997. p. 57–69.
8. Mutters R, Ihm P, Pohl S, et al. Reclassification of the genus *Pasteurella* Trevisan 1887 on the basis of deoxyribonucleic acid homology, with proposals for the new species *Pasteurella dagmatis, Pasteurella canis, Pasteurella stomatis, Pasteurella anatis,* and *Pasterella langaa.* Int J Syst Bacteriol 1985;35:309–22.
9. Botzler RG. Epizootiology of avian cholera in waterfowl. J Wildl Dis 1991;27: 367–95.
10. Hall WJ, Heddleston KL, Legenhausen DH, et al. Studies on pasteurellosis: I. A new species of *Pasteurella* encountered in chronic fowl cholera. Am J Vet Res 1955;16:598–604.
11. Korschgen CE, Gibbs HC, Mendall HL. Avian cholera in eider ducks in Maine. J Wildl Dis 1978;14:254–8.
12. Smith BJ, Higgins KF, Tucker WL. Precipitation, waterfowl densities and mycotoxins: their potential effect on avian cholera epizootics in the Nebraska rainwater basin area. Trans N Am Wildl Nat Resour Conf 1990;55:269–82.

13. Zinkl JG, Dey N, Hyland JM, et al. An epornitic of avian cholera in waterfowl and common crows in Phelps County, Nebraska in the spring, 1975. J Wildl Dis 1977; 13:194–8.

14. Friend M. Avian cholera. In: Friend M, Franson JC, editors. Field manual of wildlife diseases. Washington, DC: US Department of Interior; 1999. p. 75–92.

15. Heddleston KL, Rebers PA. Properties of free endotoxin from *Pasteurella multocida*. Am J Vet Res 1975;36:573–4.

16. Hunter B, Wobeser G. Pathology of experimental avian cholera in mallard ducks. Avian Dis 1980;24:403–14.

17. Jessup DA. Ducks, geese, swans and screamers (Anseriformes): infectious diseases. In: Fowler ME, editor. Zoo and wild animal medicine. Philadelphia: W.B. Saunders; 1986. p. 342–52.

18. Friend M. Tuberculoses. In: Friend M, Franson CJ, editors. Field manual of wildlife diseases. Washington, DC: US Dept of Interior; 1999. p. 93–8.

19. Thoen CO, Karlson AG. Tuberculosis. In: Calnek BW, Barnes HJ, Beard CW, et al, editors. Diseases of poultry. Ames (IA): Iowa State University Press; 1991. p. 172–85.

20. Mac Neil AC, Barnard T. Necropsy results in free-flying and captive *anatidae* in British Columbia. Can Vet J 1978;19:17–25.

21. Smith T, Eger A, Haagsma J, et al. Avian tuberculosis in wild birds in the Netherlands. J Wildl Dis 1987;23:485–7.

22. Ferguson SH, Wallace LJ, Dunbar F, et al. *Mycobacterium intracellulare* (*Battey bacillus*) infection in a Florida wood duck (*Aix sponsa*). Am Rev Respir Dis 1969;100:876–8.

23. Wobeser GA. Other bacteria, mycoplasmas and chlamydiae. In: Wobeser GA, editor. Diseases of Wild Waterfowl. 2nd edition. New York: Plenum Press; 1997. p. 71–91.

24. Wray C. Survival and spread of pathogenic bacteria of veterinary importance within the environment. Vet Bull 1975;45:543–7.

25. Friend M. Salmonellosis. In: Friend M, Franson JC, editors. Field manual of wildlife diseases. Washington, DC: US Dept of Interior; 1999. p. 99–109.

26. Steiniger F. *Salmonella* sp. and *Clostridium botulinum* in waterfowl and seabirds. Wildfowl Trust Ann Rep 1962;13:149–52.

27. Meyer KF. The ecology of psittacosis and ornithosis. Medicine 1942;21:175–206.

28. Anderson AA, Banrompay A. Avian chlamydiosis (psittacosis, ornithosis). In: Saif YM, editor. Diseases of poultry. 11th edition. Ames (IA): Iowa Sate University Press; 2003. p. 863–79.

29. Kaleta EF, Taday EMA. Avian host range of *Chlamydophila* spp. Based on isolation, antigen detection and serology. Avian Pathol 2003;32:435–62.

30. Anderson AA, Franson JC. Avian chlamydiosis. In: Thomas NJ, Hunter DB, Atkinson CT, editors. Infectious diseases of wild birds. Oxford: Blackwell Publishing; 2007. p. 303–16.

31. Strauss J. Microbiologic and epidemiologic aspects of duck ornithosis in Czechoslovakia. Am J Ophthalmol 1967;63:1246–59.

32. Hunter DG, Shipley A, Galvin JW, et al. Chlamydiosis in workers at a duck farm and processing plant. Aust Vet J 1993;70(5):174–6.

33. Anderson AA. Avian Chlamydiosis. OIE manual for standards for diagnostic tests and vaccines for terrestrial animals (mammals, birds and bees). France. 5th edition. Paris: Office International des Epizooties; 2004. p. 856–67.

34. Franson JC. Chlamydiosis. In: Friend M, Franson JC, editors. Field manual of wildlife diseases. Washington, DC: US Dept of Interior; 1999. p. 111–4.

35. Smith KA, Bradly KK, Stobierski MG, et al. Compendium of measures to control *Chlamydophila psittaci* (formerly *Chlamydia psittaci*) infection among humans (psittaciosis) and pet birds. J Am Vet Med Assoc 2005;226:532–9.
36. Sandhu TS. *Riemerella anatipestifer* infection. In: Saif YM, editor. Diseases of poultry. 11th edition. Ames (IA): Iowa State Press; 2003. p. 676–82.
37. Bisgaard M. Salpingitis in web-footed birds: prevalence, aetiology and significance. Avian Pathol 1995;24:443–8.
38. Eleazer TH, Blalock HG, Harrell JS. *Paseurella anatipestifer* as a cause of mortality in semiwild pen-raised mallard ducks in South Carolina. Avian Dis 1973;17:855–7.
39. Pickrell JA. Pathological changes associated with experimental *Pasteurella anatipestifer* infection in ducklings. Avian Dis 1966;10:281–8.
40. Asplin FD. A septicaemic disease of ducklings. Vet Rec 1955;67:854–8.
41. Sandhu TS, Dean WF. Effect of chemotherapeutic agents on *Pasteurella anatipestifer* infection in white Pekin ducklings. Poult Sci 1980;59:1027–30.
42. Layton HW, Sandhu TS. Protection of ducklings with a broth-grown *Pasteurella anatipestifer* bacterin. Avian Dis 1984;28:718–26.
43. Sandhu TS. Immunogenicity and safety of a live *Pasteurella anatipestifer* vaccine in white Pekin ducklings: laboratory and field trials. Avian Pathol 1991;20:423–32.
44. Roche TE, Friend M. Avian botulism. In: Friend M, Franson JC, editors. Field manual of wildlife disease. Washington, DC: US Dept of Interior; 1999. p. 271–81.
45. Wobeser G. Botulism. In: Wobeser GA, editor. Diseases of Wild Waterfowl. 2nd edition. New York: Plenum Press; 1997. p. 149–61.
46. Barnes JH, Vaillancourt JP, Gross WB. Colibacillosis. In: Saif YM, editor. Diseases of poultry. 11th edition. Ames (IA): Iowa State Press; 2003. p. 631–52.
47. Wolcott MJ. Erysipelas. In: Thomas NJ, Hunter DB, Atkinson CT, editors. Infectious diseases of wild birds. Oxford: Blackwell Publishing; 2007. p. 332–40.
48. Friend M. Mycopolasmosis. In: Friend M, Franson JC, editors. Field manual of wildlife diseases. Washington, DC: US Dept of Interior; 1999. p. 115–9.
49. Szep I, Pataky M, Bogre I. Recent practical and experimental observations on the infectious inflammatory disease of the cloaca and penis in geese. Acta Vet Acad Sci Hung 1979;27:195–202.
50. Stipkovits L, Glavits R, Ivanics E. Additional data on mycoplasma disease of goslings. Avian Pathol 1993;22:171–6.
51. McDonald ME. Catalog of Helminths of Waterfowl (anatidae). No.126. Washington, DC: US Bureau of Sport Fisheries and Wildlife Special Science Report Wildlife; 1969.
52. McDougald LR. Cestodes and trematodes. In: Saif YM, editor. Diseases of poultry. 11th edition. Ames (IA): Iowa State Press; 2003. p. 961–71.
53. Rupiper DJ, Carpenter JW, Mashima TY. Formulary. In: Olsen GH, Orosz SE, editors. Manual of avian medicine. St. Louis (MO): Mosby, Inc.; 2000. p. 553–89.
54. McDonald ME. Key to Acanthocephala in waterfowl. Washington, DC: US Dept of Interior Fish and Wildlife Service Resource Publication 173; 1988.
55. Cole RA. Acanthocephaliosis. In: Friend M, Franson JC, editors. Field manual of wildlife diseases. Washington, DC: US Dept of Interior; 1999. p. 241–3.
56. McDonald MEIn: Key to Trematodes reported in Waterfowl, 142. Washington, DC: US Dept of Interior Fish and Wildlife Service Resource Publication; 1981.
57. Oosthuizen JH, Davies RW. A new species of *Theromyzon* (Rhynchodellida: Glossiphonidae), with review of the genus in North America. Can J Zool 1993; 71:1311–4.

58. Tuggle BN. Nasal leeches. In: Friend M, Franson JC, editors. Field manual of wild-life diseases. Washington, DC: US Dept of Interior; 1999. p. 245–51.

59. Atkinson CT. Hemosporidiosis. In: Friend M, Franson JC, editors. Field manual of wildlife diseases. Washington, DC: US Dept of Interior; 1999. p. 193–9.

60. McDougal LR. Coccidiosis. In: Salf YM, editor. Diseases of poultry. 11th edition. Ames (IA): Iowa State Press; 2003. p. 974–91.

61. Friend M, Franson JC. Intestinal coccidiosis. In: Friend M, Franson JC, editors. Field manual of wildlife diseases. Washington, DC: US Dept of Interior; 1999. p. 207–13.

62. Cole RA. Renal coccidiosis. In: Friend M, Franson JC, editors. Field manual of wildlife diseases. Washington, DC: US Dept of Interior; 1999. p. 215–8.

63. Cole RA. Heartworm of swans and geese. In: Friend M, Franson JC, editors. Field manual of wildlife diseases. Washington, DC: US Dept of Interior; 1999. p. 233–4.

# Management of Select Bacterial and Parasitic Conditions of Raptors

Michelle Willette, DVM*, Julia Ponder, DVM, Luis Cruz-Martinez, DVM,
Lori Arent, MS, Irene Bueno Padilla, DVM, Olga Nicolas de Francisco, DVM,
Patrick Redig, DVM, PhD

**KEYWORDS**

- Bird of prey • Bacterial disease • Parasitic disease
- Emerging disease • Pododermatitis • Bumblefoot

The term raptor, or bird of prey, is used to describe a group of carnivorous birds whose features include keen eyesight, a hooked beak, and strong feet with sharp talons. Raptors include owls in the order Strigiformes, and eagles, hawks, falcons, vultures, osprey, and secretary birds in the order Falconiformes. Raptors are an incredibly diverse group of birds. They are found on every continent except Antarctica and occupy nearly all types of terrestrial habitat. They take various prey, including invertebrates, fish, herpetiles, birds, bats, and other mammals, carrion, and some fruit.

Raptor medicine encompasses birds exhibited in aviaries in zoologic institutions, permanently disabled "ambassadors" used in educational facilities, free-living individuals presented for wildlife rehabilitation, and hunting or breeding birds used in falconry and conservation efforts. A permit is required to maintain any native raptor species in captivity, even for rehabilitation. The husbandry and feeding practices for these raptors vary widely depending on the facility and diet availability, and the species and purposes for which they are kept. Given this breadth of circumstances, medical issues should be approached methodically. A minimum database for a raptor would include: history and signalment; visual observations before restraint; a complete physical examination, including the eyes; a complete blood count; ventrodorsal and lateral whole-body radiographs; and fecal cytology and ova and parasite check. Second-tier diagnostics could include: chemistries, including bile acids; appropriate serology; ultrasonography or endoscopy; and bacterial and fungal cultures, including any wounds and the respiratory tract (deep tracheal swab).[1]

In 1631, Burt Latham, a falconer in London, wrote the following:

*Hawkes have divers infirmities and diseases, as Feavers, Palsey, Imposthumes, Sore eyes, and Nares, Megums, Pantas, casting her Gorge, fouleness of Gorge.*

---

The Raptor Center, College of Veterinary Medicine, University of Minnesota, 1920 Fitch Avenue, St. Paul, MN 55108, USA
* Corresponding author.
*E-mail address:* wille203@umn.edu (M. Willette).

Vet Clin Exot Anim 12 (2009) 491–517
doi:10.1016/j.cvex.2009.06.006
1094-9194/09/$ – see front matter © 2009 Published by Elsevier Inc.

*Wormes, Fillanders, ill liver, or Goute, Pinne in the foot, breaking the pounce. Bones out of ioynt, Bones broken, Bruises, Lice, Colds, Frounce, Fistulaes, Stone, much gaping, more foundring, privy evill, taint in the feathers, loste of appetite, broken wind, blow on wing, wounds, swellings, eating their owne feet, taking up of veines in Hawkes, Crampe, and a world of others.[2]*

Today we recognize these conditions as aspergillosis, pododermatitis, sour crop, trichomoniasis, and "a world of others." Clearly raptors are susceptible to a wide variety of conditions, including a broad array of bacterial and parasitic infections, some of which are carried by prey items. Numerous comprehensive reviews of bacteria and ectoparasites, helminths, protozoa, and hemoparasites recovered from raptors have been published (see later discussion).

There are many host and pathogen factors that determine susceptibility to an infection. Host factors may include species and immune status, concurrent illness, conditions of captivity and management, and nutritional status. Pathogen factors include life cycle and virulence, number of infectious organisms, and opportunity. Opportunity may be of paramount importance. The vast majority of bacteria and parasites are not pathogenic under normal circumstances. Organisms detailed here are significant in raptors because of their frequency, pathogenicity, or uniqueness. This article outlines the significance, diagnosis and management, and prevention of these infections.

## FALCONRY TERMINOLOGY

Falconry is the hunting of wild quarry with trained raptors; it has been practiced for more than four millennia. Historically and today, falconers have contributed to our knowledge of disease, captive management and breeding, and reintroduction techniques, and they continue to play a vital role in the global conservation of birds of prey (Redig, in press). A unique set of terms has arisen with the sport, many of which are still heard today. Veterinarians whose practice includes falconry birds should be familiar with the more common medical and management terms (**Box 1**).

## BACTERIAL CONDITIONS OF RAPTORS

Bacterial agents are rarely reported in the literature as primary disease agents for raptors but can occur in debilitated or chronically ill individuals in poor body condition. Often the diagnosis is obtained on postmortem examination. Chlamydiosis, clostridiosis, avian mycobacteriosis, pasteurellosis (fowl cholera), and salmonellosis are discussed here. Mycoplasmosis, erysipelas, yersiniosis (pseudotuberculosis), and other gram-negative bacteria have also been described in raptor species[3,4,5,6] (H.L. Shivaprasad, DVM, PhD, personal communication, April 2009).

### Chlamydiosis

Infection with *Chlamydophila psittaci* is referred to as psittacosis, ornithosis, or chlamydiosis depending on species affected. According to Andersen,[7] this disease is most often diagnosed in wild birds in cases of epizootic mortality, during surveillance for other diseases, or when transmission occurs to humans. Reports of its occurrence in raptors in North America are scarce and its prevalence seems to be lower than that reported in the Eastern hemisphere.[8] In 1983, *C psittaci* was isolated from a group of captive red-tailed hawks (*Buteo jamaicensis*) in California; four birds were found dead and the survivors were subsequently tested. In addition, chlamydiosis was the cause of death of a free-ranging red-tailed hawk that had respiratory signs, diarrhea, and emacitation. At postmortem, splenomegaly and a fibrinous exudate on the liver were

---

**Box 1**
**Falconry terminology**

Bate: a tethered raptor's attempt to fly off a gloved hand or perch

Buteo: group of medium-sized raptors of the genus *Buteo* with broad wings for soaring and a large, fan-shaped tail

Casting or pellet: the indigestible portion of a raptor's meal, including bone, feathers, or fur; to cast is the act of regurgitating

Coping: trimming and reshaping a raptor's beak and talons; to cope is the process of trimming

Cramps: clinical signs seen with metabolic bone disease

Croaks or kecks: sounds referable to respiratory disease

Free loft: to allow to fly free within an enclosure

Frounce: trichomoniasis in raptors

Gape: corner of the mouth

Mute: to defecate; mutes are the voided cloacal contents, including urine, urates, and feces

Imping: the process of replacing broken or damaged feathers

Pinne in the foot: pododermatitis or bumblefoot

Mews: a raptor housing area that provides protection from the weather

Rangle: a medieval term whereby small stones are given orally to encourage a raptor to cast

Slice: the normal projectile defecation of eagles, hawks, and accipiters

Tiercel or tercel: the male of a raptor species, originally used for peregrine falcons; from the diminutive of Latin *tertius* or third; in general the male is about one third smaller than the female

*Data from* Refs.[2,13,14,15]

---

observed. In addition, chlamydia-like organisms were seen using Gimenez-stained impression smears of the liver.[5] Although serologic tests and polymerase chain reaction analysis are available for chlamydiosis, demonstration of the organism either by isolation and identification, or by staining of tissue or fecal smears, is the preferred method for diagnosis.[7]

## Clostridiosis

Clostridial organisms, in particular *Clostridium perfringens*, are anaerobic organisms commonly found in free-ranging raptors as part of the normal intestinal flora. Endogenous clostridia can proliferate, however, resulting in enterotoxemia in birds in poor condition or being treated with antibiotics (Patrick Redig, DVM, PhD, personal communication, April 2009). Signs of gastrointestinal disturbances include anorexia and diarrhea; radiographically, enlarged intestinal loops can be evident. Diagnosis is often done using direct fecal smears in which moderate to heavy occurrence of gram-positive rods with an intracellular spore are observed. Treatment with metronidazole (30 mg/kg every 12 hours for 5 days) provides an acceptable treatment.[1] In addition, *C perfringens* has proved to be pathogenic in food items that have not been properly frozen, allowing for an abundant growth of clostridial organisms and the production of endotoxins. When such food is fed to raptors, there is an almost immediate response with affected birds becoming moribund and most dying.

Treatment options include immediate emptying of the stomach, administration of activated charcoal, and supportive care.

Infections with *Clostridium tetani* are rarely seen and are associated with puncture wounds that introduce the bacteria deep into the tissues.[9] Treatment has been unrewarding in the few cases experienced at The Raptor Center.

### Mycobacteriosis

Mycobacteriosis in birds is distributed worldwide; it has been reported in poultry, in domestic and free-ranging birds, and in captive situations (ie, zoologic collections).[10,11] The organisms most commonly associated with disease are *Mycobacterium avium* and *M genavense*.[11] In free-ranging raptors, *M avium* serotype 2[12] has been described in buteo hawks (see **Box 1**), owls, and bald eagles (*Haliaeetus leucocephalus*); the prevalence is reported to be low.[10,11] In raptors, ingestion, inhalation, and skin abrasions have been described as routes of infection. Infections are usually disseminated and are associated with debilitation.[3]

Clinical signs are primarily those of starving birds. In addition, weight loss and diarrhea have been described, as well as the pathognomonic "punch-out" lesions in long bones.[1] A lepromatous form of mycobacteria, characterized by nodular subcutaneous lesions, has also been described.[3] These lesions have been seen in a free-ranging great horned owl (*Bubo virginianus*) and a gyrfalcon (*Falco rusticolus*) (The Raptor Center, unpublished data, 2009).

Diagnosis can be challenging and not well established in vivo.[12] Hematologic values are those of a chronic, inflammatory leukogram with or without changes in biochemistry panels.[3] The use of radiography, ultrasonography, coelomoscopy, and biopsy or fine-needle aspiration with acid-fast staining can provide a presumptive diagnosis. Because of the nonspecific nature of the clinical signs and a lack of a specific antemortem test,[16] definitive diagnosis requires culture or polymerase chain reaction testing from tissue samples (ie, liver).[16]

Treatment for mycobacteriosis in free-ranging raptors is generally not undertaken because of the often advanced stage of debilitation. In addition, zoonotic considerations have been reported, especially affecting immunocompromised patients (ie, AIDS).[17] No reports describing transmission of an *M avium* infection from a wild raptor to a human are known to the authors. In contrast, zooanthroponotic transmission of *M tuberculosis* acquired from its owner has been reported in a pet bird.[18]

### Pasteurellosis

Avian cholera is a disease caused by *Pasteurella multocida*. Serotypes 1 and 3 seem to be most commonly isolated from disease outbreaks.[19,20] In raptors it has been reported in 19 Falconiformes and 11 Strigiformes species.[21] Its occurrence in free-living raptors has been related to the ingestion of infected prey during avian cholera outbreaks[22] in areas where epizootics are known to occur (ie, western United States),[1] and from cat bite wounds.[21] Infected birds die acutely showing signs of septicemia.[21] A unique presentation involving esophageal abscesses attributable to chronic pasteurellosis in buteo hawks was reported by Morishita and colleagues.[21]

In a group of osprey chicks (*Pandion haliaetus*)[4] all birds were found dead within an outbreak area. In the case of one gyrfalcon[22] trained for falconry, the only clinical sign noted was anorexia 24 hours before death. For falconry birds, vaccination is recommended for species used to hunt ducks in regions where epizootics occur; a polyvalent killed Al hydroxide adjuvanted vaccine (Poultry Health Laboratories, Davis, California; http://www.phlassociates.com/general_info.htm) has proved both safe and effective (William Farrier, DVM, MS, personal communication, April 2009). In addition, this disease can rapidly spread inside a facility and can be deadly across species lines. It does not require direct bird–bird transmission; therefore, disinfection of equipment (ie, falconry gloves and hoods) is important (William Farrier, DVM, MS, personal communication, April 2009). In an improved methodology for disinfectant testing, Advatange 256 (Preserve Chemical Co., Zephyr Cover, Nevada), a phenolic compound, and hydrogen peroxide 3% (Kmart Corp., Troy MI) resulted in total bacterial inhibition after less than 0.5 minutes of contact time.[23]

## Salmonellosis

The presence of *Salmonella* spp organisms in free-living raptors has been associated with ingestion of the bacteria when eating infected prey, and it is presumed that these birds of prey can be carriers of the organism.[6,24] Heidenreich[9] proposes that these bacteria may be transiently carried by raptors, however. The presence of *Salmonella* spp in fecal cultures should therefore be interpreted carefully. Results should be evaluated in light of clinical signs and other diagnostic tests. Clinical signs of salmonellosis include dehydration, greenish urates, and depression, along with elevated liver enzymes.[9] Intestinal salmonellosis (*S newport*) was diagnosed postmortem as the cause for clinical deterioration in a bald eagle undergoing rehabilitation at The Raptor Center. This case was characterized by acute diphtheritic enteritis and hepatitis (The Raptor Center, unpublished data). Zoonotic considerations regarding salmonellosis in raptors have been suggested.[6] Outbreaks of salmonellosis in children have been reported after dissection of pellets from captive, healthy owls.[25] Good hygiene and sanitation practices are recommended to reduce the occurrence of these incidents. Many institutions autoclave owl pellets before these types of activities.

## INFECTIOUS PODODERMATITIS
### Significance

Long recognized among falconers, "bumblefoot" is the vernacular name for inflammatory pododermatitis, a disease commonly seen in captive raptors but only rarely in wild birds of prey. In captivity, it is most often associated with inadequate management techniques, whereas in the wild traumatic events, such as bites from prey animals, chemical or heat burns, or territorial disputes with conspecifics, may play a role. In either situation, there is compromise of the epithelium subsequent to trauma, followed by infection and abscessation. Although infection is secondary, bacteria play a significant role in the pathogenesis of the disease. Without intervention, the infection can spread to underlying deep tendons and bone resulting in loss of toe or foot function.

Essentially, there are two pathways to the development of pododermatitis. The first is a process of progressive epithelial devitalization resulting from chronic pressure on or repeated contusion of the metatarsal pad. This devitalization can result from standing long term on inappropriate perches or from hard landings when a falcon, confined to a small space, jumps from perch to perch rather than fly. Heavy-bodied falcons, especially gyrfalcons, are prone to this process, although it can be found in any raptor. The second pathway is foreign body penetration either from self-inflicted puncture wounds from sharp talons or sharp objects, such as cactus thorns. Once the skin integrity is compromised and infection sets in, there is a progressive loss of vascularity to the central foot pad that compounds the situation and complicates treatment.

### Diagnosis

Diagnosis of pododermatitis is made on history and physical examination. Pressure wound cases begin with superficial changes to the skin of the foot, such as flattened papilla or thinning and erythema of the epithelium. As the disease progresses, pressure necrosis leads to loss of skin integrity, bacterial infection, ulceration, swelling, and abscessation of the metatarsal pad. The foot becomes painful and the bird shifts its weight to the other leg often times leading to an induction of the same process in the other foot. Foreign body penetration cases follow a similar pathway after puncture of the skin. In severe cases, the falcon may present sitting on its hocks or recumbent. Several authors have presented classification schemes for pododermatitis with the number of categories varying from three to seven.[2,9,26,27] The Raptor Center uses the following classification scheme:

Type I: thinning of papilla, reddening and thinning of epithelium of metatarsal pad
Type II: devitalization of epithelium or low-grade infection with no gross swelling
Type III: gross swelling with accumulation of exudate in the wound, often encapsulated
Type IV: massive swelling of foot and involvement of deeper structures (tendon or bone)
Type V: swelling, osteomyelitis, and gross deformity of toe or foot; prognosis is poor, euthanasia or toe amputation often the only option

Depending on the severity of the condition, appropriate therapy includes management changes along with medical and surgical interventions. Because of the poor vascularity of the affected area and slow healing times, treatment can be prolonged. Treatment of mild cases and long-term prevention require the management changes discussed here.

### Management

Protecting the feet from further insult is a critical first step. Pododermatitis in the affected foot continues to progress if pressure is not removed from the damaged tissue, and the contralateral foot is at high risk for developing pododermatitis from uneven weight-bearing (see later discussion). In Type I disease, both feet benefit from protective interdigitating wraps, whereas Types II, III, and IV require the use of ball bandages or some type of protective shoe to remove weight from the metatarsal pad.[1,28] Skin irritants, such as camphor spirits, followed by tincture of benzoin are used and additional protection is provided by the application of a liquid bandage (Skin Shield, Walgreens) to the thin and reddened epithelium associated with Type I pododermatitis. As the disease progresses to swelling and ulceration of epithelium, treatment expands to include antibacterial therapy and wound management. Systemic antibiotic choice is based on culture and sensitivity results. In addition to systemic antibiosis, the use of topical antibiotics during the acute phase can be beneficial. For example, a combination of dimethylsulfoxide (0.5 mL), a steroid (0.2 mL 4 mg/mL dexamethasone), and an antibiotic (0.2 mL 100 mg/mL Enrofloxacin or other broad-spectrum antibiotic) can be applied sparingly on swollen areas of the foot. In the presence of open or surgical wounds, antibiotic-impregnated methylmethacrylate beads have been successfully used to provide local concentrations of antibacterial medications.[29,30] In addition, a nonsteroidal anti-inflammatory medication, such as meloxicam, is used for pain management and reduction of inflammation.

In addition to medical treatment, Types II, III, and IV pododermatitis often require surgical intervention to débride necrotic material and establish drainage, allowing the foot to heal by secondary intention or delayed primary intention healing. Although surgical treatment is beyond the scope of this article, it is well addressed in the literature.[1] Successful treatment of these more advanced cases of pododermatitis without surgery has been accomplished by housing birds on sand and using twice-daily foot soaks (standing for 30 minutes to 1 hour in a warm 1:250 solution of F10 [Jaime Samour, MVZ, PhD, Dipl ECAMS, personal communication, April 2009]).

### Prevention

Husbandry practices for raptors in rehabilitation, education, falconry, or breeding purposes can be challenging, because each species has specific needs. To maintain foot health in raptors, it is important to understand the biology of each species to meet their specific needs. It is also critical to monitor the birds carefully for any signs of injury or discomfort. The most common management-related causes of bumblefoot and guidelines for prevention are listed here:

#### Uneven weight-bearing due to injury
When a raptor sustains injuries, such as a fractured leg or pelvis, pododermatitis to one foot, nerve damage resulting in weakness of the posterior limbs, extensive soft tissue damage to a leg or foot, or even a broken toe, load sharing is no longer equal between the feet and increased weight-bearing occurs to the unaffected side. The result is increased pressure on one foot and the potential for breakdown of the epithelium. In this situation, a preventive bandage should be applied to the unaffected foot to keep it healthy, especially in raptors weighing more than 300 g. A thick interdigitating bandage alternating with a "shoe" as need dictates is recommended during the healing phase[31] (Patrick Redig, DVM, PhD, personal communication, April 2009).

#### Inadequate perches
One of the most common causes of pododermatitis in captive raptors is improper perches. Perches vary in shape, diameter, and surface texture, and if all three components are not suitable for a particular individual, pododermatitis will result.

**Shape** A raptor's foot is anatomically designed to use a specific shape of perching surface. Raptor species that live on bluffs, such as peregrine falcons (*Falco peregrinus*) and gyrfalcons, or spend a great deal of time on the ground, such as snowy owls (*Bubo scandiaca*), burrowing owls (*Athene cunicularia*), and vultures, have tendon structures that allow for prolonged perching on flat surfaces. Other species, especially those using trees (eg, red-tailed hawks, bald eagles), are designed to perch on rounded structures. If a raptor is maintained on an inappropriate type of perch for an extended period of time, pododermatitis often results.

**Size** If a raptor requires a rounded perch, diameter is the next consideration. The use of a perch of unsuitable diameter results in inappropriate load-bearing on different parts of the foot. Perches that are too large can result in damage to the hallices, tips, and pads of the toes, or the major pad at the base of the second digit. Perches that are too small can damage the center of the metatarsal pad. In a convalescent cage, perches with slightly different diameters should be alternated every few days to prevent pododermatitis in birds recovering from injury. In a flight pen, perches of varying diameters should be provided according to guidelines written for different species.[13]

**Surface texture** Smooth surfaces must be avoided, because they result in wearing and breakdown of the metatarsal pad epithelium. A rough texture, such as artificial turf (Monsanto, Monsanto Solutia, Inc., St. Louis, Missouri), should cover the top of block style perches and rounded perches can be made out of dowels, conduit, or specially angled 2 × 4s covered with three-strand manila or sisal rope.[13] Natural oak branches also work well but must be replaced when the bark wears off revealing a smooth surface.

### Inadequate housing structure

Active birds that are housed in small free-lofts are prone to bruising their metatarsal pads as they can only jump, not fly, from perch to perch. To prevent this, standards for raptor housing should be followed.[13] In addition, outdoor free-loft spaces constructed with some types of fencing, such as chicken wire or metal chain link, must be avoided because tissue and tendon damage can occur if birds repeatedly grab it. Outdoor pens should be constructed with dowels, conduit, solid sides, wooden slats, or a combination thereof.[9]

If a bird is tethered to a perch and repeatedly bates (see **Box 1**) onto a hard surface, metatarsal pad bruising and skin necrosis can result. A tethered bird should only have access to a soft surface, such as grass, pea gravel, sand, or a cushioned mat.

### Self-inflicted puncture wounds

In the wild, raptors maintain the length and shape of their talons by wearing them on natural surfaces. In captivity, the surfaces they have access to are limited and their talons continually grow. Overgrown talons often result in puncture wounds to the metatarsal pads. These small punctures often lead to infection, as evidenced by severe swelling and abscess formation. Regular talon trims prevent this. A cat nail trimmer works well for small raptors; use a dog nail trimmer for medium-sized and large raptors. Golden eagles have especially long quicks in their talons and a rotary tool (with a silicon bit) works best to avoid bleeding during trimming.

### Obesity

In captivity, raptors are relatively sedentary and their inactivity, along with an ample food supply, can lead to obesity; this is often a concern for birds undergoing rehabilitation or those used in educational settings. Obesity can lead to life-threatening illness and also increases the probability of pododermatitis.[32] To prevent this, a weight management plan should be established that includes a target weight range. Regular weight checks should be conducted to ensure that a raptor stays within the designated range as its metabolism changes throughout seasonal and activity variations. For raptors in breeding chambers, this strategy is not practical because they need an abundance of food to stimulate and maintain them during the breeding effort, and handling is often contraindicated. In this case, foot health should minimally be monitored with regular observations, looking for foot swelling, uneven weight-bearing, limping, or other indications of potential foot discomfort or pathology.

### Poor living conditions

An inadequate diet lacking sufficient vitamins A and D and limited exposure to sunlight or access to water contribute to poor quality skin. Raptors kept under these conditions are more susceptible to developing pododermatitis lesions. To maintain long-term health, a varied diet with vitamin supplementation if needed, and outdoor housing facilities that provide exposure to sunlight and water are critical. In addition, a clean living environment is essential to minimize the presence of bacteria that could invade a small cut or puncture, causing a foot infection.

Pododermatitis is better prevented than treated. It occurs more commonly in captive raptors that are relatively sedentary and provided limited housing and diet choices. The key to keeping raptor feet healthy is to follow established management practices. Housing and perch design, talon maintenance, diet, and clean living conditions are all crucial factors in keeping raptor feet free of wear spots and infection, as are preventative measures during convalescence of injured raptors. On recognition of a foot problem, treatment must be undertaken immediately and be suitably aggressive to meet the prevailing circumstance.

## PARASITIC CONDITIONS OF RAPTORS
### Ectoparasites

Birds of prey are host to a wide variety of external arthropod parasites, including numerous species of lice, a few species of flies, mosquitos, and an occasional species of flea, mite, or tick. Several comprehensive reviews have been published.[33,34,35] Most of the ectoparasites identified in wild birds cause no clinical disease.[36] In a study by Samour,[34] only 5 of the 12 species of arthropods found in 150 falcons were true ectoparasites; the rest were opportunistic inhabitants within the plumage. Healthy birds keep ectoparasite populations under control, so a heavy infestation may be a sign of debilitation or disease. True ectoparasites can cause irritation to skin and mechanical damage to feathers, and hematophagous species can cause anemia and be vectors or intermediate hosts for hemosporidia,[37] viral diseases,[38] and helminths, such as *Serratospiculum*.[39] This finding is especially true of ticks because ticks transmit a greater variety of infectious organisms than any other group of blood-sucking arthropods.[40]

Heavy infestations of ectoparasites may contribute to a debilitated state, especially in nestlings. Smith and colleagues[41] showed that the cumulative effects of blackfly (Simuliidae) infestation on nestlings, including physical harassment, *Leucocytozoon* infection, and direct loss of blood and body fluids from biting flies, produced mortality in 14% of the red-tailed hawk nests studied.

The diagnosis of ectoparasitism is generally done by visual examination. This examination can be challenging, especially with some of the smaller species, such as mites. Parasites vary in their anatomic preferences. Ticks prefer unfeathered areas of the skin, cere, the gape of the mouth (see **Box 1**), and eyelids. Mites and lice can often be located on the underside of feathers and around the vent of young birds. Occasionally infestations are picked up by detecting eggs or larvae in a fecal sample. Treatment for flies, lice, mites, ticks, or fleas includes mechanical removal, ivermectin, and topical pyrethrin- or carbaryl-based insecticides.[29]

Preventing an infestation by ectoparasites in captive raptors requires routine cleaning and disinfection of enclosures and performing physical examinations on a regular schedule.[13] Most of the ectoparasites of raptors have a direct transmission. Close contact between birds in captivity is likely to favor a build-up of ectoparasites, especially if it is coupled with poor hygiene. If one bird has parasite problems, all others in close association should also be examined and treated. Most lice in raptors belong to the suborder Mallophaga and are usually host specific.[42] Arthropod eggs are generally resistant to most insecticides, so all birds should be examined 1 to 2 weeks after the initial infestation to control any new hatched individuals. Control of flying arthropods, such as flies or mosquitoes, involves eliminating exposure to wild birds and the use of mosquito netting to cover housing and weathering areas.

### Hippoboscid flies

A common raptor ectoparasite that is unfamiliar to most private practitioners is the louse fly or flat fly in the Hippoboscidae family (**Fig. 1**). Interest in louse flies has increased recently because of their potential as a vector for West Nile virus; vector competency has not been established.[43,44] These are large flies (2 cm) that skirt around under the feathers and frequently startle handlers and veterinarians. A recent study at The Raptor Center noted an overall prevalence of 19%, peaking in late

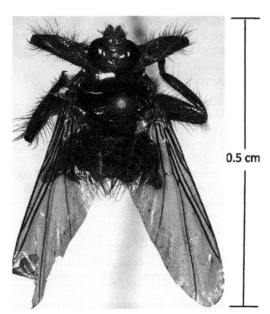

0.5 cm

**Fig. 1.** *Icosta americana* adult female. (*Courtesy of* Roger Moon, PhD, St. Paul, MN; with permission.)

summer, with great horned owls, broad-winged hawks (*Buteo platypterus*), and red-tailed hawks most likely to be carriers.[45] Raptors presented at The Raptor Center with flat flies are treated as previously discussed and kept isolated until all flies are removed to prevent infestation of other birds.

### Myiasis

Blowflies (*Calliphora* spp) are a necrophagous fly species that, in the larval stage, consume carrion or decaying flesh in wounds.[46] Maggot infestation, or myiasis, is generally only a problem for nestling raptors,[47] but infestations are occasionally observed in birds of prey secondary to open traumatic injuries.[48]

Myiasis can be a problem during the summer months or in regions where it is fairly warm or humid. Mechanical removal of maggots in an open wound can be performed using a flush with warm water or saline. The use of a topical medication, such as dilute hydrogen peroxide or an oil base liquid (Panalog; Fort Dodge Animal Health, Fort Dodge, Iowa) can make maggots more mobile and can aid in their removal.[49] Ivermectin should also be administered.

Larval *Protocalliphora*, however, are hematophagous parasites that commonly feed on nestlings of altricial species; they are frequently found in the external auditory canal of hawks.[50] Despite the presumed heavy blood loss, studies of *Protocalliphora* in 48 species of birds indicate that the larval populations are usually too small to kill or seriously injure most nestlings.[51] A drop of mineral oil or saline in ear forces the worms to stretch, facilitating their removal with forceps.[1]

### Endoparasites

Helminths are parasitic worms, such as nematodes, trematodes, cestodes, and acanthocephalans. There are excellent, comprehensive reviews in the literature.[2,9,28,52] Diagnosis of most helminth parasites is by microscopic examination of feces, or occasionally urine or other bodily fluids. A direct or sedimentation method and a flotation method should be used. Cestode infestations are diagnosed by noting characteristic proglottids in mutes (see **Box 1**) or around the vent of a bird. Treatment of helminth parasites is generally with avermectins or benzimidazoles. Note that fenbendazole has been reported to be toxic in some vulture species; administration caused profound leukopenia, depression, and death.[28,29] Fenbendazole has also been noted to cause feather abnormalities if administered during a molt and adverse effects if used during the breeding season.[28] Praziquantel is generally recommended for cestodes and trematodes.[29]

Nematodes represent the largest group of these endoparasites that infect birds of prey, and include ascarids, capillarids, spirurids, and tracheal and air sac nematodes. They can be found in almost any organ, but are most common in the gastrointestinal and respiratory systems. They are the most potentially pathogenic of the helminths. Life cycles of only a few nematode species are known completely, but in general they have indirect cycles.

Capillariasis is the most common type of nematode parasitizing both free-living and captive birds of prey. Infections are usually asymptomatic, but heavy infestations can cause diarrhea, anorexia, emaciation, and even death. In falconry birds, poor flying performance may be a sign of capillaria infection.[53] The location of the infection depends on the species of *Capillaria* and host.[28] The life cycle is usually direct,[28] but some species use an earthworm as an intermediate host.[54] Diagnosis is based primarily on the recovery of lemon-shaped ova in fecal samples. The most used successful treatment is fenbendazole (see previous discussion for cautions) at 20 to 25 mg/kg every 24 hours for 5 days with a single dose repeated in 10 days.[54]

Serratospiculiasis is a disease caused by a group of spirurids of the genus *Serratospiculum*. Within this genus, *Serratospiculum seurati* is the most widespread species affecting falcons in the Middle East.[55] A different species, *Serratospiculoides amaculata*, has been found in North America, mainly in prairie falcons (*Falco mexicanus*).[56] These parasites typically inhabit the air sacs (**Fig. 2**), but can also affect the central nervous system.[57] The life cycle is believed to be indirect, with grasshoppers and

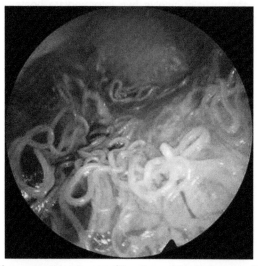

**Fig. 2.** *Serratospiculum seurati* in air sacs. (*Courtesy of* Jamie Samour, DVM, Riyadh, Saudi Arabia; with permission.)

locusts as intermediate hosts,[52] but it is unclear if the falcons become infected by feeding on arthropods directly or by feeding on other infected birds. Clinical signs include dyspnea and regurgitation. Infestation can predispose birds to other infections, such as aspergillosis or pneumonia.[55] Diagnosis is based on the finding of embryonated ova with a fecal flotation (**Fig. 3**). Parasite eggs can also be detected in the saliva or in regurgitated pellets. Radiographs can show evidence of parasites in the abdominal or thoracic air sacs.[58] The parasite can also be found incidentally at necropsy. Treatment is difficult because of the location of the nematode within the air sac membranes.[9] There have been different approaches to treatment throughout the years. Current recommended treatment is ivermectin at a suggested dosage of 0.2 mg/kg.[59] Experience gained in the Middle East shows that this dose of ivermectin is ineffective against *Serratospiculum*.[59] Instead, ivermectin at 1 mg/kg subcutaneously, followed by a second dose about 1 week later, seems to be effective.[55] Once the worms are dead, endoscopic removal of the parasites from the air sacs should be considered, because the dead parasites may cause significant inflammatory air sac disease as they decay.[9] Recently, melarsomine, an organic arsenical, was tried in combination with ivermectin. Melarsomine was administered at 0.25 mg/kg intramuscularly on 2 consecutive days followed in 10 days by ivermectin at 1 mg/kg intramuscularly. This protocol was effective in eliminating clinical signs and parasites.[60] Prevention against the transmission of *Serratospiculum* includes good hygiene and vector exclusion in aviaries.

There are several types of trematodes or flukes affecting raptors. Their life cycle requires several intermediate hosts, which makes it more difficult to be transferred from one bird to another in an aviary. They mainly affect the small intestine, but can also be found in a broad variety of organs depending on the species. Trematodes are rarely pathogenic, but there have been a few descriptions of parasitism caused by flukes with severe infections; weight loss, weakness, anemia, enteritis, and diarrhea were the main clinical signs.

Cestodes have a low prevalence of parasitism and pathogenicity in raptors. Rare cases of debilitation, diarrhea, and obstruction of the lumen of the intestine have been noted when affected by large numbers of cestodes. Cestodes have complicated indirect life cycles that usually involve two intermediate hosts, including rodents, crustaceans, and fish.[52]

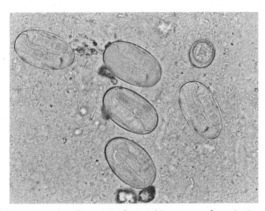

**Fig. 3.** *Serratospiculum seurati* embryonated ova. (*Courtesy of* Jamie Samour, DVM, Riyadh, Saudi Arabia; with permission.)

## Coccidiosis

### Significance

Coccidia are cyst-forming protozoa that are typically species specific in their host selection. More than 250 species of coccidia from four genera have been associated with raptors: *Eimeria*, *Caryospora*, *Sarcocystis*, and *Frenkelia*.[52] The disease has been reported in Falconiformes and Strigiformes.[1,61] *Caryospora* spp commonly cause disease in falcons in breeding chambers.[62]

Raptors can be used as definitive hosts or intermediate hosts by coccidia, which may have either direct or indirect lifecycles. Transmission of *Eimeria* and *Caryospora* is primarily through direct infection, although *Caryospora* is capable of using a rodent intermediate host (heteroxenous transmission).[2,63] The sexual stage of the coccidian organism invades the gastrointestinal epithelium of the host and multiplies, with oocysts being shed in the host bird's feces. Within days, the oocyst sporulates, and then can remain viable in the environment for months. An infected falcon can pass up to 500,000 oocysts per gram of fecal material; in a captive situation, this can result in a highly contaminated enclosure.[9] In addition to enteric coccidial infections, raptors have been reported to have tissue cysts from coccidian infection in muscle tissue (asymptomatic) and the brain (encephalitis).[64]

Most coccidian infections are asymptomatic in birds of prey. Under captive conditions, however, both *Eimeria* and *Caryospora* are associated with disease, especially in juvenile or subadult Falconiformes.[1,39] The highest incidence of disease is at 3 to 6 months of age, although adults can also show clinical signs of disease during times of stress or food scarcity, such as weight reduction during falconry training.[52] Clinical signs are typically vague and nonspecific, including lethargy, depression, weight loss, and anorexia. If the bird is being flown, falconers often complain of a reduced flight effort. Stools are abnormal in infected birds, ranging from a green stringy mass to bloody, foul-smelling diarrhea. Young merlins (*Falco columbarius*) are reported to be especially susceptible to *Caryospora* with acute death sometimes being the only sign.

### Diagnosis/management

Diagnosis of coccidiosis is easy because numerous spherical oocysts are typically found on a fecal flotation examination. *Caryospora* can be distinguished by its single sporocyst with eight sporozoites. Although *Eimeria* and *Sarcocystis* can be treated with sulfonamides (sulfadimethoxine, 25–55 mg/kg every 24 hours for 3–7 days), toltrazuril (Baycox, 10 mg/kg once daily for 2 doses) is the preferred treatment for *Caryospora*;[1] unfortunately, it is not currently available in the United States. Direct administration of toltrazuril often causes regurgitation; this can be mitigated by placing it in a gelatin capsule for administration. Clazuril (Appertex, 5–10 mg/kg every 24 hours for two doses) is also reported as being safe and effective.[9]

### Prevention

Control of coccidiosis is extremely difficult in a captive environment because of the volume and persistence of oocysts. Good hygiene and management techniques to minimize fecal contamination of food reduces exposure. A clean, dry environment with an appropriate substrate, such as pea gravel, is important. Careful attention should be paid to perch and food platform cleaning. In heavily infected breeding facilities, Forbes and Fox[62] suggest treating during prepatent period in young chicks (9–12 days), which stops shedding yet allows an immune response to develop. Techniques such as raising young by foster parents or away from infected parents can also be used.

## Trichomoniasis

### Significance

Trichomoniasis is the most clinically significant parasitic disease in birds of prey. It is a concern in wild birds and captive birds because it can cause morbidity and mortality in some species, especially those that eat pigeons. Not a native disease, trichomoniasis arrived in North America in the early 1600s with the importation of the rock dove, *Columba livia*. It has the dubious distinction of being possibly associated with the demise of the passenger pigeon, *Ectopistes migratorius*, which went extinct in 1914 with the death of Martha at the Cincinnati Zoo.[65] The parasite is enzootic in pigeons and doves, with infection rates ranging from 16% in mourning doves (*Zenaida macroura*) to 98% in white-winged doves (*Z asiatica*).

Trichomoniasis has been documented to cause mortality in several species of raptors, especially in young birds that may be less immunologically competent. An Arizona study on prevalence of trichomoniasis in Cooper's hawks found nestlings from an urban setting had an 85% prevalence rate and experienced a 41% mortality rate; nonurban nestlings had a much lower prevalence at 9%. In the urban study area, columbids, which were documented to provide 83% of the diet of Cooper's hawks, had a 98% prevalence rate of trichomonas infection.[66] The Raptor Center has seen an increase in Cooper's hawks admissions and incidence of trichomoniasis.

In falconry literature, trichomoniasis has long been referred to as frounce. The feeding of pigeons has been recognized since the sixteenth century as a cause of this parasitic condition.[65] Of 5360 falcons examined in one study in Bahrain, 31.2% had lesions of trichomoniasis.[67] Although most falconers in North America are familiar with the risk for trichomoniasis associated with feeding fresh pigeons, birds that have clinical symptoms are still presented for veterinary care on a routine basis.

The causative agent of trichomoniasis, *Trichomonas gallinae*, is a flagellated protozoan commonly found in the epithelium of the upper digestive and respiratory tracts of Columbiformes. Columbids are the primary host and reservoir. Although they do occasionally manifest clinical disease with classical ulcerative lesions of the oropharynx and upper gastrointestinal system ("crop canker"), infection is typically asymptomatic in pigeons and doves. Transmission through direct contact or ingestion of contaminated food or water is associated with the social nature of these species. In addition to horizontal transmission within social groups, the reservoir is also maintained by vertical transmission of the organism through the feeding of crop milk to the young. It has been speculated that transmission can occur to other avian species through contaminated water, but this has not been proved. In raptors, transmission is primarily through ingestion of infected prey species.

### Diagnosis

Trichomoniasis is routinely encountered in several species of bird-eating raptors, including barn owls (*Tyto alba*), barred owls (*Strix varia*), great horned owls, peregrine falcons, prairie falcons, gyrfalcons, Cooper's hawks, sharp-shinned hawks (*Accipiter striatus*), and Northern goshawks (*Accipiter gentilis*).[2,68] Although columbids provide a food source for many of these raptors year-round, trichomoniasis tends to have its peak incidence in young birds during the late spring and summer. Adult birds seem to be more immune to infection, as do peregrine falcons that are seemingly resistant to infection despite high consumption of pigeons. Trichomoniasis is more common in migrating arctic peregrines as they traverse the continent. *T gallinae* infection has also been found in American kestrels (*Falco sparverius*), merlins, and Eastern screech owls (*Megascops asio*), presumably as a result of ingesting infected passerines. In one report, a late summer epidemic in American kestrels and Eastern screech owls was speculated to occur from the ingestion of passerines that acquired infection from congregating at contaminated water sources with pigeons and doves.[69]

Clinical signs of infection are related to the upper gastrointestinal and respiratory systems. If untreated, the disease is progressive. Raptors that have mild or early infection often shows signs of food flicking when presented with food, stringy tenacious saliva, slow eating, and oral ulcers. As the disease progresses, birds develop plaque-like to nodular growths on the mucous membranes of the oral cavity, often extending into the crop and upper esophagus. There is often a foul odor noted coming from the mouth. In addition to the caseous lesions of the upper gastrointestinal system, localized infections may be found in the choanal slit, nasal cavity, infraorbital sinus and, rarely, the trachea. Lesions in the nasal cavity or infraorbital sinus may cause bulging of the palate and surrounding soft tissues. The parasite can become extremely invasive locally, extending into adjacent soft tissues and bone. Depending on the size and location of the lesions, they can also be obstructive, blocking the pharynx and even preventing swallowing. Partial to complete anorexia can result from dysphagia or obstruction and leads to emaciation, starvation, and death.

A presumptive diagnosis of *T gallinae* infection can often be made based on clinical signs and history, and then confirmed with direct visualization of the protozoan. Confirmation is critical because there are several differential diagnoses for trichomoniasis, including fungal infections (candidiasis, aspergillosis), vitamin A deficiency, avian pox, and pseudomonas stomatitis. It is commonly cited in the literature that capillariasis presents in a similar situation based on earlier reports;[70] clinicians at The Raptor Center, however, have not appreciated this as a significant differential for oral lesions in the mouth. A saline wet mount is made by swabbing the oropharynx and crop with a moistened cotton tip applicator, then rolling the swab on a slide with warm saline. Immediate examination of the slide under light microscopy (100×) reveals the motile trophozoite stage of the protozoan, which is slightly larger than an erythrocyte. It is important to be sure that everything is warm when used because the organism is susceptible to drying and chilling and quickly loses its characteristic movement.

Another option for diagnosis is the use of the In Pouch TF culture pack (BioMed Diagnostics, White City, Oregon). Developed as a screening tool for *Tritrichomonas fetus* in cattle, this test has been found to be reliable for *T gallinae* in birds. Studies have shown it to be much more sensitive than a wet mount microscopy examination.[71] In one study of 45 birds, 27 were positive using the In Pouch TF system and only 12 on wet mount examination.

### Management

Nitro-imidazoles provide the basis for treatment of trichomoniasis, with supportive care (nutritional and fluid support) and surgical débridement also playing an important role. Historically, metronidazole (30–50 mg/kg every 24 hours for 2–3 days) has been recommended for treatment,[29] although resistance has been reported and is commonly found at The Raptor Center. Samour[34] recommends a dose of 100 mg/kg daily for 3 days, which has shown much more consistent results in patients at The Raptor Center, as does carnidazole (30 mg/kg every 24 hours for two doses). Mild lesions usually disappear in a couple of days. Larger, caseous plugs often require surgical débridement, which is typically done 3 to 5 days after treatment when blunt dissection can easily separate the plug from the underlying, ulcerated mucous membrane. Because of the invasive nature of the protozoan, the removal of large plugs often leaves a significant cavity or opening into the nasal area or sinuses. Chronic food impaction and infection complicated by pseudomonas infection are common postoperative sequela.

## Prevention

Freezing pigeons before feeding them to falconry birds is commonly recommended as prevention for trichomoniasis; however, it is safest to avoid feeding pigeons to captive raptors because pigeons can also be a source of herpesvirus in addition to *T gallinae*.

## Hemoparasites

Many raptors have hemoparasites. *Atoxoplasma*, *Babesia*, *Hemoproteus*, *Leukocytozoon*, *Plasmodium*, trypanosomes, and microfilaria have been reported in raptors (H.L. Shivaprasad, DVM, PhD, personal communication, April 2009). An excellent review of intracellular hematozoa in raptors was published by Remple[72] in 2004.

The three most common blood parasites belong to Apicomplexa order: *Hemoproteus* spp, *Leucocytozoon* spp, and *Plasmodium* spp. They are transmitted by different arthropod vectors. The reported prevalence of hematozoa varies considerably depending on captive or wild status, species, age, time of year, and geographic area.[73] Some of the variability in these surveys result from multiple hematozoa infections, misidentification of organisms, and method of detection. Improved molecular biologic techniques offer new tools to determine parasite specificities, life cycles, and prevalence. These improved techniques make the accurate diagnosis of hemosporidia easier, even in the early stages or in chronic infections when parasitemia is low.[74]

The effects of these hemoparasites on free-living individuals is poorly understood and the pathogenicity difficult to assess. Unfortunately, only 5% of all the records of mortality and pathogenicity due to avian hematozoa have been described from free-living birds.[28] Although there are reports linking hemoparasites with differences of various biologic parameters,[75] in general the effects of hematozoa are believed to be low. *Leucocytozoon* have been pathogenic in young raptors; *Hemoproteus* have been pathogenic in snowy owls.[76] Even though most hematozoa are not treated, a diagnosis of hematozoa should be given attention, especially in captivity, because these birds are undergoing periods of stress. One study of raptors undergoing rehabilitation indicates the incidence of infection with hemoparasites increases with length of time in captivity; possible reasons include increasing population density of susceptible hosts or immunosuppression due to captivity.[77]

## Avian malaria

**Significance** Although most hemoparasites are incidental findings in raptors, avian malaria is an exception because it is usually pathogenic. Avian malaria is caused by protozoa in the genus *Plasmodium*. Approximately 11 species have been identified in Falconiformes and Strigiformes.[74] Many species of *Plasmodium* are capable of infecting a wide range of hosts, although prevalence rates in raptors are low: 6.8% in owls and 4.9% in falcons.[72] The organism is transmitted by *Culicine* mosquitos; passerines are considered the reservoir. Pathogenicity depends on the virulence of malarial species, the level of parasitemia, and the species and immune status of the host. Among North American raptors, young gyrfalcons, gyr-hybrids, and snowy owls are the most susceptible (Patrick Redig, DVM, PhD, personal communication, April 2009).

**Diagnosis** The diagnosis of avian malaria is based on history, presentation, and time of year (mosquito season), and confirmed by visualization of the protozoa with a thin blood smear made without anticoagulant. Some species of avian malaria may be confused with *Hemoproteus* and concurrent infections are common. Distinguishing characteristics of malaria include the presence of both gametocytes and schizonts in peripheral blood, parasite stages within thrombocytes and leukocytes, and gametocytes that cause marked displacement of the erythrocyte nucleus.[78] Clinical signs include anorexia, lethargy, depression, and the passage of jade-green mutes; labored respirations and concurrent anemia may occur in later stages of the disease.

**Management** Management includes the use of antimalarial drugs and supportive therapy, such as oxygen, fluids, and blood transfusions as needed. Mefloquine hydrochloride (Lariam; Hoffman-La Roche Pharmaceuticals, Nutley, New Jersey) is active against erythrocytic and tissue schizonts of some species of *Plasmodium*.[72,79] Currently at The Raptor Center, infections are treated with oral mefloquine at 30 mg/kg at 0, 12, 24, and 48 hours; timing is critical to affect all phases of the malarial organism.

**Prevention** Prevention of malaria includes vector exclusion, such as mosquito netting over exhibits or bringing birds inside when mosquitos are active. Prophylactic treatment of highly susceptible species with oral mefloquine at 30 mg/kg once a week during mosquito season should also be considered.

## EMERGING CONDITIONS IN RAPTORS

Emerging diseases are newly recognized or evolved, or have occurred previously but show an increase or an expansion in geographic, host, or vector range.[80] Emerging diseases have been described for both humans and animals. It has been estimated that approximately 73% of emerging infectious disease has a wildlife component.[81] Protozoa seem to be the most likely to account for emerging parasitic infections.[82] Often diseases emerge because of changing transmission dynamics that bring people or animals into novel, closer, or more frequent contact with pathogens. New strains of known pathogens occur from natural genetic variations, recombinations, and adaptions. Improved molecular diagnostic capabilities have contributed to a significantly better understanding of taxonomy and zoonoses.[83,84,85,86]

### *Cryptosporidiosis*

#### *Significance*
*Cryptosporidium* species are apicomplexan parasites that infect a wide range of vertebrate hosts, including fish, reptiles, birds, rodents, ruminants, and humans. The pathogenicity of *Cryptosporidium* varies with the species of the parasite and several host factors, including species, age, and immune status.[87] The life cycle is direct. Endogenous sporulation occurs leading to autoinfection; oocysts shed from the host are immediately infective.[88] A new cycle begins with ingestion or inhalation of these oocysts. Encysted oocysts are highly resistant and are considered ubiquitous in the environment.[89]

Cryptosporidiosis has been diagnosed from more than 30 avian species. Only three avian *Cryptosporidium* spp have been named: *C meleagridis*, *C baileyi*, and *C galli*. Each can infect a broad range of bird species (and humans), but differ in predilection site.[84] *C meleagridis* is found in the intestines and bursa; *C galli* only infects the proventriculus. *C baileyi* is the most common species of cryptosporidium isolated from birds and can cause either gastrointestinal or respiratory disease. High morbidity and mortality are often associated with *C baileyi* respiratory infections of birds, especially broiler chickens.[84,90]

#### *Diagnosis*
Recently, respiratory cryptosporidiosis caused by *C baileyi* in falcons has been reported.[91,92] All cases to date have been in falcons; most fatalities have occurred in young birds (The Raptor Center, unpublished data; H.L. Shivaprasad, DVM, PhD, personal communication, April 2009; Fern Van Sant, DVM, personal communication,

April 2009). Clinical signs are referable to the upper respiratory tract and include nasal discharge, sinusitis, conjunctivitis, respiratory stridor, dyspnea, anorexia, and death; edema of the glottis may be noted on physical examination. Otitis media was noted in one case (H.L. Shivaprasad, DVM, personal communication, April 2009). Diagnosis is made by cytologic examination of affected tissues. A sample from a nasal or ocular discharge, sinus aspirate, nasal flush, or pharyngeal or tracheal swab can be placed on a slide and examined as a wet mount or stained with Wright's or acid-fast stain; oocysts are 4 to 6 mcm, thick walled, and translucent (**Fig. 4**). Biopsied material can be submitted for histopathology (Helen Michael, DVM, personal communication, April 2009). The diagnosis can be confirmed and speciated with polymerase chain reaction[93] (Jim Wellehan, DVM, MS, DACZM, DACVM, personal communication, April 2009). Additional diagnostic tests, including hematology, radiology, bacteriology, and fecal examination, should be performed to rule out other diseases or diagnose concurrent conditions.

### Management

Treatment of cryptosporidiosis in general is unreliable. In humans, most infections are self-limiting and only supportive therapy is recommended; however, severe and disseminated disease can result in immunosuppressed individuals. Nitazoxanide is approved by the Food and Drug Administration for children older than 12 months and adults who have diarrhea due to cryptosporidiosis; it inhibits the growth of *C parvum* sporozoites.[94] Paromomycin alone or with azithromycin has also been used with inconsistent results. Paromomycin has been administered by inhalation therapy for human respiratory cryptosporidiosis with positive results.[95,96]

Paromomycin (Humatin) is an aminoglycoside antibiotic. Its antiprotozoal action is presumably by inhibition of protein synthesis and it seems to reduce the elimination of new infective oocysts.[91] Paromomycin is poorly absorbed from the intestinal tract, which may explain its poor efficacy for protozoal infections of the respiratory or renal systems. Treatment with paromomycin with or without azithromycin was tried in several falcons but most were unsuccessful[92] (The Raptor Center, unpublished data). Rodriguez reported a successful treatment in two falcons that had mild respiratory cryptosporidiosis with paromomycin at 100 mg/kg by mouth every 12 hours; marbofloxacin, meloxicam, and itraconazole were administered concurrently in one of the falcons.[91] Treatment with paromomycin at 100 mg/kg by mouth every 12 hours with

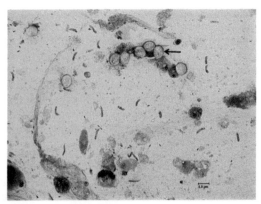

**Fig. 4.** *Cryptosporidium baileyi* oocysts. (*Courtesy of* Helen Michael, DVM, St. Paul, MN; with permission.)

additional paromomycin mixed with ophthalmic ointment and instilled into the nares twice a week failed to clear a falcon that had sinusitis caused by *C baileyi*; nebulization with paromomycin was not done (The Raptor Center, unpublished data).

Ponazuril is a triazine anticoccidial drug approved for the treatment of equine protozoal myeloencephalitis. Its mechanism of action may involve the plastid body that functions in amino acid synthesis, electron transport, and energy metabolism.[97] Compounded ponazuril at 20 mg/kg by mouth every 24 hours was used as a treatment for suspected respiratory cryptosporidium infection in two young falcons; clinical improvement was noted within 24 hours and was continued for 7 days (Fern Van Sant, DVM, personal communication, April 2009).

### Prevention

It is assumed that the organism is introduced with the falcon's food source, captive-raised coturnix and bobwhite quail, although there are no definitive studies demonstrating transmission (Helen Michael, DVM, personal communication). Once the infection is established, it is spread through direct exposure to contaminated materials or from contact with oculonasal discharges. Isolation of affected individuals and good hygiene should help limit additional cases. Oocysts are resistant in the environment. Desiccation of the oocysts has proved the most effective; bleach at standard concentrations may be somewhat effective.[98] Because there is a clear relationship between immune status and the development and severity of clinical signs in other species, proper husbandry and management are paramount, especially with juveniles, color morphs, and other high-stress situations or individuals.

In general, most species of *Cryptosporidium* are host adapted and have a narrow spectrum of natural hosts.[85,86] *C meleagridis* is the third most common *Cryptosporidium* parasite in humans,[84] and there has been at least one case of *C baileyi* in a human.[99] Even immunocompetent people can be infected.[84]

### Babesiosis

#### Significance

First described in the blood of cattle in 1891 by Romanian microbiologist Babes, organisms of the genus *Babesia* are piroplasms—small intracellular blood parasites of ticks, birds, and mammals.[83] More than 100 species have been described. Babesiosis or piroplasmosis is an intraerythrocytic protozoal infection transmitted through the bite of a tick vector into a broad array of vertebrates. The resulting hemolysis leads to anemia and other host-mediated pathologies. It is often pathogenic in livestock and therefore of major economic importance worldwide.[100] Recently, *Babesia* was listed as one of The Deadly Dozen—one of 12 pathogens that could spread as a result of climate change with the potential to affect wildlife health.[83,101]

Approximately 18 species of *Babesia* have been described from birds although there is still some confusion regarding identification;[102] some were previously described as *Nuttalia* and *Aegyptianella*. Each species of *Babesia* seems to be host specific at the family level; researchers have been unable to experimentally transmit *Babesia* except within the same family of birds.[100] Two species of *Babesia* have been described in raptors: *Babesia moshkovskii* from griffon vultures (*Gyps fulvus*), believed to be specific to Accipitridae; and *Babesia shortii*, believed to be specific to Falconidae.[72] Unknown *Babesia* species were noted in a great horned owl and barn owls.[103,104] The degree of pathogenicity of *Babesia* spp in birds is unclear.

There is little information on the natural history of *Babesia* in birds. As with *Cryptosporidium* spp, it is hoped that improved molecular diagnostic techniques will augment the detection and identification of *Babesia* spp and delineate life cycles.

The vector for babesiosis infections in mammals is generally an ixodid tick. It is assumed that the same holds true for avian babesiosis, although there is some circumstantial evidence that argasid ticks may host some avian species of *Babesia*.[72,100]

## Diagnosis

Diagnosis of babesiosis is based on identification of the organism in thin blood smears by the presence of fan-shaped or cruciform tetrad nonpigmented schizonts in a Maltese cross formation in red blood cells. The two *Babesia* spp in raptors are well described in Peirce.[100] Diagnosis can be difficult and it is impossible to speciate by morphology alone.[105] The University of Florida College of Veterinary Medicine offers polymerase chain reaction testing for piroplasms.[93] Babesiosis is probably more common than reported. Low levels of parasitemia may be missed because of concurrent hematozoa infections or misdiagnosed as *Hemoproteus*, *Plasmodium*, or *Rickettsia*-like organisms.[72] An accurate diagnosis is paramount to institute appropriate therapy.

There are several clinical case reports involving *B shortii* in Falconidae, including Saker falcon (*Falco cherrug*),[106,107] peregrine falcon,[108] steppe eagle(*Aquila rapax*),[109] and European kestrel (*Falco tinnunculus*).[110] Clinical signs included partial anorexia, weight loss, and metallic green urates; some birds also had hematologic changes reflecting anemia and liver disease.

The Raptor Center has noted babesiosis in great horned owl[103] and several other raptor species (The Raptor Center, unpublished data). All had concurrent disease; some had concurrent infections with *Hemoproteus* sp and *Leucocytozoon* sp. Occasionally small ixodid ticks were recovered.[111] Until recently, only *B shortii* was believed to be pathogenic.[106] In 1993, Peirce and colleagues[112] described *B kiwiensis*, which is pathogenic in kiwi chicks (*Apteryx australis mantelli*). Given the prevalence of pathogenic *Babesia* spp in mammals it would seem that there should be numerous pathogenic species in birds also.[100]

In what appears to be the largest study to date, *B shortii* was diagnosed in 1.54% of 1360 ill falcons presented to the International Veterinary Hospital in Ahmadi, Kuwait in 2003 and 2004; of these, tick infestation was reported in 19%.[113] It was generally found on immature birds; adult birds may represent a relapse. All had various clinical signs that resolved with treatment and *Babesia* organisms were no longer noted. Clinical signs included somnolence or lethargy, weight loss, anorexia or decreased appetite, vomiting, and blood in the feces. The degree of parasitemia was not recorded.[113]

## Management

All the above clinical cases were treated with supportive therapy and imidocarb dipropionate (Imizol). Dosages ranged from 5 to 7 mg/kg intramuscularly; the dose was repeated 1 week later and some used 3 total doses. Many clinicians report regurgitation after the first injection but not subsequent doses. The Raptor Center has no reports of regurgitation, but lacrimation, salivation, mental dullness, and "shock" have been described. No deaths have been attributed to treatment.

## Prevention

Because babesiosis can only be contracted from the bite of a tick, tick control is important. Birds should be examined on a regular basis to monitor for ectoparasites. Ticks prefer to attach to unfeathered areas of skin, including the cere, the gape of the mouth, and eyelids. Individual ticks can be removed and an anti-acaricide program instituted. The mew (see **Box 1**) and surrounding area should also be addressed. Removing brush and controlling rodents decreases opportunities for ticks to move onto birds.

## SUMMARY

Raptors are susceptible to a broad array of established and emerging bacterial and parasitic diseases. Many of these conditions are opportunistic and can be easily managed or averted with proper preventive measures. These measures include: the quarantine of new individuals as practical; prompt and periodic diagnostic examinations; regular evaluation for ecto- and endoparasites, including hemoparasites, with appropriate follow-up; proper management to reduce stress; species-appropriate husbandry; proper diet selection and preparation; maintenance of a clean environment; and vector exclusion techniques to reduce exposure to pathogens.

Once infected and clinically ill, these pathogens can easily overwhelm the raptor patient, especially those that are young, immunosuppressed, or suffering from concurrent illness or trauma. Treatment must be prompt, appropriate, and judicious, and involve both medical and management issues.

## ACKNOWLEDGMENTS

The authors thank the staff of The Raptor Center; Matt Blandford, Purdue University of School of Veterinary Medicine, Class of 2009 for his assistance; and Dr. Jamie Samour for his contributions regarding the medical management of pododermatitis.

## APPENDIX 1: CONSERVATION OF RAPTORS

Raptors are susceptible to a broad array of established and emerging bacterial and parasitic diseases. The long-term effects of these infectious diseases on population numbers of free-living raptors are unknown. For example, the introduction of West Nile virus to North America in 1999 led to a dramatic decline in many avian species, but some have rebounded.[114] Although accurate global raptor population numbers are limited, data suggest that overall, birds of prey are declining.[115] We do know that changes in the environment, especially those brought about by man, can affect raptor populations, at least on a regional level.

> In India, vulture populations in the genus *Gyps* have been severely affected by the anti-inflammatory diclofenac administered to cattle and subsequently fed on as carrion.[116]
>
> California condors (*Gymnogyps californianus*) are frequently poisoned by lead fragments from spent ammunition, further jeopardizing the recovery efforts for this species.[117]
>
> In Europe, the prohibition of muladares, or carcass dumps, to prevent the spread of bovine spongiform encephalopathy has resulted in widespread starvation of many vulture species.[118]
>
> Worldwide, habitat loss and degradation are ongoing challenges for many species; persecution of raptors by humans by shot, trap, and poison are ongoing. Collisions with vehicles and wind turbines and electrocution on power lines are inadvertent effects of human activities.

Recently, both the peregrine falcon and the bald eagle have been removed from the endangered species list. Both species had declined in the mid-twentieth century because of the use of organochlorine pesticides (DDT), which were subsequently banned. Veterinarians involved in raptor medicine, especially those involved in wildlife rehabilitation, can play a critical role in monitoring the health of free-ranging raptor populations. These veterinarians are in a unique position to observe changes in the ecology and its effects on wildlife health, monitor for emerging diseases, and advocate on behalf of these significant creatures.[119]

## REFERENCES

1. Redig PT, Cruz-Martinez L. Raptors. In: Tully TN, Dorrestein GM, Jones AK, editors. Avian medicine. 2nd edition. Edinburgh (UK): Saunders Elsevier; 2009. p. 209–42.
2. Cooper JE, editor. Birds of prey: health and disease. Oxford (UK): Blackwell Science; 2002.
3. Heatley JJ, Mitchell MM, Roy A, et al. Disseminated Mycobacteriosis in a bald eagle (*Haliaeetus leucocephalus*). J Avian Med Surg 2007;21(3):201–9.
4. Hindman LJ, Costanzo GR, Converse KA, et al. Avian cholera in Ospreys: first occurrence and possible mode of transmission. J Field Ornithol 1997;68: 503–8.
5. Mirande LA, Howerth EW, Poston RP. Chlamydiosis in a red-tailed hawk (*Buteo jamaicensis*). J Wildl Dis 1992;28(2):284.
6. Tizard I. Salmonellosis in wild birds. J Exotic Pet Med 2004;13(2):50–66.
7. Andersen AA, Vanrompay D. Avian chlamydiosis. Rev Sci Tech 2000;19(2): 396–400.
8. Gerbermann H, Korbel R. The occurrence of *Chlamydia psittaci* infections in raptors from wildlife preserves. Tierarztl Prax 1993;21(3):217–24.
9. Heidenreich M. Birds of prey. medicine and management. Oxford (UK): Blackwell Science; 1997.
10. Tell LA, Ferrell ST, Gibbons PM. Avian mycobacteriosis in free-living raptors in California: 6 cases (1997–2001). J Avian Med Surg 2004;18(1):30–40.
11. Tell LA, Woods L, Cromie RL. Mycobacteriosis in birds. Rev Sci Tech 2001;20(1): 180–203.
12. Lumeij JT, van Nie GJ. Tuberculosis in raptorial birds (II). Review of the literature and suggestions for clinical diagnosis and vaccination. Tijdschr Diergeneeskd 1982;107(15–16):573–9.
13. Arent LR. Raptors in captivity. Guidelines for care and management. Blaine (WA): Hancock House Publishers; 2007.
14. Joseph V. Raptor medicine: an approach to wild, falconry, and educational birds of prey. Vet Clin North Am Exot Anim Pract 2006;9(2):321–45.
15. Beebe FL, Webster HM. North American falconry and hunting hawks. Denver (CO): North American Falconry and Hunting Hawks; 1994.
16. Tell LA, Woods L, Foley J, et al. A model of avian mycobacteriosis: clinical and histopathologic findings in Japanese quail (*Coturnix coturnix japonica*) intravenously inoculated with *Mycobacterium avium*. Avian Dis 2003;47(2):433–43.
17. Biet F, Boschiroli ML, Thorel MF, et al. Zoonotic aspects of *Mycobacterium bovis* and *Mycobacterium avium-intracellulare* complex (MAC). Vet Res 2005;36: 411–36.
18. Schmidt V, Schneider S, Schlömer J, et al. Transmission of tuberculosis between men and pet birds: a case report. Avian Pathol 2008;37(6):589–92.
19. Brogden KA, Rhoades KR. Prevalence of serologic types of *Pasteurella multocida* from 57 species of birds and mammals in the United States. J Wildl Dis 1983; 19(4):315.
20. Heddleston KL, Goodson T, Leibovitz L, et al. Serological and biochemical characteristics of *Pasteurella multocida* from free-flying birds and poultry. Avian Dis 1972;16:729–34.

21. Morishita TY, Lowenstine LJ, Hirsh DC, et al. Lesions associated with *Pasteurella multocida* infection in raptors. Avian Dis 1997;41:203–13.
22. Williams ES, Runde DE, Mills K, et al. Avian cholera in a gyrfalcon (*Falco rusticolus*). Avian Dis 1987;31:380–2.
23. Sander JE, Hofacre CL, Cheng IH, et al. Investigation of resistance of bacteria from commercial poultry sources to commercial disinfectants. Avian Dis 2002; 46(4):997–1000.
24. Lamberski N, Hull AC, Fish AM, et al. A survey of the choanal and cloacal aerobic bacterial flora in free-living and captive red-tailed hawks (*Buteo jamaicensis*) and Cooper's hawks (*Accipiter cooperii*). J Avian Med Surg 2003;17(3):131–5.
25. Smith KE, Anderson F, Medus C, et al. Outbreaks of salmonellosis at elementary schools associated with dissection of owl pellets. Vector Borne Zoonotic Dis 2005;5(2):133–6.
26. Halliwell WH. Bumblefoot infections in birds of prey. J Zoo Wildl Med 1975;6: 8–10.
27. Oaks JL. Immune and inflammatory responses in falcon staphylococcal pododermatitis. In: Redig PT, Cooper JE, Remple JD, Hunter DB, editors. Raptor biomedicine. University of Minnesota Press; 1993. p. 72–87.
28. Samour JH. Avian medicine. 2nd edition. Edinburgh (UK): Mosby; 2008.
29. Carpenter JW. Exotic animal formulary. Philadelphia: Elsevier Saunders; 2005.
30. Remple JD, Al-Ashbal AA. Raptor bumblefoot: Another look at histopathology and pathogenesis. In: Redig PT, Remple JD, Cooper JE, editors. Raptor biomedicine. University of Minnesota Press; 1993. p. 92–8.
31. Remple JD. A multifaceted approach to the treatment of bumblefoot in raptors. J Exotic Pet Med 2006;15(1):49–55.
32. Jones R, Redig PT. Fattening up for the molt. Hawk Chalk 2000;3(39):44–9.
33. Proctor H, Owens I. Mites and birds: diversity, parasitism and coevolution. Trends Ecol Evol 2000;15(9):358–64.
34. Samour JH. *Pseudomonas aeruginosa* stomatitis as a sequel to trichomoniasis in captive saker falcons (*Falco cherrug*). J Avian Med Surg 2000;14(2):113–7.
35. Price RD, Palma RL, Hellenthal RA. New synonymies of chewing lice (Phthiraptera: Amblycera, Ischnocera) described from the Falconiformes (Aves). Eur J Entomol 1997;94:537–46.
36. Friend M, Franson JC. Field manual of wildlife diseases. General field procedures and diseases of birds. Madison (WI): Storming Media; 1999.
37. Greve JH. Parasites of the skin. Knemidokoptosis. In: Rosskopf WJ, Woerpel RW, editors. Diseases of cage and aviary birds. Baltimore (MD): Lippincott Williams & Wilkins Comp; 1996. p. 623.
38. Kettle DS. Medical and veterinary entomology. Wallingford (UK): CAB International; 1995.
39. Zucca P. Infectious diseases. In: Samour J, editor. Avian medicine. 2nd edition. Edinburgh (UK): Mosby; 2000. p. 219–52.
40. Sonenshine DE, Lane RS, Nicholson WL. Ticks (Ixodida). In: Mullen G, Durden L, editors. Veterinary medical entomology. Oxford (UK): Academic Press; 2002. p. 518.
41. Smith RN, Cain SL, Anderson SH, et al. Blackfly-induced mortality of nestling red-tailed hawks. Auk 1998;115:368–75.
42. Redig PT. Medical management of birds of prey: a collection of notes on selected topics. University of Minnesota; 1985.
43. Farajollahi A, Crans WJ, Nickerson D, et al. Detection of West Nile virus RNA from the louse fly *Icosta americana* (Diptera: Hippoboscidae). J Am Mosq Control Assoc 2005;21(4):474–6.

44. Pollock CG. West Nile virus in the Americas. J Avian Med Surg 2008;22(2):151–7.
45. Latchman S. Hippoboscid flies on raptors in the Upper Midwest. Lanham (MD): Entomological Society of America; 2008.
46. Proudfoot GA, Usener JL, Teel PD. Ferruginous pygmy-owls: a new host for *Protocalliphora sialia* and *Hesperocimex sonorensis* in Arizona. Wilson Bull 2005; 117:185–8.
47. Smith SA. Parasites of birds of prey: their diagnosis and treatment. J Exotic Pet Med 1996;5:97–105.
48. Cooper JE. Veterinary aspects of captive birds of prey. Saul, Gloucestershire, England: Standfast Press; 1978.
49. Burke HF, Swaim SF, Amalsadvala T. Review of wound management in raptors. J Avian Med Surg 2002;16(3):180–91.
50. Smith SA. Diagnosis and treatment of helminths in birds of prey. In: Redig PT, Cooper JE, Remple JD, et al, editors. Raptor biomedicine. University of Minnesota Press; 1993. p. 21–7.
51. Whitworth TL, Bennett GF. Pathogenicity of larval Protocalliphora (Diptera: Calliphoridae) parasitizing nestling birds. Revue canadienne de zoologie 1992;70: 2184–91.
52. Lacina D, Bird DM. Endoparasites of raptors—a review and an update. In: Lumeij JT, Remple DJ, Redig PT, et al, editors. Raptor biomedicine III. Lake Worth (FL): Zoological Education Network; 2000. p. 65–99.
53. Jones MP. Selected infectious diseases of birds of prey. Journal of Exotic Pet Medicine 2006;15(1):5–17.
54. Redig PT. Falconiformes (vultures, hawks, falcons, secretary bird). In: Fowler ME, Miller RE, editors. Zoo and wild animal medicine. 5th edition. Philadephia: Saunders; 2005. p. 150–61.
55. Samour JH, Naldo J. Serratospiculiasis in captive falcons in the Middle East: a review. J Avian Med Surg 2001;15(1):2–9.
56. Bigland CH, Liu SK, Perry ML. Five cases of *Serratospiculum amaculata* (Nematoda: Filarioidea) infection in prairie falcons (*Falco mexicanus*). Avian Dis 1964;8:412–9.
57. Hawkins MG, Couto S, Tell LA, et al. Atypical parasitic migration and necrotizing sacral myelitis due to *Serratospiculoides amaculata* in a prairie falcon (*Falco mexicanus*). Avian Dis 2001;45(1):276–83.
58. Ward FP, Fairchild DG. Air sac parasites of the genus *Serratospiculum* in falcons. J Wildl Dis 1972;8(2):165–8.
59. Lierz M. Evaluation of the dosage of ivermectin in falcons. Vet Rec 2001;148(19): 596–600.
60. Tarello W. Serratospiculosis in falcons from Kuwait: incidence, pathogenicity and treatment with melarsomine and ivermectin. Parasite 2006;13(1):59.
61. Hoberg EP, Cawthorn RJ, Hedstrom OR. Enteric coccidia (Apicomplexa) in the small intestine of the northern spotted owl (*Strix occidentalis caurina*). J Wildl Dis 1993;29(3):495.
62. Forbes NA, Fox MT. Field trial of a *Caryospora* species vaccine for controlling clinical coccidiosis in falcons. Vet Rec 2005;156(5):134–8.
63. Cawthorn RJ. Cyst-forming coccidia of raptors: significant pathogens or not?. In: Redig PT, Cooper JE, Remple DJ, et al, editors. Raptor biomedicine. University of Minnesota Press; 1993. p. 14–20.
64. Wunschmann A, Rejmanek D, Cruz-Martinez L, et al. Sarcocystis falcatula-associated encephalitis in a free-ranging great horned owl (*Bubo virginianus*). J Vet Diagn Invest 2009;21(2):283.

65. Stabler RM. Trichomonas gallinae: a review. Exp Parasitol 1954;3(4):368–402.
66. Boal CW, Mannan RW, Hudelson KS. Trichomoniasis in Cooper's hawks from Arizona. J Wildl Dis 1998;34(3):590.
67. Samour JH, Bailey TA, Cooper JE. Trichomoniasis in birds of prey (order Falconiformes) in Bahrain. Vet Rec 1995;136(14):358–62.
68. Pokras MA, Wheeldon EB, Sedgwick CJ. Trichomoniasis in owls: report on a number of clinical cases and a survey of the literature. In: Redig PT, Cooper JE, Remple DJ, editors. Raptor biomedicine. University of Minnesota Press; 1993. p. 88–91.
69. Ueblacker SN. Trichomoniasis in American kestrels (Falco Sparverius) and Eastern screech-owls (Otus asio). In: Lumeij JT, Remple JD, Redig PT, et al, editors. Raptor biomedicine III. Lake Worth (FL): Zoological Education Network; 2000. p. 59–63.
70. Trainer DO, Folz SD, Samuel WM. Capillariasis in the gyrfalcon. Condor 1968;70: 276–7.
71. Cover AJ, Harmon WM, Thomas MW. A new method for the diagnosis of Trichomonas gallinae infection by culture. J Wildl Dis 1994;30(3):457.
72. Remple JD. Intracellular hematozoa of raptors: a review and update. J Avian Med Surg 2004;18(2):75–88.
73. Lierz M, Hafez HM, Krone O. Prevalence of hematozoa in falcons in the United Arab Emirates with respect to the origin of falcon hosts. J Avian Med Surg 2008; 3(22):208–12.
74. Krone O, Waldenström J, Valkiūnas G, et al. Haemosporidian blood parasites in European birds of prey and owls. J Parasitol 2008;94(3):709–15.
75. Dawson RD, Bortolotti GR. Effects of hematozoan parasites on condition and return rates of American kestrels. Auk 2000;117(2):373–80.
76. Evans M, Otter A. Fatal combined infection with Haemoproteus noctuae and Leucocytozoon ziemanni in juvenile snowy owls (Nyctea scandiaca). Vet Rec 1998;143(3):72–6.
77. Ziman M, Colagross-Schouten A, Griffey S, et al. Haemoproteus spp. and Leukocytozoon spp. in a captive raptor population. J Wildl Dis 2004;40(1):137–40.
78. Campbell TW, Ellis CK. Avian, exotic animal hematology and cytology. Ames (IA): Blackwell Publishing Professional; 2007.
79. Tavernier P, Sagesse M, Wettere A, et al. Malaria in an Eastern screech owl (Otus asio). Avian Dis 2005;49(3):433–5.
80. World Health Organization. Emerging diseases. Available at: http://www.who.int/ topics/emerging_diseases/en/. Accessed April 10, 2009.
81. Jones KE, Patel NG, Levy MA, et al. Global trends in emerging infectious diseases. Nature 2008;451(7181):990–3.
82. Weiss LM. Zoonotic parasitic diseases: emerging issues and problems. Int J Parasitol 2008;38(11):1209–10.
83. Hunfeld KP, Hildebrandt A, Gray JS. Babesiosis: recent insights into an ancient disease. Int J Parasitol 2008;38(11):1219–37.
84. Xiao L, Fayer R, Ryan U, et al. Cryptosporidium taxonomy: recent advances and implications for public health. Clin Microbiol Rev 2004;17(1):72–97.
85. Xiao L, Fayer R. Molecular characterization of species and genotypes of Cryptosporidium and Giardia and assessment of zoonotic transmission. Int J Parasitol 2008;38(11):1239–55.
86. Xiao L, Feng Y. Zoonotic cryptosporidiosis. FEMS Immunol Med Microbiol 2008; 52(3):309–23.
87. Sreter T, Varga I. Cryptosporidiosis in birds—a review. Vet Parasitol 2000;87(4): 261–79.

88. Bryan S, Latimer KS. An overview of cryptosporidiosis. Available at: http://www. vet.uga.edu/VPP/clerck/bryan/index.php. Accessed July 30, 2009.

89. Kansas State University. Parasitology laboratory. Basic biology of Cryptosporidium. Available at: http://www.k-state.edu/parasitology/basicbio. Accessed April 11, 2009.

90. Lindsay DS, Blagburn BL. Prevalence of encysted apicomplexans in muscles of raptors. Vet Parasitol 1999;80(4):341–4.

91. Rodriguez R, Forbes NA. Use of paromomycin in the treatment of a cryptosporidium infection in two falcons. 2007:191–7.

92. Van Zeeland YRA, Schoemaker NJ, Kik MJL, et al. Upper respiratory tract infection caused by *Cryptosporidium baileyi* in three mixed-bred falcons (*Falco rusticolus× Falco cherrug*). Avian Dis 2008;52(2):357–63.

93. University of Florida, Research UF College of Veterinary Medicine. Available at: http://www.vetmed.ufl.edu/college/departments/sacs/research/Accessed. Accessed April 11, 2009.

94. Sureshbabu J, Venugopalan P, Kourtis AP. Cryptosporidiosis. Available at: http://emedicine.medscape.com/article/996876-overview. Accessed March 31, 2009.

95. Fujita H, Mohri H, Inayama Y, et al. Successful paromomycin inhalation therapy for respiratory cryptosporidiosis in AIDS patients. Proceedings and abstracts of AIDS Congress. Yokohama: 1994.

96. De la Tribonniere X, Valette M, Alfandari S. Oral nitazoxanide and paromomycin inhalation for systemic cryptosporidiosis in a patient with AIDS. Infection 1999; 27(3):232.

97. Lech PJ. Ponazuril. Compendium on continuing education for the practicing veterinarian 2002;24(6):484–5.

98. Fayer R, Xiao L. Cryptosporidium and cryptosporidiosis. Taylor and Francis Group, LLC; 2008.

99. Ditrich O, Palkovič L, Štěrba J, et al. The first finding of *Cryptosporidium baileyi* in man. Parasitol Res 1991;77(1):44–7.

100. Peirce MA. A taxonomic review of avian piroplasms of the genus *Babesia starcovici* (Apicomplexa: Piroplasmorida: Babesiidae). J Nat Hist 2000;34(3):317–32.

101. Wildlife Conservation Society. The deadly dozen. Available at: http://www.wcs. org/deadly-dozen/wcs_deadly_dozen. Accessed April 10, 2009.

102. Jefferies R, Down J, McInnes L, et al. Molecular characterization of *Babesia kiwiensis* from the brown kiwi (*Apteryx mantelli*). J Parasitol 2008;94(2): 557–60.

103. Beaufrère H, Cruz-Martinez L, Redig PT. Diagnostic challenge. Journal of Exotic Pet Medicine 2007;16(1):55–7.

104. Mohammed AHH. Systematic and experimental studies on protozoal blood parasites of Egyptian birds. Cairo: Cairo University Press; 1958.

105. Homer MJ, Aguilar-Delfin I, Telford SR, et al. Babesiosis. Clin Microbiol Rev 2000;13(3):451–69.

106. Samour JH, Peirce MA. Babesia shortii infection in a saker falcon (Falco cherrug). Vet Rec 1996;139:167–8.

107. Ghazaei C. Babesiosis in a steppe saker falcon (*Falco cherrug*)—a case report. J Appl Anim Res 2007;31(2):183–4.

108. Samour JH, Naldo JL, John SK. Therapeutic management of *Babesia shortii* infection in a peregrine falcon (*Falco peregrinus*). J Avian Med Surg 2005; 19(4):294–6.

109. Tarello W. Babesiosis in a steppe eagle (*Aquila rapax*). Revue de Médecine Vétérinaire 2005;156(1):11–2.

110. Munoz E, Molina R, Ferrer D. *Babesia shortii* infection in a common kestrel (*Falco tinninculus*) in Catalonia (Northeastern Spain). Avian Pathol 2005;28: 207–9.
111. Arent LR. Bugs in the blood: the rise of blood parasites in raptors. Wildlife Rehabilitation Bulletin 2008;26(1):38.
112. Peirce MA, Jakob-Hoff R, Twentyman C. New species of haematozoa from Apterygidae in New Zealand. J Nat Hist 2003;37(15):1797–804.
113. Tarello W. Effective imidocarb dipropionate therapy for *Babesia shortti* in falcons. Vet Rec 2006;158(7):239–40.
114. Nemeth NM, Kratz GE, Bates R, et al. Clinical evaluation and outcomes of naturally acquired West Nile virus infection in raptors. J Zoo Wildl Med 2009;40(1): 51–63.
115. The peregrine fund. Global raptor information network. Avalable at: http://www.globalraptors.org/grin/SiteMap.asp?sm=6. Accessed April 11, 2009.
116. Oaks JL, Gilbert M, Virani MZ, et al. Diclofenac residues as the cause of vulture population decline in Pakistan. Nature 2004;427:630–3.
117. Cade TJ. Exposure of California Condors to lead from spent ammunition. J Wildl Manage 2007;71(7):2125–33.
118. Diary Planet. Planet diary archive 2009-fauna—Spain's vultures are starving. Available at: http://www.phschool.com/science/planetdiary/archive09/faun1040409.html. Accessed May 28, 2009.
119. Sleeman JM, Clark EE. Clinical wildlife medicine: a new paradigm for a new century. J Avian Med Surg 2003;17(1):33–7.

# Bacterial and Parasitic Diseases of Rabbits

Angela M. Lennox, DVM, DABVP–Avian[a], Susan Kelleher, DVM[b],*

KEYWORDS

• Rabbit • Bacteria • Parasites • Dental abscesses
• *Encephalitozoon cuniculi*

## BACTERIAL DISEASES

Bacterial disease is common in pet rabbits, and successful resolution depends on careful and accurate diagnosis, correction of underlying husbandry deficits, and management of concurrent disease processes. Bacteria can invade any body system; however, this article addresses the more common presentations seen in clinical practice.

### Respiratory Disease

Respiratory disease is common in rabbits and commonly involves bacterial pathogens, although other etiologies should be considered as well (eg, viral, neoplastic, foreign body, other). Bacterial infection may involve the upper or lower respiratory tract. A survey of conjunctival flora from normal rabbits demonstrated the following organisms: DNase–negative *Staphylococcus* sp, *Micrococcus* sp, and *Bacillus* sp. Other less frequently seen organisms included *Stomatococcus* sp, *Neisseria* sp, *Pasteurella* sp, *Corynebacterium* sp, *Streptococcus* sp, and *Moraxella* sp.[1]

Rabbits are a common model for research on rhinitis and sinusitis in humans, and infection is established after mechanical blockage of the ostium between the nasal and sinus cavities.[2] Infection is considerably more difficult to produce when the nasal cavity is functionally normal. A recent study of 121 rabbits with upper respiratory tract disease (nasal discharge and sneezing) indicated that the most common bacterial isolates from nasal samples were *Pasteurella multocida* (54.8%), *Bordetella bronchiseptica* (52.2%), *Pseudomonas* spp (27.9%), and *Staphylococcus* sp (17.4%). Mixed infections were common.[3] Another study demonstrated that damage to the maxillary premolar roots reliably produced varying degrees of sinusitis in laboratory rabbits (see section on dental disease).[4] Otitis media can be associated with respiratory disease in

[a] Avian and Exotic Animal Clinic of Indianapolis, 9330 Waldemar Road, Indianapolis, IN 46268, USA
[b] Broward Avian and Exotic Animal Hospital, 1730 University Drive, Coral Springs, FL 33071, USA
* Corresponding author.
*E-mail address:* auntnoon@snappydsl.net (S. Kelleher).

Vet Clin Exot Anim 12 (2009) 519–530
doi:10.1016/j.cvex.2009.06.004
1094-9194/09/$ – see front matter © 2009 Published by Elsevier Inc.

rabbits, because infection can spread by way of the Eustachian tube to the tympanic bulla and middle and possibly inner ear.[5]

Surveys of rabbits with confirmed pulmonary lesions demonstrated the following isolates in this order of frequency: *Pasteurella* spp, including *P multocida*, *Escherichia coli*, *B bronchiseptica*, and *Pseudomonas aeruginosa*.[6] Pure culture of any organism in ill rabbits should be considered a potential pathogen.

*P multocida* is a common respiratory pathogen and can produce several disease processes, including rhinitis, sinusitis, conjunctivitis, nasolacrimal duct infections, otitis, tracheitis, pneumonia, and abscesses. Many pet rabbits harbor *P multocida*. Rabbits may remain symptom-free or exhibit symptoms in response to stress (weaning, transport, purchase from the pet store, poor sanitation, poor ventilation, and concurrent illness.)[7] The organism gains entry to the host through the nares (aerosolization, direct contact, or fomites) or through wounds. Rabbits can resist infection, become infected, or develop subclinical infections. In laboratory animals, rhinitis occurs 1 to 2 weeks after intranasal infection. After nasal infection, the organism spreads to the sinuses, nasolacrimal duct, Eustachian tubes, trachea, lungs, and middle ear.[7]

Although older literature suggests that *B bronchiseptica* is not pathogenic in rabbits, this organism is often isolated in pure culture in ill rabbits. Some suspect that it may be a predisposing factor to development of *P multocida* infections. Severe infection has been reported in the absence of *P multocida* in a colony of inbred laboratory rabbits, suggesting that more pathogenic strains might exist (Deeb and DiGiacomo, unpublished data).

Several unusual organisms have been implicated as a cause of respiratory disease in rabbits, including *Mycoplasma* spp described in a group of laboratory rabbits housed in close proximity to rats[8] and *Mycobacterium* spp. Kelleher[9] described a case of nasal mycobacteriosis in a rabbit (**Fig. 1**).

Treatment success of bacterial infections relies on accurate diagnosis and identification of the pathogen in question, plus treatment and resolution of concurrent

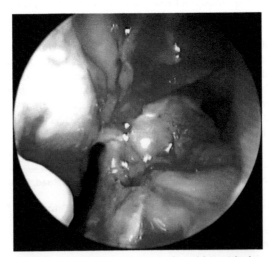

**Fig. 1.** Endoscopic view of a mass in the nasal cavity of a rabbit with chronic nasal discharge. Multiple debridement with biopsy revealed acid-fast bacteria identified as Mycobacterium avium.

disease processes. In the case of abscess (nasal, pulmonary, or aural), resolution is unlikely without excision of the granuloma and affected tissue. One of the authors (A.M.L.) has had success in treating chronic rhinitis nonresponsive to medical therapy with rhinotomy, debridement and flushing, and placement of a nasal catheter for intermittent infusion of antibiotics.

## Gastrointestinal Disease

Clinical experience shows that true bacterial gastroenteritis is rare in rabbits. In many cases, bacterial enteritis is seen in extremely young rabbits or in animals undergoing stress (eg, overcrowding, poor husbandry, concurrent illness). According to a recent study, the predominant organisms in the lower gastrointestinal tract include streptococci and enterobacteria in normal young rabbits and *Bacteroides* spp in adult rabbits. Low gastric pH in rabbits produces a relatively sterile stomach.[10]

Organisms implicated in primary bacterial enteritis include *Salmonella* spp, *E. coli*, *Campylobacter* spp, and others. Proliferative enteropathy with confirmed *Lawsonia intracellularis* has been diagnosed in rabbits with diarrhea.[11]

Epizootic rabbit enteropathy, first recognized in 1997, is an enteric disease of particular importance to rabbits under intensive production conditions. Elucidation of an etiology is problematic, but recent studies suggest a bacterial pathogen.[12]

Inappropriate antibiotic use in rabbits (eg, oral penicillin, lincomycin, clindamycin, erythromycin, cephalosporins) is linked to destruction of normal bacterial flora and overgrowth of *Clostridium* sp, with exotoxin formation. Although not every rabbit that is exposed to these drugs develops gastrointestinal disease, the risk completely precludes the use of these drugs.[10]

Treatment of bacterial enteritis is based on results of culture and sensitivity. Underlying husbandry issues and concurrent illnesses must be addressed as well.

## Urogenital Tract Disease

Disease of the urinary tract is often related to mineral accumulation (calcium sludge) or urolithiasis.[13] In some but not all cases, bacterial organisms may be contributory. As in other species, urine for culture and sensitivity testing should be collected by means of cystocentesis to prevent sample contamination. Bacterial analysis of calculi may be useful as well.

Bacterial nephritis is reported in the literature. Disease presentations include abscesses, staphylococcal nephritis, pyelonephritis, and pyelitis.[14]

Pyometra and uterine abscess have also been reported. Some rabbits may produce mucopurulent vaginal discharge. *Pasteurella* sp are common isolates.[13] Ovariohysterectomy with appropriate antibiotic therapy is recommended for treatment of bacterial uterine disease.

*Treponema cuniculi* (rabbit syphilis) produces lesions of the genitalia, lips, eyelids, and anus, in order of frequency.[15] Maternally acquired infections commonly produce facial lesions.

## Otitis

Bacterial otitis can occur in any rabbit but is most frequent in the lop-eared rabbit breed because of altered skull anatomy. The authors have noted that otoscopic or endoscopic otic examination of older lop-eared rabbits frequently reveals a stenotic horizontal ear canal filled with debris. Introduction of bacteria from the external ear canal or as an extension of upper respiratory disease can result in an accumulation of pus. Pus and debris are easily differentiated on cytology. Infection is often difficult to manage medically (eg, ear flushing, appropriate antibiotics). Surgical management includes lateral ear canal resection, which has been described in rabbits.[16]

### Dental Disease

A common consequence of acquired dental disease in rabbits is periapical infections and abscess. Any disease processes leading to loosening or fracture of teeth can permit food and bacteria to enter the alveolar socket. The rabbit is a model for dental-related sinusitis in humans.[4] In one study, disease was created by damaging and exposing the roots of maxillary premolars, allowing normal mouth microflora to enter the periodontal space. When the damaged site was left open, the result was varying degrees of alveolar widening, bone reaction, and sinusitis. The primary bacterial pathogens isolated were gram-negative aerobes. When the damaged site was capped 1 week later by means of a root canal procedure, pathologic changes were more pronounced and bacterial pathogens were mostly anaerobes.[4]

Depending on the location of the tooth or teeth involved, periapical infection can result in the appearance of an abscess associated with the maxilla or mandible, or in the case of infection of maxillary cheek teeth three through five, accumulation of pus in the alveolar bulla and rupture into the retrobulbar space with the clinical presentation of exopthalmos.[17] Clinical experience has shown the predominance of anaerobic organisms in dental abscesses of rabbits; therefore, sample submission should include requests for aerobic and anaerobic cultures.[18]

### Septicemia

Bacterial septicemia can occur in immunocompromised animals and can involve various organisms, including *P multocida.* A 5-year-old pet rabbit was diagnosed with *Actinobacillus capsulatus* septicemia after a 3-day history of anorexia and depression.[19]

## PARASITIC DISEASE

External and internal parasites are responsible for a variety of disease presentations that affect the pet rabbit. This section covers common parasites of rabbits that affect the skin and hair, alimentary system, liver, and peritoneal cavity.

### Ectoparasites

External parasites that affect rabbits include fleas, ticks, mites, lice, and fly larvae (myiasis). In the United States, *Ctenocephalides canis* or *C felis* commonly infests rabbits.[5] In the authors' experience, fleas do not prefer rabbits and their presence indicates heavy infestation in the environment.

Mite infestation is generally limited to the common ear mite of the rabbit, *Psoroptes cuniculi*; the fur mite, *Cheyletiella parasitovorax*; and the common fur mite, *Leporacarus gibbus.*[5,20,21]

*P cuniculi* is a nonburrowing mite that causes a significant host inflammatory response (**Fig. 2**). Patients that are presented with infestations of this mite often have ear pinnae full of flaky tan exudates (**Fig. 3**). Occasionally, lesions spread to other parts of the body. The mite can cause significant irritation to the rabbit, including pain and pruritus. The client and clinician must resist the temptation to debride ear lesions because this results in discomfort and does not speed healing.[20]

*C parasitovorax* and *L gibbus* are nonburrowing fur mites that produce flaky skin usually encountered along the dorsal midline. The authors have noted that outbreaks are commonly seen in solitary rabbits and seem to be related to immunosuppression,

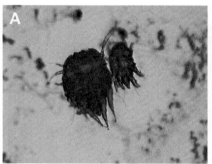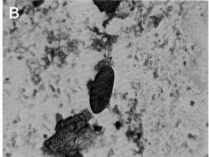

**Fig. 2.** Psoroptes cuniculi, or the common ear mite of rabbits. Mature mites (*A*) and ova (*B*).

aging, and the presence of concurrent disease. This observation implies the presence of subclinical infestations. It should be noted that *C parasitovorax* is zoonotic and can produce skin lesions in humans. Other reported mites in rabbits include *L gibbus* (common fur mite), which is not considered zoonotic. The mites can be distinguished microscopically (**Fig. 4**).[21]

Other mites reported in the literature include *Notoedres* and *Sarcoptes scabiei,* which can cause extensive lesions of the head, neck, and genitals if untreated (**Fig. 5**).[21] Lice (*Haemodipsus ventricosus)* are uncommonly encountered in pet rabbits but are seen in wild rabbits. Lice are thought to be mechanical vectors for tularemia and myxomatosis.[21]

Myiasis commonly occurs in rabbits housed outdoors. Flies are attracted to feces, moist skin, or wounds.[22] Thick- or long-furred rabbits are especially prone to matting and accumulation of feces and urine, which are ideal feeding sites for fly larvae. *Cuterebra horripilum* and *C buccata* infest rabbits housed outdoors and cause one or more raised lesions containing a single larvae.[5] One of the authors (A.M.L.) treated an endemic outbreak of *Cuterebra* infestation in rabbits housed free range in a barn that were also experiencing high mortality from an undetermined cause. It is assumed that the weakened condition of the rabbits made them prone to attack by *Cuterebra* flies.

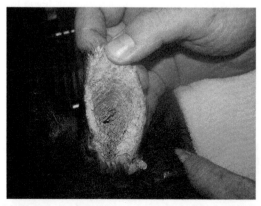

**Fig. 3.** Psoroptes otitis externa. In severe cases, the pinna fills with flaky debris. Treatment with ivermectin is usually effective. Debridement of the pinna is painful and not recommended.

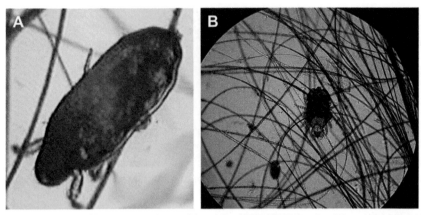

**Fig. 4.** Fur mites of rabbits. Leporacacus gibbus (*A*) and Cheyletiella parasitivorax (*B*) are easily distinguished microscopically. Note the curved claws and hook-like mouth parts of C. parasitivorax.

### Endoparasites

Although parasites present in wild rabbit populations (*Obeliscoides cuniculi, Graphidium strigosum, Trichostrongylus retortaeformis*, and others) endoparasites are uncommon in pet rabbits. An exception is the rabbit pinworm, *Passalurus ambigous*.[21] This oxyurid dwells in the cecum and large intestine and in rabbits with heavy worm burdens and may be visible through the wall of the cecum during abdominal surgery. It is a ubiquitous bacteria-feeding parasite with a direct life cycle. Adult worms are approximately 5 to 10 mm in length and readily apparent in feces. Pinworms do not usually cause significant disease in the adult rabbit, but they are of esthetic concern to owners. Heavy infestation in extremely young animals can contribute to enteritis.[21] Infestation is by means of ingestion of embryonated ova in feces or fecal-contaminated feed, water, or debris.[23]

*Trichuris leporis* is the rabbit whipworm. The adult worms are found in the cecum and large intestine. Although infections have been reported in domestic rabbits, they are uncommon.[24]

Rabbits are the intermediate host for several canine or feline tapeworms, and pet rabbits exposed to feces may become infected. *Cysticercus pisiformis* is the larval

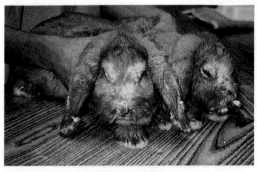

**Fig. 5.** Appearance of sarcoptic mange in two rabbits.

stage of *Taenia pisiformis,* a tapeworm of dogs and foxes. Eggs are ingested by rabbits and pass into the small intestine. The oncosphere migrates to the peritoneal cavity by way of the liver, and fluid-filled cysts form in the mesentery. Most infections are inapparent and are sometimes noted by veterinarians performing abdominal surgery; however, heavy infestation may produce abdominal discomfort. The larval form of the dog or fox tapeworm *T serialis* similarly affects rabbits, producing subcutaneous cysts. Cases of *Taenia* sp cysts have also been identified in the orbit of rabbits, and produced exophthalmos in each case.[21,25]

*Baylisascaris procyonis,* a roundworm of the raccoon, has a predisposition for central nervous system (CNS) tissue of aberrant hosts, including the rabbit. One of the authors (A.M.L.) has documented several cases of parasitic encephalitis after rabbits were housed in hutches previously occupied or contaminated by raccoons.

### Protozoa

Protozoa that infect rabbits include coccidia, *Encephalitozoon cuniculi, Toxoplasma gondii,* and cryptosporidia.[21]

Numerous species of coccidia can infect rabbits.[23] Coccidiosis is of concern in rabbit colonies and can produce diarrhea in young or immunocompromised rabbits.

*Eimeria magna, E performans, E media,* and *E irresidua* are the most common intestinal coccidia in North America.[23] Although coccidia share general microscopic characteristics, unique features allow differentiation (**Fig. 6**A). Exact identification is not essential in practice, because therapeutic options are the same for each species (**Table 1**). It should be noted that the appearance of the normal cecal yeast inhabitant *Saccharomyces guttulatus* is similar to that of coccidia and must be distinguished (see **Fig. 6**B).[23]

*E stiedae* has increased potential for pathogenicity. Infected animals are usually asymptomatic, but heavy infestation can produce anorexia, failure to gain weight, weight loss, hepatomegaly, icterus, diarrhea, debilitation, and death.[23] Although transmission is by means of ingestion of sporulated oocysts in the feces, identification through fecal parasite analysis is difficult; therefore, diagnosis is usually made at necropsy. Common lesions include irregularly shaped, raised, yellow-white nodules or cords in the liver. The gallbladder and extrahepatic ducts may be thickened and distended with yellowish green fluid as well. *E stiedae* oocysts are elongated ellipsoid bodies measuring approximately 20 μm × 37 μm. They are smooth and light yellow and have a thin micropyle and residual body.[23]

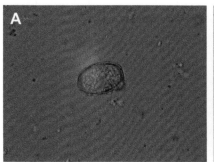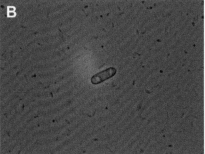

**Fig. 6.** (*A*) Typical appearance of coccidia in the rabbit. (*B*) These organisms should be distinguished from the yeast Saccharomyces guttulatus, a normal inhabitant of the rabbit cecum.

**Table 1**
Treatment of selected bacterial and parasitic diseases of domestic rabbits

| Disease | Treatment Options | Comments |
|---|---|---|
| Bacterial disease, aerobic<br>Pasteurella multocida<br>Clostridium spp<br>Treponema cuniculi | Enrofloxacin or trimethoprim sulfa is often a good empiric choice<br>Enrofloxacin: 5–15 mg/kg q 12 h[34]<br>Trimethoprim sulfa: 15–30 mg/kg PO q 12 h[34]<br>Marbofloxacin: 5 mg/kg q 12 h[35,36]<br>Metronidazole: 20 mg/kg PO q 12 h[34]<br>Injectable penicillin procaine: 42,000–84,000 IU/kg SQ q 7 d × 3[34] | Appropriate treatment is based on culture whenever possible |
| Bacterial disease, anaerobic | Injectable penicillin procaine: 40,000 IU/kg SQ[34] | Dosing interval recommendations are variable and range from q 24–72 h |
| Bacterial, dental abscess | Best results obtained from excision of abscess, capsule, and affected tooth or bone and marsupialization of the wound for repeated flushing/packing until healing occurs by second intention<br>Success reported with and without long-term antibiotic use[17] | — |
| Parasitic disease, ectoparasites<br>Fleas, ticks<br>Fly larvae (myiasis) | Imidacloprid: 10 mg/kg topically[37,38]<br>Selamectin: 6–28 mg/kg topically[39]<br>Careful individual removal and treatment of associated abscess | Control of fleas in environment and on contact animals (dogs/cats/rabbits) is essential<br>Fipronil is toxic to rabbits (do not use)[40] |
| Parasitic disease, ectoparasites<br>Ear mites and lice | Ivermectin: 0.1–0.6 mg/kg q 7–14 d × 2[39]<br>Selamectin: 6–18 mg/kg topically[41]<br>Topical permethrin | Do not attempt to debride infested ears |

| | | Comments |
|---|---|---|
| **Parasitic disease, ectoparasites** | | |
| Fur mites or Sarcoptes mites | Ivermectin: 0.6 mg/kg SQ q 7 d for 3–6 weeks<br>Ivermectin: 0.6 mg/kg SQ q 14 d[39]<br>Selamectin: 6–18 mg/kg[39] topically once monthly for 2–3 months.[41] | Cheyletiella may require additional treatments<br>Resistant cases may benefit from lime/sulfur dips q 7 d for 3–6 treatments<br>One of the authors (S.K.) recommends using dips at 25% strength |
| **Parasitic disease, endoparasites** | — | — |
| Coccidia | Trimethoprim/sulfamethoxazole: 40 mg/kg PO q 12 h[42] | — |
| Toxoplasma | No current recommendations available | — |
| Encephalitozoon cuniculi | Fenbendazole: 20 mg/kg PO q 24 h for 28 d[31] | — |
| Cryptosporidia | No current recommendations available | — |
| Pinworms | Piperazine: PO (500 mg/kg in adult, 750 mg/kg in young)[43]<br>Fenbendazole: 10 mg/kg PO q 14 d × 2[44] | — |

*Abbreviations:* d, days; h, hours; PO, per os; q, every; SQ, subcutaneous.

Control of *E stiedae* infections is best accomplished by prevention. The oocysts are extremely resistant and can remain infectious in the environment for several months. Rigid sanitation practices are necessary to eliminate the organism from the environment. Treatment is only possible during a short inapparent stage early in the asexual part of the protozoan life cycle.[23]

*E cuniculi* is a microsporidian parasite infecting a wide range of mammalian hosts. In rabbits, it can produce granulomatous disease resulting in a wide range of symptoms. Clinical experience and postmortem surveys suggest that the most commonly affected tissues are those of the brain, followed by those of the kidney and eye.[21,26] Ocular lesions include cataracts and lens-induced uveitis.[27] The disease is widespread in pet rabbits, and various surveys demonstrate high percentages of seropositive animals (31.6%–40%), including normal and apparently infected animals.[21,26,28]

Researchers are attempting to develop accurate testing for *E cuniculi.* Dr. Carolyn Cray is investigating the use of antibody ELISA combined with protein electrophoresis.[29] Results have shown that a large number of samples submitted demonstrate a titer to the organism, which concurs with other surveys of various rabbit populations. Rabbits considered by practitioners to be at high suspicion for having *E cuniculi* tended to demonstrate higher titers, along with increases in gamma-globulins. Therefore, the use of these two tests together may help to identify infected animals and help to guide treatment decisions.[29] In a 2008 study comparing cerebrospinal fluid of apparently normal rabbits versus rabbits suspected of having *E cuniculi*, suspect rabbits had higher levels of protein than normal rabbits and cytology was characterized as lymphomonocytic pleocytosis.[30] Diagnosis is enhanced by attempting to rule out other diseases processes producing similar clinical symptoms.

Several studies have focused on the use of fenbendazole for treatment of this disease.[31] In general, practitioners depend on change in clinical condition to judge response to therapy, because laboratory confirmation of successful treatment is problematic.

*T gondii* can potentially infect any mammalian host, including rabbits.[21] Infection is usually subclinical, but outbreaks of disease have been seen in young rabbits and in commercial rabbits. Various surveys have demonstrated antibodies to *Toxoplasma* sp in 18% to 19% of normal rabbits.[32] Although this disease has zoonotic potential, as in other nonprimary hosts, oocytes are not shed in the feces of rabbits.

*Cryptosporidium* spp have been confirmed in pet rabbits, primarily in those with diarrhea. One study identified two types of oocytes, recovered at rates of 16.7% and 13.6% in rabbits with diarrhea and at rates of 3.3% and 0% in normal control rabbits. Symptoms include anorexia, fever, CNS symptoms, and death.[33] Zoonotic risk must be considered.

## SUMMARY

Bacterial and parasitic diseases in rabbits are common. An understanding of pathogens known to infect or likely to infect rabbits plus a thorough diagnostic approach facilitate diagnosis and enhance treatment.

## REFERENCES

1. Cooper SC, McLellan GJ, Rycroft AN. Conjunctival flora observed in 70 healthy domestic rabbits (Oryctolagus cuniculus). Vet Rec 2001;149(8):232–5.
2. Broome RL, Brooks DL. Efficacy of enrofloxacin in the treatment of respiratory pasteurellosis in rabbits. Lab Anim Sci 1991;41:572–6.

3. Rougier S, Galland D, Boucher S, et al. Epidemiology and susceptibility of pathogenic bacteria responsible for upper respiratory tract infections in pet rabbits. Vet Microbiol 2006;115(103):192–8.
4. LegertGarming K, Melen I, Heimdah A, et al. Development and characterization of an animal model of dental sinusitis. Acta Oto-Laryngologica. 2005;125(11): 1195–202.
5. Harcourt-Brown F. Skin diseases. In: Harcourt-Brown F, editor. Textbook of rabbit medicine. Philadelphia: Elsevier Science Limited; 2002. p. 224–48.
6. Marlier D, Mainil J, Linde A, et al. Infectious agents associated with rabbit pneumonia: isolation of amyxomatous myxoma virus strains. Vet J 2000;159:171–8.
7. Deeb BJ, DiGiacomo RF, Bernard BL, et al. *Pasteurella multocida* and *Bordetella bronchiseptica* infections in rabbits. J Clin Microbiol 1990;28:70–5.
8. Deeb B. Respiratory disease and pasteurellosis. In: Quesenberry KE, Carpenter JW, editors. Ferrets, rabbits and rodents clinical medicine and surgery. 2nd edition. St. Louis (MO): Elsevier; 2004. p. 172–82.
9. Kelleher S. Mycobacteriosis in a rabbit. Proc BZVA 2006.
10. Fann K, O'Rourke D. Normal bacterial flora of the rabbit gastrointestinal tract: a clinical approach. Sem Avian Exot Pet Med 2001;10(1):45–7.
11. Horiuchi N, Watarai M, Kobayashi Y, et al. Proliferative enteropathy involving Lawsonia intracellularis infection in rabbits (Oryctolagus cuniculus). J Vet Med Sci 2008;70(4):389–93.
12. Szalo IM, Lassence C, Licois D, et al. Fractionation of the reference inoculum of epizootic rabbit enteropathy in discontinuous sucrose gradient identifies aetiological agents in high density fractions. Vet J 2007;173(3):652–7.
13. Harcourt-Brown F. Urogenital disease. In: Harcourt-Brown F, editor. Textbook of rabbit medicine. Philadelphia: Elsevier Science Limited; 2002. p. 335–51.
14. Hinton M. Kidney diseases in the rabbit: a histological survey. Lab Anim 1981;15: 263–5.
15. Saito K, Hasegawa A. Clinical features of skin lesions in rabbit syphilis: a retrospective study of 63 cases (1999–2003). J Vet Med Sci 2004;66(10):1247–9.
16. Capello V. Lateral ear canal resection and ablation in pet rabbits. Available at. http://www.ivis.org/proceedings/navc/2006/SAE/617.pdf?LA=1. Proc N Am Vet Cont 2006;20:1711–3. Accessed June 15, 2009.
17. Capello V, Gracis M. Secondary diseases. In: Lennox AM, editor. Rabbit and rodent dentistry handbook. Hoboken (NJ): Wiley-Blackwell (formerly Zoological Education Network); 2005. p. 165–86.
18. Tyrrell KL, Citron DM, et al. Periodontal bacteria in rabbit mandibular and maxillary abscesses. J Clin Microbiol 2002;40(3):1044–7.
19. Meyerholz DK, Haynes JS. Actinobacillus capsulatus septicemia in a domestic rabbit (Oryctolagus cuniculus). J Vet Diagn Invest 2005;17(1):83–5.
20. Burdeau PJ. Dermatology of small mammals. In: Parasitic and infectious skin diseases in rodents and rabbits. Proceedings of the Fourth World Congress of Veterinary Dermatology. San Francisco (CA); 2000. p. 195–200.
21. Harcourt-Brown F. Infectious diseases of domestic rabbits. In: Harcourt-Brown F, editor. Textbook of rabbit medicine. Philadelphia: Elsevier Science Limited; 2002. p. 361–85.
22. Cosquer G. Veterinary care of rabbits with myiasis. In Practice 2006;28(6):342–9.
23. Harkness JE, Wagner JE. The biology and medicine of rabbits and rodents. Baltimore (MD): Williams & Wilkins; 1995.
24. Wescott RB. Helminth parasites. In: Weisbroth SH, Flatt RE, Kraus AL, editors. The biology of the laboratory rabbit. New York: Academic Press; 1974. p. 317–31.

25. O'Reilly A, McCowan C, Hardman C, et al. Taenia serialis causing exophthalmos in a pet rabbit. Vet Ophthalmol 2002;5(3):227–30.
26. Kunzel F, Gruber A, Tichy A, et al. Clinical symptoms and diagnosis of encephalitozoonosis in pet rabbits. Vet Parasitol 2008;151(2–4):115–24.
27. Giordano C, Weigt A, Vercelli A, et al. Immunohistochemical identification of Encephalitozoon cuniculi in phacoclastic uveitis in four rabbits. Vet Ophthalmol 2005;8(4):271–5.
28. Santaniello A, Dipineto L, Rinaldi L, et al. Serological survey of *Encephalitozoon cuniculi* in farm rabbits in Italy. Res Vet Sci 2009;87(1):67–9.
29. Cray C, Arcia G, Kelleher S, et al. Application of ELISA and protein electrophoresis in the diagnosis of Encephalitozoon cuniculi infection in rabbits. Am J Vet Res 2009;70(4):478–82.
30. Jass A, Matiasek K, Henke J, et al. Analysis of cerebrospinal fluid in healthy rabbits and rabbits with clinically suspected encephalitozoonosis. Vet Rec 2008;19(10):618–22.
31. Suter C, Muller-Dobilies UU, Hatt JM, et al. Prevention and treatment of Encephalitozoon cuniculi infection in rabbits with fenbendazole. Vet Rec 2001;148(15):478–80.
32. Figueroa-Castillo JA, Duarte-Rosas V, Juarez-Acevedo M, et al. Prevalence of *Toxoplasma gondii* antibodies in rabbits (Oryctolagus cuniculus) from Mexico. J Parasitol. 2006;92(2):394–5.
33. Shiibashi T, Imai T, Sato Y, et al. Cryptosporidium infection in juvenile pet rabbits. J Vet Med Sci 2006;68(3):281–2.
34. Hernandez-Diver SJ. Rabbits. In: Carpenter JW, editor. Exotic animal formulary. 3rd edition. St. Louis (MO): Elsevier/Saunders; 2005. p. 411–44.
35. Carpenter JW, Pollock CG, Koch DE, et al. Single and multiple-dose pharmacokinetics of marbofloxacin after oral administration to rabbits. AJVR 2009;70(4):522–6.
36. Carman RJ, Wilkins TD. In vitro susceptibility of rabbit strains of *Clostridium spiroforme* to antimicrobial agents. Vet Micro 1991;28(4):391–7.
37. Morrisey JK. Ectoparasites of small mammals. Proc N Am Vet Conf 1998;844–5.
38. Hutchinson MJ, Jacobs DE, Bell GD, et al. Evaluation of imidacloprid for the treatment and prevention of cat flea *(Ctenocephalides felis felis)* infestation on rabbits. Vet Rec 2001;148:695–6.
39. Jacobs DE, Hutchinson MJ. Efficacy of imidacloprid on rabbits naturally or experimentally infested with the cat flea *(Ctenocephalides felis)*. Suppl Compend Contin Educ Pract Vet 2001;23(4):11–4.
40. Bourne D. Fipronil toxicity in rabbits. Available at: http://wildlife1.wildlifeinformation.org/S/00dis/toxic/FipronilToxicityRabbits.html. Accessed June, 15 2009.
41. McTier T, Hair J, et al. Efficacy and safety of topical administration of selamectin for treatment of ear mite infestation in rabbits. J Am Vet Med Assoc 2003;223(3):322–4.
42. Harcourt-Brown F. Therapeutics. In: Harcourt-Brown F (editors) Textbook of rabbit medicine. Philadelphia: Elsevier; 2002. p. 94–120.
43. Kraus A. Arthropod parasites. In: Weisbroth SH, Flatt RE, Kraus AL, editors. Biology of the laboratory rabbit. New York: Academic Press; 1974. p. 320.
44. Hillyer EV. Pet rabbits. Vet Clin North Am Small Anim Pract 1994;24:25–65.

# Bacterial and Parasitic Diseases of Ferrets

Lauren V. Powers, DVM, DABVP–Avian

KEYWORDS

- *Mustela putorius furo* • Bacterial • *Heliobacter mustela*
- Parasitic • Heartworm Disease
- Mycobacteriosis • Ferrets

The domestic ferret, *Mustela putorius furo*, is a popular companion animal and is used in biomedical research. As a member of the family *Mustelidae*, it is closely related to mink, weasels, and otters. The European polecat (*M putorius*), the North American black-footed ferret (*M nigripes*), and the Russian polecat (*M eversmanni*) are among its closest free-ranging relatives.[1,2] When compared with other companion mammals, primary bacterial and parasitic infections are less common in domestic ferrets.[3] In countries such as the United States, pet ferrets are generally kept indoors, and the risk for exposure to primary bacterial and parasitic infectious agents is low. Companion, breeding, and working ferrets are commonly kept outdoors in other parts of the world, placing them at comparatively greater risk for exposure to infectious diseases.

## HELICOBACTER MUSTELAE

*Helicobacter mustelae* is a small, microaerophilic, gram-negative, slightly curved, urease-positive bacterial rod with four to eight sheathed flagella.[4–6] An excellent review of *H mustelae* infection in ferrets has recently been published.[7] Clinical disease caused by *H mustelae* is one of the more common bacterial diseases seen in the domestic ferret.[8] It is believed that close to 100% of domestic ferrets are infected.[6,7,9–11] Ferrets are believed to be infected at or shortly after weaning.[5] Transmission is likely fecal to oral and may be made easier through hypochlorhydria, which can be induced by oral administration of omeprazole.[5,7] An increased gastric pH may allow the bacteria to pass into the intestines and be shed into the feces.[7] *H mustelae* colonizes the gastric antrum and pyloric portion of the duodenum and can cause ulcerative gastritis and duodenitis.[6,8] Because *H mustelae* is antigenically related to *Helicobacter pylori*, the domestic ferret is used as a research model for human gastritis caused by *H pylori*.[6,8]

Ferrets infected with *H mustelae* may be at increased risk for gastric neoplasia. Gastric adenocarcinoma and mucosa-associated lymphoma tissue have been

Carolina Veterinary Specialists, Avian and Exotic Pet Service, Statesville Road, Huntersville, NC 28078, USA
*E-mail address:* miloplume@gmail.com

Vet Clin Exot Anim 12 (2009) 531–561
doi:10.1016/j.cvex.2009.06.001
1094-9194/09/$ – see front matter © 2009 Elsevier Inc. All rights reserved.

observed in infected ferrets, but a direct causal relationship between infection and neoplasia has not been fully established.[5–9,12–14] Colonized ferrets produce antibodies to gastric parietal cells.[15] Persistent gastritis, lymphoproliferation, and focal glandular atrophy of the proximal antrum are seen in infected animals.[5,16] Uncolonized stomachs are devoid of lymphoid follicles.[5,7] Hepatobiliary inflammation and hepatic hemangiosarcoma were seen in ferrets that were infected with H mustelae.[13] Lesions included chronic cholangiohepatitis with proliferative changes ranging from hyperplasia to carcinoma. Further investigation is needed to fully elucidate the role of H mustelae in cases of hepatitis or hepatic neoplasia.[7,13]

### Clinical Signs

Clinical disease is not altogether common, but may occur more frequently in stressed ferrets or those that have concurrent illness.[5,6,8,10] Clinical signs are related to the presence of ulcerative gastritis and duodenitis, and include lethargy, anorexia, ptyalism, abdominal pain, rapid weight loss, nausea, dehydration, anemia, and melena (**Fig. 1**).[5,6,8]

### Diagnosis

A tentative diagnosis can be made based on history, physical examination, and diagnostic testing to exclude similar diseases.[6,8] Fecal occult blood testing to evaluate for gastric bleeding can be performed (Hemoccult; Beckman Coulter, Fullerton, California) after dietary exclusion of heme. A convalescent care diet (Carnivore Care; Oxbow Pet Products, Murdock, Nebraska) has been evaluated and found to be free of heme.[10] Samples of gastric mucosa can be collected by endoscopy or laparotomy. Exploratory surgery can also be useful to evaluate for other causes of clinical disease, such as gastric foreign bodies.[6] Biopsy samples can be evaluated for inflammation with routine hematoxylin-eosin stain, and for the presence of Helicobacter sp using Warthin-Starry 4.0, silver, and immunohistologic stains.[5–8] Samples can also be tested using commercially available polymerase chain reaction (PCR) assays.[7,10] Appropriate samples for PCR testing include gastric biopsies and gastric or fecal swabs.[7,10] Feces and gastric biopsy samples can also be submitted for microbiologic culture.[5,7] Culture methods are not routinely used in the diagnosis of helicobacteriosis in ferrets because H mustelae requires selective media for growth.[5,6,10] Because nearly all ferrets are likely colonized,

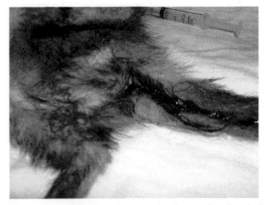

**Fig. 1.** Melena adhered to the tail and perineum of a ferret that has helicobacteriosis.

caution is advised in interpreting positive samples by PCR or culture. Serologic testing can be useful, although because of the high prevalence of infection, a positive titer does not necessarily indicate the cause of clinical disease.[6] Titers tend to increase with advancing age and chronicity of infection and decrease after effective treatment.[5,7] Serologic response does not seem to be protective, because ferrets that have confirmed infection and associated gastritis often have high titers.[5] A urea breath test has been adapted for use in ferrets in evaluating for helicobacteriosis but is not clinically practical because it requires scintigraphy and use of a metabolic chamber.[5,7,17]

### Treatment

Although the cornerstone of treatment includes appropriate antimicrobial therapy, supportive measures are also important.[8] *Helicobacter* sp is highly susceptible to bismuth, a heavy metal with antimicrobial activity linked to its effect on bacterial iron uptake.[18] Bismuth compounds also act against pepsin, a proteolytic enzyme that may contribute to ulcer formation.[8] A suggested dosage of a 262 mg/15 mL (17.5 mg/mL) bismuth subsalicylate suspension (Pepto-Bismol; Procter & Gamble, Cincinnati, Ohio) for ferrets is 1 mL/kg administered orally every 8 hours.[8] There is a concern regarding the use of salicylates in the face of gastrointestinal ulceration. Ranitidine bismuth citrate can also be used and is a component of several treatment protocols. This drug is not approved for use in the United States but it can be compounded. Other supportive agents in the treatment of gastritis and duodenitis include:

- Ulcer protection
  - Sucralfate (Carafate suspension; Axcan Scandipharm, Birmingham, Alabama) at 100 mg/kg administered orally every 8 hours[8] or 25 mg/kg administered orally every 8 hours[6]
- Proton pump inhibition for gastric acid reduction
  - Omeprazole (Prilosec; AstraZeneca, Wilmington, Delaware) at 0.7 mg/kg administered orally every 24 hours
- Histamine H2-receptor antagonism
  - Ranitidine HCl (Zantac syrup 15 mg/mL; GlaxoSmithKline, Research Triangle Park, North Carolina) 24 mg/kg administered orally every 8 hours for 14 days[7] or
  - Famotidine at 0.25 to 0.50 mg/kg administered intravenously or orally every 24 hours or
  - Cimetidine at 5 to 10 mg/kg administered intramuscularly, subcutaneously, or orally every 8 hours[6,8,9]

Specific antibiotic treatment protocols that have been developed for the treatment of helicobacteriosis in ferrets include the following:

- Amoxicillin 30 mg/kg administered orally every 12 hours, metronidazole 20 mg/kg administered orally every 12 hours, bismuth subsalicylate 17.5 mg/kg administered orally every 12 hours. Treat for 21 to 28 days.[19,20] Reportedly 71%[19] to 100%[20] effective in eradicating the organism.
- Amoxicillin 30 mg/kg administered orally every 8 hours, metronidazole 20 mg/kg administered orally every 8 hours, and bismuth subsalicylate 7.5 mg/kg administered orally every 8 hours. Treat for 21 to 28 days.[7]
- Clarithromycin (Biaxin; Abbott Laboratories, North Chicago, Illinois) 12.5 mg/kg administered orally every 12 hours, ranitidine bismuth citrate 24 mg/kg administered orally every 12 hours. Reportedly 100% effective in eradicating infection.[21] Treat for 14 days.[21,22]

- Enrofloxacin (Baytril; Bayer, Shawnee Mission, Kansas) 8.5 mg/kg/d administered orally divided every 12 hours, bismuth subcitrate 12 mg/kg/d administered orally divided every 12 hours. Treat for 14 days. Reportedly 100% effective in eradicating infection.[23]

Several treatment protocols have been shown to be ineffective.[5,24] These include:

- Chloramphenicol 50 mg/kg administered orally ever 12 hours for 21 days
- Enrofloxacin 5 mg/kg/d administered orally divided every 12 hours for 14 days
- Amoxicillin 30 mg/kg/d administered orally divided every 12 hours for 4 weeks
- Omeprazole 69 mg/kg/d, amoxicillin 30 mg/kg/d administered orally divided every 12 hours for 4 weeks
- Tetracycline 25 mg/kg administered orally every 8 hours for 4 weeks, metronidazole 20 mg/kg administered orally every 8 hours for 10 days, bismuth subsalicylate 2.1 mg/kg administered orally every 8 hours for 4 weeks.

Successful treatment does not result in protection against reinfection. Treated ferrets may be reinfected through exposure to infected animals.[5,8,20,25] Treatment failures can also occur through the development of antimicrobial resistance by the organism.[7]

### PROLIFERATIVE BOWEL DISEASE

Proliferative bowel disease of ferrets is caused by an intracellular campylobacter-like organism that resembles *Desulfovibrio* spp, and in swine and hamsters is called *Lawsonia intracellularis*.[6,9,26,27] The bacteria is gram-negative and comma- to spiral-shaped.[9] Fecal-to-oral transmission is suspected.[8,9,27] Clinical disease may occur in only a small percentage of exposed ferrets.[8] Coinfection with *Campylobacter* spp, coccidia, and *Chlamydia* sp has been recognized, but the role of each copathogen is not yet clear.[9]

### Clinical Signs

Clinical disease occurs most frequently in rapidly growing juveniles of about 10 to 16 weeks of age.[6,8] Clinical signs include chronic diarrhea (large or small bowel), lethargy, anorexia, rapid weight loss, and dehydration.[6,8,9,27] Diarrhea may be bloody or green or contain mucus.[6,8,9,27] Continuous or intermittent rectal prolapse can also occur.[6,8,9] Thickened intestinal loops may be palpable.[6,8,27] Intestinal perforation with subsequent peritonitis can occur in severe cases.[6,8] Ataxia and tremors have also been reported.[27]

### Diagnosis

A tentative diagnosis of proliferative bowel disease can be made through historical and physical examination findings.[8] Biopsy of affected tissue can demonstrate a hyperplastic mucosa, and silver staining or IFA can demonstrate the bacteria.[6,8,27] The organism is an obligate intracellular bacterium and therefore is not typically shed in high numbers in the stool and cannot be grown on traditional culture media.[6,27]

### Treatment

Most ferrets that have mild to moderate diarrhea can be treated as outpatients.[6] Successful treatment of serious cases requires appropriative supportive measures, including fluid therapy and nutritional support.[6,8,9,27] Prolapsed rectal tissue should be reduced and a purse-string suture placed until the stools have returned to normal.[6]

The antimicrobial of choice is chloramphenicol, which should be administered for at least 10 to 14 days (**Table 1**).[6,8,9,31] Metronidazole has also reportedly been effective in the treatment of proliferative bowel disease of ferrets.[6,9]

## CAMPYLOBACTERIOSIS

*Campylobacter jejuni* is a gram-negative, slender, microaerophilic, spiral to curved bacterial rod[27,32] and has a characteristic darting or corkscrew motion.[9,32] The organism can be isolated from the feces of clinically normal ferrets[6,9,27,32] but is not usually a cause of primary gastrointestinal disease in this species. *Campylobacter* spp (*C jejuni* and, less frequently, *C coli*) are a significant cause of human enteritis and can cause diarrheic illness in domestic animals, including ferrets.[9] *C coli* was isolated from the intestines of a 16-week-old female ferret in a group of ferrets housed at a commercial ferret farm that had anorexia, weight loss, diarrhea.[33] Diarrhea can be experimentally induced in ferrets through oral inoculation with *C jejuni*.[34,35] Transmission occurs through direct contact with feces or through contaminated water or foods, such as uncooked poultry.[6,9,27] Infected dogs and cats may transmit the organism to humans.[32]

### Clinical Signs

Affected ferrets often develop a self-limiting diarrhea. Diarrhea occurs more often in ferrets less than 6 months of age.[27] The diarrhea can contain mucous or be watery or bile streaked, with or without blood and leukocytes.[6,27,35] Anorexia, fever, dehydration, and tenesmus can also be observed.[6,9,27] Stress and concurrent illness may increase the likelihood of clinical disease.[6,27] Rectal prolapses in mink (*M vison*) kits have been observed in natural and experimental infections.[27] Experimental infection in pregnant ferrets led to abortion, and *C jejuni* was isolated from the uterine contents of two jills.[36]

### Diagnosis

*Campylobacter* spp may be detected in gram-stained feces or through fecal wet mount evaluation using a high phase or dark field objective.[6] Definitive diagnosis requires bacteriologic culture on selective media.[6,27,32] The organism can also be identified by PCR using primers to the 16S rDNA.[6,32]

### Treatment

Although erythromycin has been shown to clear *C jejuni* from fecal samples in humans, experimental administration in ferrets did not eliminate the carrier state in one study.[37] The authors postulated that treatment failure was because of inadequate dosage or frequency of drug delivery or through reinfection.[37] Despite these results, erythromycin in feed at 220 g/ton was successful in controlling colitis in weanling mink kits in two outbreaks.[38] Suggested drug protocols include erythromycin, chloramphenicol, neomycin, clindamycin, tetracycline, and metronidazole.[6,27] Penicillins may potentially be ineffective in treatment.[6] The isolation of *C jejuni* from asymptomatic ferrets and the fact that *Campylobacter* spp are a known cause of enteritis in humans suggest a risk for zoonotic transmission.[9]

## SALMONELLOSIS

*Salmonella* spp are gram-negative, non–spore-forming, facultative anaerobic bacteria.[6,9,27,32] *Salmonella* spp can cause enteritis and occasionally septicemia in ferrets.[6] Salmonellosis is an unusual disease in the domestic ferret, with most reported cases occurring in breeding or research ferrets or those fed undercooked meats or

**Table 1**
**Common antibiotics used in ferrets**

| Drug Name | Dosage | Specific Uses | Comments |
|---|---|---|---|
| Amikacin | 8–16 mg/kg SQ, IM, IV divided q 18–24 h<br>10–15 mg/kg SQ, IM q 12 h | — | Potentially ototoxic and nephrotoxic |
| Amoxicillin | 30 mg/kg PO q 8–12 h for 21–28 d<br>20 mg/kg PO or SQ q 12 h<br>15–30 mg/kg PO, SQ q 12 h | Helicobacter gastritis<br><br>Clostridial gastroenteritis<br>Urinary tract infections | — |
| Amoxicillin/ clavulanic acid | 12.5 mg/kg PO q 12 h<br>13–25 mg/kg PO q 8–12 h | — | — |
| Ampicillin | 5–30 mg/kg SQ, IM, IV q8–12hr | — | — |
| Cephalexin | 15–25 mg/kg PO q 12 h<br>15–30 mg/kg PO q 8 h | — | — |
| Chloramphenicol | 30–50 mg/kg PO, SQ, or IM q 12 h<br>25–50 mg/kg PO q 12 h for 5 d<br>50 mg/kg IM, SQ, or PO for at least 10–14 d | Salmonellosis<br><br>Campylobacteriosis<br><br>Proliferative bowel disease | Extreme caution is advised with human exposure Use for at least 14 days for proliferative bowel disease |
| Ciprofloxacin | 5–15 mg/kg PO q 12 h<br>10–30 mg/kg PO q 24 h | — | — |
| Clarithromycin | 12.5 mg/kg PO q 8–12 h for 14 d | Helicobacter gastritis | — |
| Clindamycin | 5.5–10 mg/kg PO q 12 h | Clostridial gastroenteritis | Also used for other anaerobic infections and for osteomyelitis and dental disease |
| Enrofloxacin | 10–20 mg/kg PO, SQ, IM q 12 h<br>5.0 mg/kg IM followed by 2.5 mg/kg PO q 12 h | Salmonellosis, urinary tract infections<br>Escherichia coli mastitis | — |
| Erythromycin | 10 mg/kg PO q 6 h for 5 d<br>220 g/ton of feed | Campylobacteriosis | — |
| Gentamicin | 2 mg/kg PO q 12 h<br>2–4 mg/kg SQ, IM, IV q 12 h<br>5 mg/kg SQ, IM q 24 h | Used for cases of proliferative bowel disease unresponsive to chloramphenicol | — |

(*continued on next page*)

| Table 1 | | | |
| (continued) | | | |
| Drug Name | Dosage | Specific Uses | Comments |
| --- | --- | --- | --- |
| Metronidazole | 15–20 mg/kg PO q 12 h for 2 wk | Giardiasis | Chloramphenicol is the drug of choice for the treatment of proliferative bowel disease |
| | 50 mg/kg PO daily for at least 5 d | | |
| | 15–20 mg/kg PO q 12 h for 5 d | Campylobacteriosis | |
| | 20 mg/kg PO q 12 h for 2 wk | Proliferative bowel disease | |
| | 15–20 mg/kg PO q 12 h | Clostridial gastroenteritis | |
| Neomycin | 10–20 mg/kg PO q 6 h for 5 d | Campylobacteriosis | — |
| Penicillin G (sodium or potassium) | 20,000 IU/kg IM q 12 h | — | — |
| | 40,000–44,000 IU/kg SQ, IM q 24 h | | |
| Tetracycline | 20 mg/kg PO q 8 h | — | — |
| | 25 mg/kg PO q 12 h | | |
| Trimethoprim-sulfamethoxazole | 15–30 mg/kg PO q 12 h | Salmonellosis Urinary tract infections | — |
| Tylosin | 5–10 mg/kg IM, IV q 12 h | — | — |
| | 10 mg/kg PO, SQ q 8–12 h | | |

*Data from* Refs.[6,8,9,28–30]

poultry products[6,8] or improperly processed pet foods or treats.[9,27] In experimental studies, ferrets showed a fairly high resistance to infection.[9] An asymptomatic carrier state is rare in ferrets.[6] Natural outbreaks have been seen with *S typhimurium*, and several strains, including *S hadar*, *S enteritidis*, *S kentucky*, *S newport*, and *S typhimurium* have been isolated from research ferrets.[8,9,27]

### Clinical Signs

Clinical signs of salmonellosis in ferrets include conjunctivitis, anorexia, lethargy, vomiting, fever, dehydration, abdominal pain, diarrhea with or without blood, tenesmus, mesenteric lymphadenopathy, weight loss, and pale mucus membranes.[6,8,9,27] With septicemia and septic shock there may be evidence of weakness, cardiovascular collapse, and disseminated intravascular coagulation.[6,27]

### Diagnosis

*Salmonella* spp can be cultured, but selective media are required for isolation.[6,8,9,27] Sampling of several fecal samples over several days may improve the chances of isolating the organism.[8] Leukocytes may be visible by fecal cytology.[6] PCR testing for *Salmonella* spp is commercially available.[39]

### Treatment

Successful treatment requires aggressive supportive care, including appropriate fluid therapy and nutritional support.[6,8,27] Hypoglycemia is common with sepsis and must be recognized immediately and corrected.[27] *Salmonella* spp isolated from ferrets have shown resistance to several antibiotics, so antimicrobial selection ideally should be based on culture and sensitivity testing.[9,27] Suggested antibiotics include trimethoprim-sulfamethoxazole, enrofloxacin, and chloramphenicol (see **Table 1**). Both clinically ill ferrets and asymptomatic carriers may serve as primary sources to humans.[6,27] Clients should be advised to avoid feeding raw meat and poultry products to ferrets and to follow sound hygiene practices.[6] As raw food and whole prey diets increase in popularity, salmonellosis should always be suspected in cases of diarrhea and septicemia in ferrets.

## ESCHERICHIA COLI

*Escherichiae* are straight, gram-negative, medium to long rods.[32] *E coli* inhabits the lower intestine of most vertebrate species.[32] It is not known if *E coli* is a normal gastrointestinal flora of domestic ferrets, although in one report of mastitis caused by *E coli* in ferrets, the organism was isolated from rectal swabs of clinically unaffected animals.[32,40] *E coli* was associated with sudden death, dehydration, anorexia, and diarrhea in a captive breeding colony of black-footed ferrets that were fed a diet consisting of mink chow, raw rabbit meat, beef liver powder, blood meal, and lard.[41] An enterotoxigenic *E coli* with genes for heat-stable toxins STa and STb was isolated from the gastrointestinal tract and viscera of ferrets that died and from rectal swabs from clinically affected ferrets. The same toxin genotype was isolated from the mixed ration.[41] In another reported outbreak, contaminated bovine meat was suspected to be the source of infection to ferrets.[9] Infection with *E coli* should be considered a differential diagnosis for ferrets with generalized illness or diarrhea that are fed raw meat or whole prey diets.

The organism can also be isolated in cases of opportunistic reproductive tract infections in ferrets, such as vaginitis, pyometra, and stump pyometra associated with adrenocortical disease. Mastitis with severe coagulative necrosis has been associated with *E coli* infections and with other coliforms and gram-positive cocci.[9,40,42]

*E coli* is a more common isolate from urinary tract infections in ferrets, along with *Staphylococcus aureus* and *Proteus* spp.[6,43] Bladder infections can be silent in ferrets, and ascending infection can lead to severe pyelonephritis and renal failure.[43] Predisposing conditions include urogenital cystic disease and urolithiasis.[6]

### Diagnosis and Treatment

*E coli* readily grows on traditional culture media.[32] Although not clinically used in ferrets, molecular assays and serotypic markers can be used to differentiate virulent isolates from those that are avirulent.[32] Because antimicrobial resistance is common, antibiotic selection should be based on results of culture and sensitivity testing.[32] Trimethoprim-sulfamethoxazole, cephalexin, amoxicillin/clavulanic acid, and enrofloxacin are appropriate empiric choices.[6] Supportive care measures should be provided as necessary. Husbandry and sanitation practices should be improved to assist in elimination of predisposing factors.[32] For cases of acute mastitis, surgical resection or débridement of affected glands may be necessary.[9] Kits from affected jills may need to be isolated and fed separately.[9]

### CLOSTRIDIAL DISEASES

Clostridia are large, sporulating, gram-positive, oxygen-tolerant to strictly anaerobic bacterial rods.[32] Sources of infection can be exogenous, such as from the soil, or endogenous, such as from the intestinal tract.[27,32] Ferrets are susceptible to infection by *Clostridium botulinum* types A and B, are susceptible to type C, and are refractory to type E.[27] Ferrets infected experimentally with types A and B toxins developed clinical signs of botulism, including lethargy, blepharospasm, photophobia, ataxia, urinary incontinence, and ascending paralysis, with death from respiratory failure occurring between 1 and 7 days after exposure.[44] Hepatic, splenic, and renal congestion with subcapsular splenic and cerebellar hemorrhage were commonly observed.[44] Deaths in ferrets due to botulism were reportedly associated with ingestion of wild bird carcasses in England.[45] Ferrets should be prevented from consuming hoarded food, and working ferrets should be kept away from animal carcasses.

*C perfringens* type A is environmentally ubiquitous and found in the intestinal contents of animals and humans.[6,8–10] Disease is considered rare in pet ferrets. Suggested predisposing factors include overeating, sudden dietary changes, excessive dietary carbohydrate, prolonged antimicrobial use, intestinal hypomotility, and the overproduction of toxin.[6,8,9] Disease can also occur through the ingestion of the toxin alone.[27,32] Two syndromes in ferrets have been suggested, including a mild to moderate diarrheic form and a gastric bloat form of disease.[6] In the diarrheic form, tenesmus with scant, small stools can be present, or there can be diarrhea, often green in color, with mucus or small amounts of fresh blood.[6] In the gastric bloat form, abdominal distension, dyspnea, and cyanosis are seen, and disease is most commonly reported in weanling ferrets.[9] Ferrets may be found dead or bloated, with a thin-walled and gas-filled stomach with acute mucosal necrosis of the gastrointestinal tract found at necropsy.[9,27] Subcutaneous emphysema may be present. Acute gastrointestinal disease has been reported on ferret farms and in weanling black-footed ferrets (*M nigripes*).[6,8,9,46] In the outbreak involving black-footed ferrets, over-eating or supplementation of liver mix was believed to have allowed rapid bacterial proliferation and toxin production.[6,46]

### Diagnosis and Treatment

The diagnosis of botulism is made through confirmation of ingestion of spoiled or contaminated food and by clinical signs, although definitive diagnosis requires demonstration of the botulinum toxin from food or from clinical samples, such as gastrointestinal contents, blood, or serum.[27] Because antitoxins are not routinely available, treatment of botulism is primarily supportive and the prognosis is guarded to poor.[27]

The diagnosis of *C perfringens* type A is made through identification of the organism. The observation of abundant gram-positive bacilli in smears of gastric and intestinal contents is suggestive of disease.[6,9] Anaerobic culture may be helpful, but results may be falsely negative because of the fastidious growth requirements of the bacterium.[6] If necessary, the toxin can be isolated through mouse protection assay.[9,27] Because clostridial gastroenteritis is so acute in nature, treatment is often unrewarding.[27] Aggressive supportive measures, including appropriate analgesic therapy, are indicated.[6] Relief of gastric accumulation of gas can be attempted through gastric decompression by orogastric feeding tube placement or gastric trocarization.[8,27] Antibiotics reported effective against *C perfringens* type A include amoxicillin, clindamycin, and metronidazole. Corticosteroids may be useful to stabilize cellular membranes and to aid in cardiovascular support and prevention of reperfusion injury.[6] Chronic disease may require prolonged antimicrobial therapy.[6] Prevention through dietary management is the best control, although prevention of infection can be difficult because of the ubiquitous nature of the organism.[8,27]

## STAPHYLOCOCCI AND STREPTOCOCCI

Staphylococci and streptococci are both gram-positive cocci. Staphylococci occur singly, in pairs, or in grapelike clusters.[32] In one study, *Staphylococcus* sp and *Corynebacterium* sp were isolated from the conjunctival sacs and eyelid margins in clinically healthy ferrets and were considered normal flora.[47] Experimental infection with influenza A virus in ferrets greatly enhances adherence of *S aureus* to respiratory epithelial cells of the anterior nasal turbinate.[48] Experimental *Streptococcus pneumonia* rhinitis, sinusitis, and otitis media were common in young ferrets infected with certain strains of human influenza virus (eg, H3N2 influenza A virus) but not others (eg, H1N1 and influenza B).[49] Ferrets had a more severe respiratory infection when coinfected with influenza virus and Group C *Streptococcus* than with either organism alone.[27] *Staphylococcus intermedius* is the organism most frequently isolated in cases of chronic mastitis in ferrets.[50] Streptococci have also been isolated in cases of vaginitis, pyometra, and stump pyometra related to adrenocortical disease in ferrets.

### Diagnosis and Treatment

Staphylococci and streptococci can be cultured routinely, although selective media are available.[32] Microscopic examination and Gram stain of infected tissue or fluid may reveal gram-positive bacteria. Antibiotic selection should be based on results of culture and sensitivity testing. The emergence of multiple-antibiotic–resistant strains, particularly for *S aureus*, is cause for great concern in veterinary medicine.[32] Culling of jills afflicted with chronic mastitis, such as that caused by *S intermedius*, has been suggested because of the reportedly poor response to antimicrobial therapy and highly infectious nature of the bacterium.[9,50]

## MYCOBACTERIOSIS

*Mycobacteria* spp are aerobic, acid-fast, non–spore-forming, gram-positive rods.[9,32] Natural and experimental infections have been well documented in domestic ferrets,[8,9] and several strains have been isolated from clinically affected animals kept as companion pets.[51] The ferret is highly susceptible to certain strains, including avian, bovine, and human forms.[27] Most historic reports of mycobacteriosis in ferrets were animals in Europe fed raw meat and poultry and unpasteurized milk.[8,9,27] Since the development of commercially prepared diets, the incidence of disease in maintained domestic ferrets has decreased considerably.[9] This decline may change with the increase in popularity of raw meat and whole prey diets for ferrets.

### Mycobacteria bovis

In New Zealand, where a robust population of feral domestic ferrets exists, infection with *Mycobacteria bovis* is a cause for great concern.[51–53] It is still uncertain if ferrets are spillover or maintenance hosts of *M bovis* in this country.[54] There is evidence to suggest that ferrets are infected by ingesting brush-tailed possums (*Trichosurus vulpecula*), which are a reservoir for *M bovis* in New Zealand. Disseminated disease in ferrets is more likely with *M bovis* than with other strains.[27] Splenomegaly, hepatomegaly, and palpable intestinal nodule formation can be detected with disseminated disease.[27] In ferrets experimentally infected with *M bovis*, weight loss, anorexia, lethargy, ascending paralysis, and subsequent death have been observed.[27] The zoonotic potential of this strain is unknown. In one case involving a 63-year-old man who had a chronic *M bovis* synovitis of the wrist, a bite from a ferret 51 years previously (and surgically treated 22 years previously) may have been the source of infection.[55]

### Mycobacterium avium

Mycobacterium avium was isolated from a pet ferret that had chronic weight loss, diarrhea, and vomiting.[56] Granulomatous enteritis with acid-fast bacilli was identified from intestinal biopsy samples. A 6-year-old neutered male ferret that had weight loss was diagnosed with lymphoma and disseminated granulomatous disease caused by M avium.[57] The source of the infection was not known. M avium has also been reported as a cause of pneumonia in ferrets kept in a zoologic garden in France.[27] Wild bird droppings may provide a source of natural infection for ferrets that are allowed outside.[27]

### Mycobacterium genavense

Disseminated infection with Mycobacterium genavense was diagnosed in two ferrets, one that had generalized lymphadenopathy and conjunctivitis and another that had conjunctival swelling, serous ocular discharge, and swelling of the subcutaneous tissues of the nasal bridge.[53] The diagnosis was based on characteristic cytology and sequence analysis of the 16S rRNA gene amplified using PCR from fresh biopsy material. One ferret was treated with rifampicin, clofazimine, and clarithromycin, and the other was treated with rifampicin alone. Clinical improvement was observed in both ferrets. Both ferrets died within 10 months of initiation of therapy, but histopathology and additional testing were not performed.[53]

### Other Mycobacterial Strains

Two ferrets from a three-ferret household that had lethargy, weight loss, and cough were diagnosed by bronchoalveolar lavage with Mycobacterium abscessus.[58] The ferrets were treated with clarithromycin and clinically improved. One of the two ferrets was diagnosed with lymphoma 6 months later.[58] M abscessus, a rapidly growing mycobacteria, is commonly present in soil, water, and decaying vegetable matter, and can colonize pipes and other fomites.[32,58] Entry through wounds, inhalation of soil, or ingestion of contaminated water or soil are likely sources of infection. The two ferrets in this report had access to an outdoor garden.[58] A 4-year-old male ferret in Norway had a 6-month history of weight loss, lethargy, and cough.[51] At necropsy there was generalized lymphadenopathy and multiple pale gray nodules present in the lungs, trachea, and liver. Acid-fast bacilli were found within granulomatous lesions. Mycobacterium celatum type 3 was isolated using 16S rDNA sequence analysis.[51] In humans, M celatum is primarily a disease associated with immunosuppression.

### Diagnosis

Diagnosis of mycobacteriosis in ferrets can be made through routine histopathology to identify characteristic granulomatous inflammatory changes, acid-fast or fluorochrome (eg, Auramine O-acridine) stains, bacteriologic culture using selective media, and DNA sequence analysis.[8,32,39] Nodular lesions can occasionally be detected radiographically.[27]

### Treatment

The zoonotic potential of mycobacteriosis in ferrets remains unknown.[27] Mycobacteriosis is a well-recognized disease in people, particularly in immunocompromised individuals. Antibiotic resistance is common to single-drug therapy, and the suggested duration of treatment is prolonged. Despite the apparent brief response to treatment with antimicrobials described in several clinical reports, euthanasia of affected ferrets must be strongly considered.[27]

## YERSINIA PESTIS

Yersiniae are facultatively anaerobic, gram-negative rods and members of the family *Enterobacteriaceae*.[32] *Yersinia pestis* is the causative agent of bubonic plague.[32] The organism resembles a safety pin when stained with Wright, Giemsa, or Wayson stains.[32] The life cycle generally is flea-rodent-flea, with occasional breakouts to other species.[32] Infection in carnivores is most likely through ingestion of infected prey, although transmission by flea bite is also possible.[59] There are no published reports of clinical disease in the domestic ferret, although ferrets are susceptible to infestation by dog and cat fleas.

In the United States, the white-tailed prairie dog (*Cynomys leucurus*) is a natural prey species for the endangered native black-footed ferret and also serves as a reservoir species for *Y pestis*.[27] Although studies have shown that seroprevalence has not been observed in free ranging black-footed ferrets, ferrets that ingest dead white-tailed prairie dogs infected with *Y pestis* can develop signs of plaque and die.[27] Multiple deaths of black-footed ferrets occurred after ingestion of prairie dog meat contaminated with *Y pestis* in one report.[59] In a separate case report,[60] a black-footed ferret died after escaping into a prairie dog enclosure. Hemorrhage and necrosis of the cervical and mesenteric lymph nodes, subcutaneous hemorrhages, and pulmonary edema were found at necropsy, and *Y pestis* bacterial sepsis was diagnosed.[60] In one study, domestic ferrets and Siberian polecats were used as models of infection for the black-footed ferret, and experimentally infected with *Y pestis*.[61] No animals developed clinical disease, and a persistently elevated serologic titer was observed.[61] In another experimental study, the Siberian polecat was shown to be susceptible to the plague with death occurring in a high (88%) percentage of infected animals.[59] Seroconversion occurred after exposure and was believed to be potentially protective against subsequent infection in polecats.[59]

### Diagnosis and Treatment

Diagnostic samples can be collected from abscesses, draining wounds, lymph node aspirates, or swabs from the oral cavity and pharynx.[32] Samples from abscess exudates can be Gram stained, and a homogenous population of bipolar coccobacilli is observed.[32] *Y pestis* grows slowly in culture.[32] Rapid testing can be accomplished using a fluorescent antibody test for the *Y pestis* F1 antigen.[32] *Y pestis* is susceptible to several classes of antibiotics.[32] Flea control is strongly advised for ferrets that go outdoors or are exposed to dogs and cats.[32]

## LISTERIOSIS

*Listeria monocytogenes* is a gram-positive, non–spore-forming, facultatively anaerobic, motile rod.[27,32] The natural habitat of *Listeria* spp is decomposing plant matter.[32] Ingestion of contaminated food and inhalation are believed to be the modes of transmission.[27] Disease typically manifests as a febrile gastroenteritis or as an influenza-like disease. Immunosuppression is associated with more severe signs, such as meningoencephalitis and bacteremia.[32] In pregnant mammals, *L monocytogenes* may cause fetal death and abortion.[32] *L monocytogenes* was isolated from pulmonary and splenic tissue from a group of ferrets inoculated with lung tissue infected with distemper virus.[62] *L monocytogenes* was believed to be the cause of pneumonia and hepatitis in an immunosuppressed ferret that had adrenocortical disease and cardiomyopathy.[63] The diagnosis is made through routine culture techniques.[32] Antimicrobial treatment should be based on culture and sensitivity results, although reportedly tetracyclines, sulfonamides, and penicillins may be effective therapeutic options.[32]

## LEPTOSPIROSIS

*Leptospira grippotyphosa* and *L icterohaemorrhagiae* have been isolated from domestic ferrets, although reports in this species are fragmentary at best.[27] Historically, ferrets were used to control rodent populations and could easily have been exposed to leptospires in rodent urine.[27] Ferrets raised in the fur industry have also contracted leptospirosis.[27] Pet ferrets exposed to infected dogs may be at risk for contracting the disease.[27] In New Zealand, despite there being a high prevalence of infection in mice and rats commonly eaten by free-living ferrets, no animals had serologic evidence of infection and culture of renal tissues was negative in one study.[64]

## MYCOPLASMA AND CHLAMYDIA

*Mycoplasma mustelidae* was isolated from normal-appearing lungs of 1- to 2-month-old mink kits from three mink farms in Denmark.[2] This bacterium was also isolated from oral and nasal cavities of clinically normal ferrets in Japan.[27] The clinical significance of *M mustelidae* remains unknown.[27] *Chlamydia* sp has been isolated from ferrets that have diarrhea, and has induced pneumonitis in ferrets challenged intranasally with the bacteria. The clinical importance of chlamydial infections in ferrets remains unclear, however.[27]

## BACTERIAL PNEUMONIA

The following bacteria have been reported as primary and secondary pathogens in cases of pneumonia in domestic ferrets: *Streptococcus zooepidemicus* and other group C and G streptococci, *E coli*, *Klebsiella pneumonia*, *Pseudomonas aeruginosa*, and *Bordetella bronchiseptica*.[6,9,27] Most isolates are believed to be opportunistic.[6] Debilitation and immunocompromise from concurrent infections, such as from human influenza virus, can predispose ferrets to opportunistic bacterial infections.[9,27] Anaerobic bacteria may be found in pulmonary abscesses and in cases of aspiration pneumonia, which can occur secondary to megaesophagus in ferrets.[6,9] Clinical signs include weight loss, lethargy, dehydration, serous or mucopurulent nasal discharge, dyspnea, lethargy, anorexia, harsh lung sounds on auscultation, cyanosis, and fever.[6,9] Sepsis and death can ensue.[9] The diagnosis of bacterial pneumonia is made from history and examination findings and assessment of a complete blood count and thoracic radiographs.[6,9,28] A definitive diagnosis is made on culture and cytology of tracheal or lung wash samples or by fine-needle lung aspiration.[6,9,28] Supportive therapy, including fluids, oxygen, and nutritional support, is warranted for moderate to severe cases. Selection of antibiotics should be based on culture and sensitivity, but should be broad spectrum and bacteriocidal, if possible.[3,9,28] A combination of antibiotics that are broad spectrum and effective against anaerobes is a suitable empiric choice.[6] Ferrets should be kept away from humans who have signs of influenza virus and should be vaccinated against canine distemper virus.[6]

## ABSCESSES AND BITE WOUNDS

Bacterial skin diseases are uncommon in ferrets, but are most often caused by *S aureus* or *Streptococcus* sp. Infections are most often caused by bite wounds, or those self-inflicted through pruritic diseases.[9,65,66] Lesions can range from superficial to deep pyodermas, abscesses, or cellulitis.[65,66] Abscesses around the mouth are most often caused by the ingestion of sharp objects, such as bone.[66] Bacteria that have been isolated from dermal infections in ferrets include *Pasteurella* spp, *E coli*, *Corynebacterium* spp, *Pasteurella* spp, and *Actinomyces* spp.[9,65–67]

*Actinomyces* spp are gram-positive, anaerobic to microaerophilic bacteria.[27,29,32] *Actinomyces* spp, or "lumpy jaw," is infrequently diagnosed in ferrets.[27,29,65,66] Although susceptibility to disease may be low, immunocompromised ferrets may be at greater risk for infection.[27] A subcutaneous granuloma caused by *Actinomyces* sp was reported in a ferret that had lymphoma.[68] Transmission is through openings or wounds in the oral mucosa or by inhalation or swallowing of the organism.[27,29,65] Cervical masses develop, often with sinus tracts containing thick, yellow to green purulent exudate.[27,29,65,66] Some masses are large enough to cause difficulty breathing. In one case, a ferret died suddenly and had firm nodules beneath the visceral pleura and mediastinal lymphadenopathy.[27]

### Diagnosis and Treatment

Cytology and gram staining of aspirates or impression smears can aid in the diagnosis of bacterial skin disease and abscesses.[9,27,66] Bacteriologic culture and sensitivity should also be performed on diagnostic samples.[29,66] Encapsulated abscesses can be surgically removed or lanced and drained if excision is not possible.[9,65,66] Topical and systemic antimicrobial therapy should be administered.[9,27,29,65,66] A broad-spectrum antibiotic can be provided pending culture results.[9,65] Penicillins and tetracycline may be effective against *Actinomyces* spp.[27,29,66]

### ANTIMICROBIAL THERAPY

Antibiotics are most commonly used in ferrets for gastrointestinal infections, wound infections, and treatment of secondary infections, such as pneumonia.[3] Selection of antibiotics should be based on results of microbiologic culture and sensitivity testing.[3] No antimicrobials are currently labeled for use in ferrets by the US Food and Drug Administration. Few antimicrobials have been studied in ferrets, so it is not surprising that treatment failure occasionally occurs.[3] Ferrets are carnivores with a simple gastrointestinal tract, and antibiotics safe for use in dogs and cats are generally considered safe to use in ferrets.[3] Antibiotics are best administered in liquid form to ferrets, which may require compounding. Palatability can be improved by combining medications with enteral feeding products (eg, Carnivore Care; Oxbow Pet Products) or supplements for ferrets such as FerreTone Skin and Coat Liquid (Spectrum Products, Atlanta, Georgia).

### PARASITIC DISEASES

The domestic ferret is naturally infected with relatively few species of parasites.[69] The most common parasites that affect ferrets are also found in other carnivores kept as pets, including dogs and cats.[69] With the exception of coccidia, intestinal parasitic infections are uncommon in ferrets. Any ferret that has diarrhea should be evaluated for parasites, however, including wet mount and fecal flotation.[8] Because parasitic diseases are infrequently reported in domestic ferrets, little information is available regarding the use of anthelmintics in ferrets.[69] As with antibiotics, all antiparasitic drugs are used in off-label fashion in ferrets.[69]

### COCCIDIA

Three different species of coccidia are reported to infect the domestic ferret: *Eimeria furonis*, *E ictidea*, and *Isospora laidlawi*.[9,69,70] In one report, asymptomatic ferret kits raised on the same premises with puppies were found to shed oocysts of *I ohioensis*.[69] The life cycles of these parasites are similar and direct.[69] Oocysts become infective 1 to 4 days after being shed in the feces.[6] Once ingested, sporozoites are released and invade intestinal epithelial cells, becoming trophozoites. Ferrets that have proliferative bowel disease have been found to be coinfected with coccidia and *L intracellularis*, but the role of the protozoa in the disease remains unclear.[6,71] Cases of hepatic and biliary coccidiosis infections have been documented.[6,72]

### Clinical Signs

Infected ferrets that are young and healthy may show no signs of disease, although clinical signs can occur if the ferrets are stressed.[69] Clinical signs include diarrhea, lethargy, dehydration, rectal prolapse, mesenteric lymphadenopathy, and palpably thickened intestines.[6,8] The diarrhea may be watery, mucoid, or bloody.[6]

### Diagnosis and Treatment

The diagnosis of coccidiosis is made through historical and examination findings and through fecal examination by wet mount and flotation.[6,8,9,69] Treatment of ferrets is similar to that for dogs and cats.[8] Treatment options include sulfadimethoxine, sulfadiazine-trimethoprim, amprolium, and decoquinate (**Table 2**).[9,69] Because oocysts sporulate rapidly, prevention of oocyst ingestion during an outbreak requires close attention to hygiene and rapid disposal of feces.[9,69]

### GIARDIASIS

Clinical reports of giardiasis in the domestic ferret are scarce, because primary infections are rare in this species.[6,69] Dogs and cats may serve as reservoirs of infection to ferrets.[6] In one report,[76] *Giardia intestinalis* was isolated from an asymptomatic ferret housed at a pet store. This *Giardia* isolate was determined through genetic analysis to be in genetic group A-I, which may have zoonotic potential.[76] Debilitated ferrets, or those that have concurrent disease, are more likely to shed *Giardia* spp.[6] Although little is known about giardiasis in ferrets, the clinical course and veterinary management are likely similar to that in the dog.[69] Giardiasis causes a malabsorption syndrome, leading to soft, voluminous, or grainy stools. Other clinical signs include weight loss and a lackluster coat.[76] The diagnosis is generally made through observation of trophozoites and cysts in fresh feces by wet mount.[6,69] Addition of an iodine stain may be helpful in parasite identification.[6] The treatment of choice is metronidazole administered for at least 5 days[69] or up to 2 weeks (see **Table 2**).[6]

### CRYPTOSPORIDIOSIS

*Cryptosporidium* spp are protozoa that inhabit the respiratory and intestinal epithelium.[9] Transmission, like other coccidian parasites, is through ingestion of sporulated oocysts from contaminated food or water.[9] Autoinfection can also occur.[9] Young ferrets can be infected with *C parvum*, but the disease is usually self-limiting and subclinical, even in animals experimentally immunosuppressed.[9,69] The oocysts can be detected in the stool of clinically normal ferrets.[8,9] Infection has been also been identified in black-footed ferrets and mink that did not show clinical signs.[9,77,78] Clinical disease is associated with eosinophilic infiltration of the small intestinal lamina propria.[8,9] Clinically ill ferrets may show signs of intractable diarrhea.[9] Young ferrets may have a persistent infection that can last for weeks.[8] The diagnosis is made by identifying the small oocysts in the feces by direct examination or through centrifugation techniques, often with the help of acid-fast, auramine, or fluorescent antibody

**Table 2**
**Common anthelmintics used in ferrets**

| Drug Name | Dosage | Specific Uses | Comments |
|---|---|---|---|
| Amitraz | Dip applied every 5–7 days until clinical resolution. Has also been applied to ears | Generalized demodicosis | Use of gloves is strongly recommended |
| Amprolium | 19 mg/kg PO for at least 2 wk | Coccidiosis | Treatment recommendation for larger groups of ferrets |
| Decoquinate | 0.50 mg/kg PO for at least 2 wk | Coccidiosis | Treatment recommendation for larger groups of ferrets |
| Fenbendazole | 50 mg/kg PO q 24 h for 3 d | Nematode infections | — |
| Fipronil | 0.2–0.4 mL of 9.7% solution topically q 30 d | Flea prevention and treatment | — |
| Imidacloprid | 1.9–3.33 µg/kg (Advantage Plus, based on imidacloprid) topically monthly | Heartworm prevention | — |
| | 10 mg/kg topically every 30 d | Flea prevention and treatment | |
| Ivermectin | 0.02 mg/kg PO monthly year-round or during heartworm season | Heartworm prevention | May require dilution in propylene glycol or olive oil |
| | 0.2–0.4 mg/kg SQ every 2 wk until mites eradicated | Sarcoptic mange | |
| | 0.2–0.4 mg/kg SQ q 14 d for three to four doses | Ear mite treatment | |
| | 0.40–0.50 mg/kg divided between both ears | Ear mite treatment | |
| | 0.2–0.4 mg/kg SQ once, repeat in 14 d | Gastrointestinal nematodes | |
| Melarsomine | For severe cases: 2.5 mg/kg IM once, then two injections 24 h apart 1 month later. For mildly affected or asymptomatic ferrets: 2.5 mg/kg IM twice, 24 h apart, followed by a single injection a month later | Heartworm adulticide therapy | For microfilaremic ferrets, pretreat with ivermectin at 50 µg/kg SQ q 30 days until clinical signs and microfilaremia resolved. Sedation for IM injection is advised. Concurrent treatment with corticosteroids is advised |

*(continued on next page)*

| Drug Name | Dosage | Specific Uses | Comments |
|---|---|---|---|
| **Table 2** | | | |
| **(continued)** | | | |
| Metronidazole | 15–20 mg/kg PO q 12 h for 5–14 d | Giardia and other protozoal infections | |
| Moxidectin | 0.17 mg SQ per ferret, once | Heartworm adulticide therapy | — |
| | 1.9–3.33 µg/kg (Advantage Multi for Cats, Bayer; based on imidacloprid) topically monthly | Heartworm prevention | |
| | 0.40 mL of imidacloprid (10%) and moxidectin (1%) topically | Flea elimination and prevention | |
| Praziquantel | 25 mg/kg PO for 3 consecutive d | Trematodes | Dosage may depend upon species of trematode |
| | 5 mg/kg PO | Cestode infections | |
| Pyrantel pamoate | 4.4 mg/kg PO, SQ, repeat in 14 d | Nematode infections | — |
| Selamectin | 18 mg/kg topically monthly | Heartworm prevention | — |
| | 6–18 mg/kg topically monthly | Fleas, ear mites | |
| | 15 mg per ferret topically | | |
| Sulfadimethoxine | 50 mg/kg PO on day 1, then 25 mg/kg PO q 24 h for 9 d | Coccidiosis | — |
| Thiabendazole | Apply topically once daily to both ears for 7 d, stop for 7 d, repeat for 7 d (Tresaderm, Merial) | Ear mite treatment | Treatment failures reportedly are common with this medication |

*Adapted from* Refs.[6,9,29,30,69,73–75]

staining.[9,69] Because of the small size of the oocysts, they are frequently mistaken for yeasts.[9] Yeasts are oval, whereas cryptosporidium oocysts are usually spherical or ellipsoidal.[9]

### Treatment

There is no effective treatment described for ferrets.[9,69] Infections are self-limiting in immunocompetent animals.[9] Paromomycin therapy may hold promise for humans and cats.[69] Caution is advised with extrapolating the cat dose (165 mg/kg administered orally every 12 hours for 5 days) to ferrets, however, because renal pathology has been described for this and lower dosages in cats.[69] Control is through elimination of infective oocysts in the environment and avoidance of contact with known sources of infection.[9] Recent studies in genetic sequencing have shown that the ferret genotype of *C parvum* is unique, but the zoonotic potential is not known.[69,79] Isolates should be considered potentially zoonotic until more data are available, and infected ferrets should be isolated from children and immunosuppressed individuals.[8,9,69]

## TOXOPLASMA GONDII

*Toxoplasma gondii* is an obligate intracellular parasite. After ingestion, sporulated oocysts rupture in the intestinal tract and release sporozoites. These enter and multiply in intestinal epithelial cells and associated lymph nodes to produce tachyzoites, which spread to other tissues of the body where they continue replication.[80] The ferret can be infected with *T gondii* oocysts, and ferrets can serve as potential intermediate hosts.[69,81] Infection in ferrets likely occurs through ingestion of food contaminated with cat feces or by eating toxoplasma encysted in raw meat.[69] Ferrets that go outside are at risk for exposure to cat feces. In one reported outbreak, 30% of neonatal ferrets raised for fur died suddenly and had multifocal necrosis in the lung, heart, and liver.[82] A congenital infection was suspected.[82] In another report, a young, free-ranging mink was found outside and had left hindlimb lameness, head tremors, ataxia, and bilateral blindness. A mild, nonsuppurative meningoencephalitis and severe chorioretinitis were identified by histopathology.[80] An epizootic of toxoplasmosis was reported in a captive population of black-footed ferrets.[83] Affected animals died quickly following a bout of anorexia and lethargy, or developed progressive hindlimb weakness and ataxia.[83] Meningoencephalitis and meningoencephalomyelitis were observed at necropsy. Frozen, uncooked rabbit meat was suspected to be the source of infection in this outbreak.[83] Histopathology and immunologic methods are used in the diagnosis of toxoplasmosis.[82] Serologic techniques can be used to establish an antemortem diagnosis.[69] Treatment guidelines for ferrets are not currently available.[69] As more owners start feeding ferrets whole prey, such as mice, this disease may become more of a clinical problem. Ferret food should be stored in airtight containers away from cats.[69] In zoos, it is recommended to house felids away from other animals, including mustelids, to avoid transmission.

## SARCOCYSTOSIS

Sarcocystosis is caused by *Sarcocystis* spp, an intracellular protozoal parasite. These parasites have an indirect life cycle, cycling between a definitive and an intermediate host. Natural sarcocystosis in ferrets is likely asymptomatic.[81] Transmission of *Sarcocystis muris* to ferrets was reported to occur after ingestion of infected mice that were infected through ingestion of food contaminated with fecal oocysts. Cysts were observed in the skeletal muscles and heart of infected ferrets. In another report, three young farmed mink in Michigan developed progressive neurologic disease.[84] Sarcocysts were found in skeletal muscle of one mink, and nonsuppurative meningoencephalitis and meningomyelitis were present in all three animals.[84] The source of infection was not determined.[84] This species is another parasite of concern for ferrets fed whole rodent prey and raw meat diets.

## NEOSPOROSIS

Dogs are the definitive host for *Neosporum caninum* and young animals can develop an ascending paralysis.[85] Oocysts are shed unsporulated in the feces. *N caninum* can be experimentally transmitted to mice through the ingestion of oocysts.[85] Rodents are believed to be a potential reservoir of infection to other species.[86] There are no reports of natural or experimental infection of ferrets with *N caninum*, although *N caninum* has historically been mistaken for *T gondii*.[81] In one experimental study, *N caninum* oocysts were not detected in the feces of ferrets despite oral inoculation of between 150 and 350 tissue cysts.[85] Ferrets remained asymptomatic and did not mount a serologic response to infection.[85] In a separate study of wild carnivores in Spain,[86] one of two polecats (*M putorius*) was serologically positive for *N caninum*. As more owners begin feeding uncooked meats, such as whole rodent prey, cases of neosporosis in domestic ferrets may become documented.

## HEARTWORM DISEASE

The nematode of primary importance in the domestic ferret is the heartworm *Dirofilaria immitis*.[69] Ferrets are susceptible to natural and experimental infection with *D immitis*,[9,69,81,87–91] with ferrets living in endemic areas most susceptible.[87,91] A low worm burden can lead to life-threatening or fatal disease.[87–91] In fact, sudden death in ferrets in heartworm-endemic areas is often attributed to pulmonary thromboembolism due to dirofilariasis.[88] The heartworm life cycle is similar to the dog and cat, in that L3 larvae are introduced through a mosquito bite and then migrate into the vasculature.[9,69,81,87] L5 larvae can be found in the smaller pulmonary vessels.[87] Larvae can reach the heart in as little as 70 days in ferrets, developing into adult worms.[69] Although worm burdens from 1 to 21 worms have been reported,[6,87] severe clinical disease can be seen with just one or two adult worms.[6,87,91] Worms can be found in the pulmonary arteries and right heart (**Fig. 2**),[6,69,87] although most live worms reside in the cranial and caudal venae cavae in ferrets. This finding may be due to the relatively large size of the adult worm and relatively small size of the pulmonary artery and right heart chambers in the ferret.[88]

### Clinical Signs

Clinical signs of heartworm disease in ferrets are similar to those in dogs, but the disease tends to progress more rapidly.[88,90] Ferrets may be presented with signs of mild to fulminant congestive heart failure.[6,88,92] Common historical and physical examination findings include coughing, dyspnea, exercise intolerance, cyanosis, pleural effusion, heart murmur, anorexia and weight loss, posterior paresis, ascites, and vomiting.[6,9,69,81,88,92] In one study that evaluated naturally infected ferrets, hematologic and biochemical abnormalities included anemia, monocytosis, and mild hyperchloremia.[92] Bilirubinuria was observed in 83% of ferrets and trace hematuria was seen in 67% of infected animals.[92] One of seven ferrets (14.3%) had caval

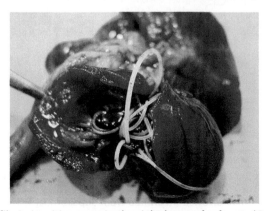

**Fig. 2.** Adult *Dirofilaria immitis* worms in the right heart of a ferret. (*Courtesy of* Stephen Hernandez-Divers, BVetMed, MRCVS, DZooMed, DACZM, Athens, GA.)

syndrome.[92] In one experimental study, circulating eosinophil counts were higher in infected ferrets, but no other abnormalities were found on hematology, serum biochemistry, or urinalysis.[93]

### Diagnosis

Radiographic findings in ferrets that have heartworm disease differ from those in dogs and cats.[88] Whereas dogs and cats typically have enlargement of the pulmonary arteries, ferrets often have right-sided heart enlargement and pleural effusion without radiographic changes to the pulmonary artery system.[6,81,88,91,94,95] Adult heartworms can be observed as filling defects in the venae cavae, azygous vein, and left caudal lobar pulmonary artery when selective angiography is used (**Fig. 3**).[95] Although radiographic findings can be consistent with heartworm disease, definitive diagnosis requires additional testing, such as ultrasound, selective angiography, and evaluation for circulating antigen and microfilaria.[69,87,89] Adult worms can be observed by ultrasonographic evaluation as early as 5 months after experimental infection.[88,94]

Diagnostic testing used in the dog and cat are appropriate in the evaluation for heartworm disease in the ferret.[88] Microfilaremia is reportedly observed but is an inconsistent finding in infected animals.[9,87] In experimental infections, microfilaria can be found after the seventh month of infection.[93,96] Concentration tests, such as the modified Knott test, may be unreliable as screening tests in ferrets because of intermittent microfilaremia and low worm burden in ferrets.[81,88,89] ELISA heartworm antigen detection tests for circulating female worm antigen can be useful in ferrets but can be falsely negative with low worm burdens of single to low numbers of male worms.[9,87,88,91] In experimental studies, 40% to 80% of ferrets were antigen-positive 4 months after inoculation and 100% were positive 6 months after inoculation.[93,96] In the future, PCR-based assays may hold promise in the diagnosis of ferret dirofilariasis. In one study involving feral cats, 63% of positive cats were positive by PCR analysis.[97] In a separate study, all feral cats that tested positive by ELISA were positive by PCR analysis.[98]

### Treatment

Ferrets that have pleural effusion due to heartworm disease may benefit from therapeutic thoracocentesis.[6] Strict cage rest for 4 to 6 weeks following adulti-

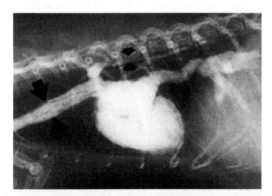

**Fig. 3.** Right lateral recumbent angiogram of a male ferret infected with *Dirofilaria immitis*. Worms are visible in the enlarged cranial vena cava (*large arrows*). A worm can also be seen in the azygous vein (*small arrows*). (*Reprinted from* Supakorndej P, Lewis RE, McCall JW, et al. Radiographic and angiographic evaluation of ferrets experimentally infected with *Dirofilaria immitis*. Vet Radiol Ultrasound 1995;36:27; with permission.)

cide treatment is essential.[6,87] Treatment of congestive heart failure, such as with furose-mide and enalapril, may be of clinical benefit in reducing cardiac afterload and preload.[6,69]

There are currently no approved drugs available in the treatment of heartworm disease in ferrets.[89,90] Adulticide treatments options include melarsomine (Immiticide; Merial, Duluth, Georgia), ivermectin, and moxidectin (ProHeart 6; Fort Dodge Animal Health, Fort Dodge, Iowa) (see **Table 2**).[6,69,87,99] For mild to moderate cases, melarso-mine can be administered at 2.5 mg/kg administered intramuscularly 24 hours apart, followed by a single injection 1 month later.[6] Sedation for injection of melarsomine is recommended.[6] For microfilaremic ferrets, initial treatment with ivermectin is advised at 50 μg/kg administered subcutaneously every 30 days until clinical signs and micro-filaremia are resolved, followed by melarsomine at 2.5 mg/kg administered intramus-cularly, then two doses of 2.5 mg/kg 24 hours apart 30 days later.[6,69,87] Adulticidal treatment safety and efficacy in ferrets has been marginal at best.[88,91,92,100] The risk for pulmonary thromboembolism following adulticidal therapy is high,[6,92] and throm-boembolic disease can be observed up to 3 months after treatment.[6,81] In one study of naturally infected ferrets, only two of five ferrets (40%) survived after adulticide treatment with melarsomine.[91] In another study, only two of six ferrets (33.3%) survived after treatment with melarsomine and ivermectin and only two of four ferrets (50%) survived after treatment with ivermectin alone.[92] In one experimental study, 28 ferrets inoculated with infective larvae tolerated high doses of melarsomine (3.25 mg/kg), but therapy was only 35.3% effective for single doses and only 63.2% to 80.3% effective for two- and three-dose protocols.[88] Two of seven ferrets (14.3%) receiving one to two injections died, as did three of seven ferrets (42.9%) receiving three injections,[88] of pulmonary thromboembolism.

Moxidectin adulticide therapy was reported in 10 ferrets naturally infected with heartworm disease.[99] Moxidectin was administered subcutaneously at 0.17 mg per ferret.[99] All ferrets survived treatment except one that died from unrelated causes, and four ferrets that were monitored after treatment were reportedly subsequently antigen-negative.[99] Monthly preventative doses of ivermectin and treatment with corticosteroids (eg, prednisone 0.50 mg/kg administered orally every 12–24 hours) may lead to higher long-term survival rates for infected ferrets that have few or no clin-ical signs of disease.[6,91] Corticosteroid use is recommended during the treatment period and until clinical signs resolve, or for at least 4 months.[6,69,87] Posttreatment testing should be done at 3 months and then monthly until negative and prophylaxis resumed.[9,91]

### Prevention

Preventative therapy is recommended for ferrets, even for those living exclusively indoors in nonendemic areas. Year-round preventative therapy is strongly advised in heartworm-endemic areas.[9,69] No drug is yet approved for heartworm chemopro-phylaxis in ferrets.[88–90] Single oral doses of ivermectin at 50 and 200 μg/kg were 100% effective in preventing infection 1 month after experimental inoculation of infec-tive L3 larvae.[88] In another report,[93] ivermectin administered at 3.0 and 6.0 μg/kg was 100% protective. Monthly oral administration of ivermectin at 0.02 mg/kg is recom-mended by one author.[91] Dilution of commercially available ivermectin products may be required. Reportedly, ivermectin in a propylene glycol base (Ivomec 10%; Merial) can be diluted in propylene glycol[91] or olive oil for use as a heartworm preven-tative, although stability data for diluted ivermectin have not been published and are not available from the manufacturer. Monthly oral administration of ivermectin in a chewable form (eg, Heartgard for Cats, 55 μg per tablet; Merial) has been advocated,[87,91] but not all ferrets may find the tablet palatable, the drug may not be evenly distributed across the tablet if the tablet is to be divided, and the remaining portion of a divided tablet must be used immediately or discarded.[91]

Imidacloprid (10%) with moxidectin (1%) (Advantage Multi; Bayer) applied topically at 1.9 to 3.33 μg/kg was completely effective in preventing heartworm disease in ferrets.[90] Monthly topical application throughout the heartworm season in endemic areas was recommended by the authors of this study.[90] Selamectin (Revolution; Pfizer Animal Health, New York), a semisynthetic avermectin, applied topically at 6 mg/kg and 18 mg/kg, was 99.5% and 100% effective in preventing heartworm infection.[73] Injectable moxidectin (ProHeart 6) may also prove to be an effective preventative for heartworm disease in ferrets. Control involves keeping ferrets indoors and effective mosquito control.[81]

## OTHER ENDOPARASITES
### Nematodes

Infection by nematodes apart from *D immitis* is rare in ferrets.[8] *Toxocara cati, T canis, Toxascaris leonina, Ancylostoma* sp, *Trichinella spiralis, Filaroides martis,* and *Spiroptera nasicola* have all been isolated from ferrets.[8,9,81] The ferret may be an accidental host to cat and dog nematodes, however.[2] Most infected ferrets may be asymptomatic,[101] although diarrhea, vomiting, and weight loss can occur with heavy worm burdens.[101] The diagnosis is usually made by microscopic observation of parasite ova in the feces.[101] Fenbendazole and ivermectin are effective anthelmintics against nematodes (see **Table 2**).[101] In New Zealand, *F martis* was isolated from lung nodules in two adult male ferrets.[102] The life cycle of the parasite was indirect, with snails and slugs as intermediate hosts and mice as paratenic hosts.[102]

A previously undescribed filarial parasite was reported in a reintroduced group of black-footed ferrets.[103] Twelve percent of animals screened were positive for *D immitis* on an antigen-based ELISA test but all were PCR-negative for *D immitis* using a highly sensitive PCR-based assay. Genetic analysis showed that the parasite shared only 76% identity with *D immitis* but the worm shared 97% sequence similarity with *Acanthocheilonema viteae.*[103] One hundred percent of positive ferrets in one group were microfilaremic, suggesting the black-footed ferret is a suitable host for life cycle completion.[103]

### Cestodes and Trematodes

Species reportedly isolated from ferrets include *Mesocestoides* spp, *Atriotaenia procyonis, Dipylidium caninum,* and *Taenia mustelae.*[9,81,104] Ferrets cohabitating with dogs and cats and their fleas may become infected with the tapeworm *D caninum.*[2] Cestode infections are rare in ferrets, but can effectively treated with praziquantel (see **Table 2**). Praziquantel has been used to effectively treat wild mustelids with trematode infections, although the dosage may depend upon the species of tremadode.[2]

## FLEAS

Ferrets living in homes infested with the cat flea (*Ctenocephalides felis*) or dog flea (*C canis*) are at risk for infestation.[29,66,74,105] *Pulex irritans* can also affect exposed ferrets,[29,74] as can the badger flea (*Paracaras melis*), the squirrel flea (*Ceratophyllus sciurorum*), and the mink flea (*Ceratophyllus vison*).[105] Transmission is by direct contact or exposure in an infested environment.[9,29,69,73] Ferrets react to fleas with mild to intense pruritus, particularly on the back or nape of the neck.[6,29,66,69,74,81] Ferrets can develop a flea bite hypersensitivity, leading to papulocrustous dermatitis and self-induced alopecia over the tail base, ventral abdomen, and caudomedial thighs.[6,29,69,74,81,105] Severe flea infestations may cause anemia.[6] The diagnosis is made based on clinical signs and identification of fleas or flea dirt on the animal.[6,9,69,74,81]

## Treatment and Prevention

No flea treatment products are labeled for use in ferrets by the US Department of Agriculture.[29] For effective eradication of fleas, the animal and the environment must be treated at the same time.[29,66,69,74,81] Although pyrethrins are relatively safe, the effect is short-lived and frequent treatments are often required.[6,9,29] Organophosphates and dichlorvos-impregnated collars can be toxic to ferrets and are not recommended.[6,29,81]

Lufenuron (Program; Novartis Animal Health, Greensboro, North Carolina) at 45 mg orally once monthly has been suggested for use in ferrets.[29] Lufenuron prevents flea eggs from hatching but requires the bite of a flea to be effective.[6]

Fipronil 9.7% solution (Frontline Top Spot; Merial) at 0.2 to 0.4 mL topically every 30 days has also been suggested as a safe and effective topical flea product.[6,29,74]

Imidacloprid (Advantage; Bayer) administered topically to ferrets at 10 mg/kg using a 10% weight/volume solution removed the adult flea population and provided a high level of protection against reinfection for 1 week in one study. No adverse effects were observed.[75] In one clinical study in ferrets,[105] 0.40 mL of a combination of imidacloprid (10%) and moxidectin (1%) in a spot-on formulation (Advantage Multi for Cats; Bayer) was 100% effective in eliminating fleas and was more than 90% effective in preventing reinfestation 4 weeks after treatment. No local or systemic adverse effects were observed.[105]

Selamectin (Revolution) has been advocated for use in the treatment of flea infestations in ferrets.[6,29] In one clinical trial, selamectin was topically applied to ferrets at 6 or 18 mg/kg. Both doses were 100% effective in eliminating flea infestation for between 7 and 21 days after treatment.[73] Monthly topical application of 15-mg selamectin per ferret has also been suggested to control flea infestations.[73]

## OTODECTES CYNOTIS

The common ear mite of dogs and cats (*Otodectes cynotis*) can also be a clinical problem for ferrets.[9,29,66,69,74,106,107] The life cycle is direct and requires 3 weeks for completion.[9,69] Transmission is through direct contact with infected animals or contaminated debris.[9,66,69] Most ferrets are asymptomatic, but some ferrets may scratch at their ears or shake their heads.[6,9,29,66,69,74] Dark brown waxy to crusty ear debris is frequently present in unaffected ferrets but can be a sign of infection (**Fig. 4**).[6,29,66,74] Secondary otitis interna with head tilt, circling, and signs of Horner syndrome has been reported with heavy infestations or overzealous ear cleanings.[6,9,29,69,74] Mites can also spread to other anatomic locations, such as the perineum.[74] The diagnosis is made through direct visualization of moving adults in the ear canal or aural debris, or by microscopic visualization of the mites, larvae, or eggs in the ear debris (**Fig. 5**).[9,29,66,69,74] With disseminated infections, skin scrapings may be necessary to obtain a diagnosis.[6]

## Treatment

If the aural debris is excessive, the ear canals can be gently cleaned.[9,74] All affected and in-contact animals should be treated.[9,69,74] Ivermectin administered parenterally every 2 weeks for three to four treatments can eradicate infections.[6,74] Ivermectin has

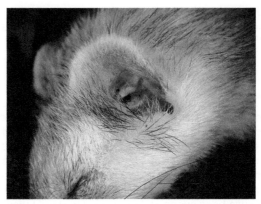

**Fig. 4.** Left ear canal of a ferret demonstrating a small amount of brown ceruminous exudate. *Otodectes cynotis* mites and eggs were identified in the exudate.

been found to be more effective when applied topically to the ear canals than when administered systemically.[6,9,66,69,74] A commercially available ivermectin 0.01% suspension (Acarexx; IDEXX Pharmaceuticals, Greensboro, North Carolina) for use in cats and kittens against *O cynotis* has not been evaluated in ferrets but may hold promise in future studies. When one 0.50-mL ampule was applied to each ear, 94% of cats and kittens were cleared of adult ear mite infestations within 7 to 10 days. Repeat treatment may be necessary with this product.

The ferret ear canal is narrow and flanked by long hairs. As such, it can be challenging to administer medications directly to the ear canal. Several topical spot-on medications are effective against ear mites. Selamectin has been reported to be safe and effective when used topically at 45 mg per ferret,[107] at 15 mg per ferret,[73] or at 6 mg/kg 28 days apart.[6,29,74] Although thiabendazole (Tresaderm; Merial) has historic use in the treatment of ear mite infestations in ferrets, treatment failures reportedly are common with this product.[6] Several other effective topical treatments labeled for use in cats and dogs for the treatment of ear mites, including MilbeMite Otic (0.1% milbemycin oxime; Novartis Animal Health) and Advantage Multi for Cats (Bayer) may also prove effective in ferrets but have yet to be studied in this species.

## SARCOPTIC MANGE

Sarcoptic mange is rare in ferrets, especially in animals kept indoors.[6,69] The mite, *Sarcoptes scabiei*, is the same organism that affects dogs and cats[9,29,74] and dogs

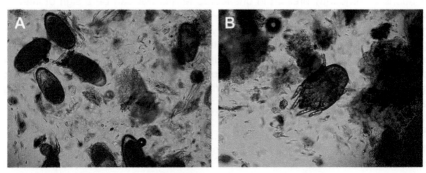

**Fig. 5.** *Otodectes cynotis* eggs (A) and an adult mite (B) from a ferret.

can provide a natural source of infection to ferrets.[6,66] Transmission is by direct contact with an infected host or through fomites.[9,69] There are two clinical forms of disease: a generalized form and a pedal form.[6,66,69] In the generalized form, there is focal to generalized alopecia with intense pruritus often involving the face, pinnae, and ventrum. In the pedal form, lesions are present only on the feet.[9,29,66,69,74] The paws and toes are often inflamed, swollen, crusted, and intensely pruritic.[6,69] Nails can become deformed and even slough if left untreated.[6,9,29,74] Although mites, larvae, ova, and nymphs can be observed on skin scraping samples, false negatives are common.[6,9,29,66,74] The collection of multiple skin scrapes from less excoriated areas is recommended.[69]

## Treatment

All affected and in-contact animals must be treated.[66,74] Cages and bedding should be thoroughly cleaned every 3 to 4 days during treatment.[66,74] Secondary bacterial skin infections should be treated with appropriate antibiotics.[6,9,29] In the pedal form, affected paws should be treated with soaking, nail trimming, and careful removal of crust.[9,74] Ivermectin can be administered subcutaneously every 7 to 14 days until the mites are eradicated.[29,66,69,74] A whole-body lime sulfur dip every 7 days until 2 weeks after clinical resolution may be effective.[6,9] Anecdotally, topical selamectin has been reported effective, although trials have not been done in ferrets.[6] Clients should be cautioned regarding the zoonotic potential of this disease.[66]

## DEMODICOSIS

Demodex sp is present in the skin of many mammal species and is generally not considered contagious.[9] Clinical signs in ferrets include alopecia and seborrhea of the skin behind the ears, in the inguinal area, and on the tail. A brown ceruminous aural exudate may be present.[9,29,108] Demodex mites can be observed on deep skin scrapings, biopsy samples, and in aural debris.[29] Observation of a substantial number of mites, eggs, and immature forms is required to make a diagnosis.[9,108] In chronic cases, the skin may be so thickened that skin scrapings may be unrewarding, requiring biopsy for diagnosis.[9] A potentially new species of Demodex was discovered in skin scrapings and biopsies from two ferrets with localized alopecia, yellowish skin, and pruritus.[69] Both ferrets had been treated repeatedly for ear mites with an ointment containing the immunosuppressive glucocorticoid triamcinolone acetate, which was considered a potentially predisposing factor for these animals. The ferrets responded to a series of amitraz dips and topical application to the ears.[69] In dogs, there is good evidence for recommending treatment with macrocyclic lactones, including ivermectin (0.3–0.60 mg/kg every 24 hours), milbemycin oxime (2 mg/kg every 24 hours), and moxidectin (0.4 mg/kg every 24 hours).[100] Although these drugs may hold promise in the treatment of generalized demodicosis in ferrets, clinical trials have not been performed in this species.

## OTHER MITES AND TICKS

The fur mite, Lynsacarus mustelae, was observed in five ferret kits that had ulcerative dermal lesions on the face. The infection responded to topical application of a permethrin powder and cage cleansing with a permethrin-containing shampoo.[29] Ticks are common in ferrets used for hunting and those housed outdoors and can potentially transmit zoonotic diseases to exposed humans.[29,66] Heavy infestations can cause anemia.[66] Ixodes ricinus is an important tick of ferrets.[66] Ticks can be removed manually or treated with systemic ivermectin at 0.40 mg/kg.[66] Sprays labeled for use in cats can generally be used safely on ferrets.[29]

## MYIASIS

The natural hosts for *Cuterebra* larvae include rabbits, squirrels, chipmunks, and mice. Ferrets are rarely affected but may become exposed if they are housed outdoors in warm weather.[29,74] The diagnosis is generally made when the fly larvae pupate in the subcutaneous tissues, resulting in the appearance of palpable subcutaneous swellings about 1 to 3 cm in diameter, most commonly over the back and in the axillary, inguinal, and ventral cervical regions.[29,74] The larva produces a distinct breathing hole visible through the fur. To remove the larvae, the ferret should be anesthetized and a small incision made over the site. The larva should be carefully removed intact.[74] Broad-spectrum antibiotics should be administered to prevent or treat secondary bacterial infections. Larval forms of *Hypoderma bovis* reportedly have been associated with the formation of granulomatous masses in the cervical area in ferrets.[29] Fly strike caused by the flesh fly *Wohlfahrtia vigil* has been reported in ferret ranches and ferrets housed outdoors.[29] Kits are generally attacked during the summer months at 4 to 5 weeks of age.[29] The eggs are laid on face, neck, and flanks, and the larvae bore through the skin, leading to the formation of subcutaneous abscesses.[29]

## ACKNOWLEDGMENTS

The author thanks Pam Sessoms for assistance in obtaining many of the referenced articles and Kim Hull for graciously providing subject material for photography.

## REFERENCES

1. Church RR. Ferret-polecat domestication: genetic, taxonomic and phylogenetic relationships. In: Lewington LH, editor. Ferret husbandry, medicine & surgery. Philadelphia: WB Saunders; 2008. p. 122.
2. Salih MM, Friis NF. Arseculeratne. *Mycoplasma mustelae*, a new species from mink. Int J Syst Bacteriol 1983;33:476–9.
3. Rosenthal KL. Antibiotic treatment protocols for small mammal bacterial diseases. Proceedings of the North American Veterinary Conference. Orlando (FL); 2007. p. 1676–768.
4. O'Rourke J, Lee A, Fox JG. An ultrastructural study of *Helicobacter mustelae* and evidence of a specific association with gastric mucosa. J Med Microbiol 1992;36(6):420–7.
5. Fox JG, Marini RP. *Helicobacter mustelae* infection in ferrets: pathogenesis, epizootiology, diagnosis, and treatment. Semin Avian Exotic Pet Med 2001; 10(1):36–44.
6. Oglesbee BL. The 5-minute veterinary consult: ferret and rabbit. Ames (IA): Blackwell Publishing; 2006.
7. Johnson-Delaney CA. The ferret gastrointestinal tract and *Helicobacter mustelae* infection. Vet Clin North Am Exotic Anim Pract 2005;8:197–212.
8. Hoefer HL, Bell JA. Gastrointestinal diseases. In: Carpenter JW, Quesenberry KE, editors. Ferrets, rabbits, and rodents: clinical medicine and surgery. 2nd edition. St. Louis (MO): Saunders; 2000. p. 25–40.
9. Marini RP, Otto G, Erdman S, et al. Biology and diseases of ferrets. In: Fox JG, Anderson LC, Loew FM, et al, editors. Laboratory animal medicine. 2nd edition. Amsterdam: Academic Press; 2002. p. 483–517.

10. Lennox A. Working up gastrointestinal disease in the ferret. Presented at the CVC East Proceedings. Baltimore, MD, April 18–21, 2008.

11. Solnick JV, Schauer DB. Emergence of diverse *Helicobacter* species in the pathogenesis of gastric and enterohepatic disease. Clin Microbiol Rev 2001;14(1): 59–97.

12. Erdman SE, Correa P, Coleman LA, et al. *Helicobacter mustelae*-associated gastric MALT lymphoma in ferrets. Am J Pathol 1997;151(1):273–80.

13. Garcia A, Erdman SE, Xu S, et al. Hepatobiliary inflammation, neoplasia, and argyrophilic bacteria in a ferret colony. Vet Pathol 2002;39(2):173–9.

14. Erdman SE, Correa P, Li X, et al. *Helicobacter mustelae*-associated gastric lymphoma in four ferrets. Lab Anim Sci 1996;46:455–6.

15. Croinin TO, Clyne M, Appelmelk BJ, et al. Antigastric autoantibodies in ferrets naturally infected with *Helicobacter mustelae*. Infect Immun 2001;69(4):2708–13.

16. Fox JG, Dangler CA, Sager W, et al. *Helicobacter mustelae*-associated gastric adenocarcinoma in ferrets (*Mustela putorius furo*). Vet Pathol 1997; 34:225–9.

17. McColm AA, Bagshaw JA, O'Malley CF. Development of a 14C-urea breath test in ferrets colonised with *Helicobacter mustelae*: effects of treatment with bismuth, antibiotics, and urease inhibitors. Gut 1993;34:181–6.

18. Bland MV, Ismail S, Heinemann JA, et al. The action of bismuth against *Helicobacter pylori* mimics but is not caused by intracellular iron deprivation. Antimicrob Agents Chemother 2004;48(6):1983–8.

19. Blanco MC, Fox JG, Palley LS. Eradication of *Helicobacter mustelae* infection in the ferret: efficacy of multiple antibiotic therapies [abstract]. Contemp Top Lab Anim Sci 1993;32:15.

20. Batchelder M, Fox JG, Hayward A, et al. Natural and experimental *Helicobacter mustelae* reinfection following successful antimicrobial eradication in ferrets. Helicobacter 1996;1:34–42.

21. Marini RP, Fox JG, Taylor NS, et al. Ranitidine bismuth citrate and clarithromycin alone or in combination, for eradication of *Helicobacter mustelae* infection in ferrets. Am J Vet Res 1999;60(10):1280–6.

22. Alder JD, Ewing PJ, Mitten MJ, et al. Relevance of the ferret model of *Helicobacter*-induced gastritis to evaluation of antibacterial therapies. Am J Gastroenterol 1996;91:2347–54.

23. Stables R, Campbell CJ, Clayton NM, et al. Gastric antisecretory, mucosal protective, anti-pepsin and anti- *Helicobacter* properties of ranitidine bismuth citrate. Aliment Pharmacol Ther 1993;7:237–46.

24. Otto G, Fox JG, Wu P, et al. Eradication of *Helicobacter mustelae* from the ferret stomach: an animal model of *Helicobacter (Campylobacter) pylori* chemotherapy. Antimicrob Agents Chemother 1990;34(6):1232–6.

25. Czinn SJ, Bierman JC, Diters RW, et al. Characterization and therapy for experimental infection by *Helicobacter mustelae* in ferrets. Helicobacter 1996;1(1):43–51.

26. Fox JG, Dewhirst FE, Fraser GJ, et al. Intracellular *Campylobacter*-like organism from ferrets and hamsters with proliferative bowel disease is a *Desulfovibrio* sp. J Clin Microbiol 1994;32(5):1229–37.

27. Fox JG. Bacterial and mycoplasmal diseases. In: Fox JG, editor. Biology and diseases of the ferret. 2nd edition. Baltimore (MD): Williams & Wilkins; 1998. p. 321–54.

28. Rosenthal KL. Respiratory disease. In: Carpenter JW, Quesenberry KE, editors. Ferrets, rabbits, and rodents: clinical medicine and surgery. 2nd edition. St. Louis (MO): Saunders; 2000. p. 72–8.

29. Orcutt C. Dermatologic diseases. In: Carpenter JW, Quesenberry KE, editors. Ferrets, rabbits, and rodents: clinical medicine and surgery. 2nd edition. St. Louis (MO): Saunders; 2000. p. 107–14.

30. Carpenter JW. Exotic animal formulary. 3rd edition. St. Louis (MO): Elsevier Saunders; 2001. p. 447–51.

31. Kreuger KL, Murphy JC, Fox JG. Treatment of proliferative colitis in ferrets. J Am Vet Med Assoc 1989;194(10):1435–6.

32. Songer JG, Post KW. Veterinary microbiology: bacterial and fungal agents of animal disease. St. Louis (MO): Saunders; 2005. p. 95–109.

33. Larson DJ, Hoffman LJ. Isolation of Campylobacter coli from a proliferative intestinal lesion in a ferret. J Vet Diagn Invest 1990;2(3):238–9.

34. Fox JG, Ackerman JI, Taylor NS, et al. Campylobacter jejuni infection in the ferret: an animal model of human campylobacteriosis. Am J Vet Res 1987; 48(1):85–90.

35. Bell JA, Manning DD. Pathogenicity of Campylobacter jejuni in intraperitoneally or intravenously inoculated ferrets. Curr Microbiol 1990;21:47–51.

36. Bell JA, Manning DD. Reproductive failure in mink and ferrets after intravenous or oral inoculation of Campylobacter jejuni. Can J Vet Res 1990;54(4): 432–7.

37. Fox JG, Moore R, Ackerman JI. Canine and feline campylobacteriosis: epizootiology and clinical and public health features. J Am Vet Med Assoc 1983; 183(12):1420–4.

38. Hunter DB, Prescott JF, Hoover DM, et al. Campylobacter jejuni colitis in ranch mink in Ontario. Can J Vet Res 1986;50(1):47–53.

39. Lennox AM. Novel exotic animal diagnostics. Exotic DVM 2005;7(4):27–30.

40. Liberson AJ, Newcomer CE, Ackerman JI, et al. Mastitis caused by hemolytic Escherichia coli in the ferret. J Am Vet Med Assoc 1983;183(11):1179–81.

41. Bradley GA, Orr K, Reggiardo C, et al. Enterotoxigenic Escherichia coli infection in captive black-footed ferrets. J Wildl Dis 2001;37(3):617–20.

42. Fox JG, Pearson RC, Bell JA. Diseases of the genitourinary system. In: Fox JG, editor. Biology and diseases of the ferret. 2nd edition. Baltimore (MD): Williams & Wilkins; 1998. p. 247–72.

43. Woods JB, Schmitt CK, Darnell SC, et al. Ferrets as a model system for renal disease secondary to intestinal infection with Escherichia coli O157:H7 and other shiga toxin–producing E. coli. J Infect Dis 2002;185(4):550–4.

44. Moll T, Brandly CA. Botulism in mouse, mink and ferret with special reference to susceptibility and pathological alterations. Am J Vet Res 1951;12(45): 355–63.

45. Harrison SG, Borland ED. Deaths in ferrets (Mustela putorius) due to Clostridium botulinum type C. Vet Rec 1973;93(22):576–7.

46. Schulman FY, Montali RJ, Hauer PJ. Gastroenteritis associated with Clostridium perfringens type A in black-footed ferrets (Mustela nigripes). Vet Pathol 1993; 30(3):308–10.

47. Montiani-Ferreira F, Mattos BC, Russ HHA. Reference values for selected ophthalmic diagnostic tests of the ferret (Mustela putorius furo). Vet Ophthalmol 2006;9(4):209–13.

48. Sanford BA, Ramsay MA. In vivo localization of Staphylococcus aureus in nasal tissues of healthy and influenza A virus-infected ferrets. Proc Soc Exp Biol Med 1989;191(2):163–9.

49. Peltola VT, Boyd KL, McAuley JL, et al. Bacterial sinusitis and otitis media following influenza virus infection in ferrets. Infect Immun 2006;74(5):2562–7.

50. Bell JA. Periparturient and neonatal diseases. In: Carpenter JW, Quesenberry KE, editors. Ferrets, rabbits, and rodents: clinical medicine and surgery. 2nd edition. St. Louis (MO): Saunders; 2000. p. 50–7.

51. Valheim M, Djonne B, Heiene R, et al. Disseminated *Mycobacterium celatum* (type 3) infection in a domestic ferret (*Mustela putorius furo*). Vet Pathol 2001; 38(4):460–3.

52. de Lisle GW, Kawakami RP, Yates GF, et al. Isolation of *Mycobacterium bovis* and other mycobacterial species from ferrets and stoats. Vet Microbiol 2008; 132:402–7.

53. Lucas J, Lucas A, Furber H, et al. *Mycobacterium genavense* infection in two aged ferrets with conjunctival lesions. Aust Vet J 2000;78:685–9.

54. Caley P, Hone J, Cowen PE. The relationship between prevalence of *Mycobacterium bovis* infection in feral ferrets and possum abundance. N Z Vet J 2001; 49(5):195–200.

55. Jones JW, Pether JVS, Rainey HA, et al. Recurrent *Mycobacterium bovis* infection following a ferret bite. J Infect 1993;26:225–6.

56. Schultheiss PC, Dolginow SZ. Granulomatous enteritis caused by *Mycobacterium avium* in a ferret. J Am Vet Med Assoc 1994;204(8):1217–8.

57. Saunders GK, Thomsen BV. Lymphoma and *Mycobacterium avium* infection in a ferret (*Mustela putorius furo*). J Vet Diagn Invest 2006;18:513–5.

58. Lunn JA, Martin P, Zaki S, et al. Pneumonia due to *Mycobacterium abscessus* in two domestic ferrets (*Mustelo putorius furo*). Aust Vet J 2005;83(9):542–6.

59. Castle KT, Biggins D, Carter LG, et al. Susceptibility of the Siberian polecat to subcutaneous and oral *Yersinia pestis* exposure. J Wildl Dis 2001;37(4): 746–54.

60. Williams ES, Mills ESK, Kwiatkowski DR, et al. Plague in a black-footed ferret (*Mustela nigripes*). J Wildl Dis 1994;30(4):581–5.

61. Williams ES, Thorne ET, Quan TJ, et al. Experimental infection of domestic ferrets (*Mustela putorius furo*) and Siberian polecats (*Mustela eversmanni*) with *Yersinia pestis*. J Wildl Dis 1991;27(3):441–5.

62. Twigg GI, Cuerden CM, Hughes DM. Leptospirosis in British wild mammals. Symp Zool Soc London 1968;24:75–98.

63. Fox JG, Garibaldi BA, Goad MEP, et al. Hyperadrenocorticism in a ferret. J Am Vet Med Assoc 1987;191(3):343–4.

64. Hathaway SC, Blackmore DK. Failure to demonstrate the maintenance of leptospires by free living carnivores. N Z Vet J 1981;29(7):115–6.

65. Pilny AA, Hess L. Ferrets: wound healing and therapy. Vet Clin North Am Exotic Anim Pract 2004;7(1):105–21.

66. Paterson S. Skin diseases of exotic pets. Ames (IA): Blackwell Science; 2006. p. 204–9.

67. Collins BR. Dermatologic disorders of common small non-domestic animals. In: Nesbitt GH, editor. Topics in small animal medicine: dermatology. Volume 8. New York: Churchill Livingstone; 1987. p. 235–394.

68. Erdman SE, Moore FM, Rose R, et al. Malignant lymphoma in ferrets: clinical and pathological findings in 19 cases. J Comp Pathol 1992;106(1):37–47.

69. Patterson M, Fox JG. Parasites of ferrets. In: Baker DG, editor. Flynn's parasites of laboratory animals. 2nd edition. Ames (IA): Blackwell Publishing; 2007. p. 501–8.

70. Abe N, Tanoue T, Ohta G, et al. First record of *Eimeria furonis* infection in a ferret, Japan, with notes on the usefulness of partial small subunit ribosomal RNA gene sequencing analysis for discriminating among *Eimeria* species. Parasitol Res 2008;103:967–70.

71. Li X, Pang J, Fox JG. Coinfection with intracellular *Desulfovibrio* species and coccidia in ferrets with proliferative bowel disease. Lab Anim Sci 1996;46(5):569–71.
72. Williams BH, Chimes MJ, Gardiner CH. Biliary coccidiosis in a ferret (*Mustela putorius furo*). Vet Pathol 1996;33(4):437–9.
73. Fisher M, Beck W, Hutchinson MJ. Efficacy and safety of selamectin (Stronghold/Revolution) used off-label in exotic pets. Intl J Appl Res Vet Med 2007;5: 87–96.
74. Hoppmann E, Barron HW. Ferret and rabbit dermatology. J Exotic Pet Med 2007; 16(4):225–37.
75. Hutchinson MJ, Jacobs DE, Mencke N. Establishment of the cat flea (*Ctenocephalides felis felis*) on the ferret (*Mustela putorius furo*) and its control with imidacloprid. Med Vet Entomol 2001;15:212–4.
76. Abe N, Read C, Thompson RCA, et al. Zoonotic genotype of *Giardia intestinalis* detected in a ferret. J Parasitol 2005;91(1):179–82.
77. Gómez-Couso H, Méndez-Hermida F, Ares-Mazás E. First report of *Cryptosporidium parvum* 'ferret' genotype in American mink (*Mustela vison* Shreber 1777). Parasitol Res 2007;100(4):877–9.
78. Fayera R, Morgan U, Upton SJ. Epidemiology of *Cryptosporidium*: transmission, detection and identification. Int J Parasitol 2000;30(12–13):1305–22.
79. Abe N, Iseki M. Identification of genotypes of *Cryptosporidium parvum* isolates from ferrets in Japan. Parasitol Res 2003;89(5):422–4.
80. Jones YL, Fitzgerald SD, Sikarske JG, et al. Toxoplasmosis in a free-ranging mink. J Wildl Dis 2006;42(4):865–9.
81. Fox JG. Parasitic diseases. In: Fox JG, editor. Biology and diseases of the ferret. 2nd edition. Baltimore (MD): Williams & Wilkins; 1998. p. 375–91.
82. Thornton RN, Cook TG. A congenital *Toxoplasma*-like disease in ferrets (*Mustela putorius furo*). N Z Vet J 1986;34(3):31–3.
83. Burns R, Williams ES, O'Toole D, et al. *Toxoplasma gondii* infections in captive black-footed ferrets (*Mustela nigripes*), 1992–1998: clinical signs, serology, pathology, and prevention. J Wildl Dis 2003;39(4):787–97.
84. Ramos-Vera JA, Dubey JP, Watson GL, et al. Sarcocystosis in mink (*Mustela vison*). J Parasitol 1997;83(6):1198–201.
85. McAllister M, Wills RA, McGuire AM, et al. Ingestion of *Neospora caninum* tissue cysts by Mustela species. Int J Parasitol 1999;29(10):1531–6.
86. Sobrino R, Dubey JP, Pabon M, et al. *Neospora caninum* antibodies in wild carnivores from Spain. Vet Parasitol 2008;155(3–4):190–7.
87. Petrie JP, Morrisey JK. Cardiovascular and other diseases. In: Carpenter JW, Quesenberry KE, editors. Ferrets, rabbits, and rodents: clinical medicine and surgery. 2nd edition. St. Louis (MO): Saunders; 2000. p. 58–71.
88. McCall JW, Genchi C, Kramer LH, et al. Heartworm disease in animals and humans. Adv Parasitol 2008;66:193–285.
89. McCall JW. Dirofilarisis in the domestic ferret. Clin Tech Small Anim Pract 1998; 13:109–12.
90. Schaper R, Heine J, Arther RG, et al. Imidacloprid plus moxidectin to prevent heartworm infection (*Dirofilaria immitis*) in ferrets. Parasitol Res 2007;101:S57–62.
91. Kemmerer DW. Heartworm disease in the domestic ferret. Recent Advances in Heartworm Disease Symposium. Tampa (FL): 1998. p. 87–9.
92. Antinoff N. Clinical observations in ferrets with naturally occurring heartworm disease and preliminary evaluation of treatment, with ivermectin and with and without melarsomine. Recent Advances in Heartworm Disease Symposium. San Antonio (TX): 2001. p. 45–7.

93. Supakorndej P, McCall JW, Lewis RE, et al. Biology, diagnosis and prevention of heartworm infection in ferrets. Proceedings of the Heartworm Symposium. Batavia (IL): 1992. p. 60–9.

94. Sasaik H, Sasaki KT, Koyamat S, et al. Echocardiographic diagnosis of dirofilariasis in a ferret. J Small Anim Pract 2000;41(4):172–4.

95. Supakorndej P, Lewis RE, McCall JW, et al. Radiographic and angiographic evaluation of ferrets experimentally infected with *Dirofilaria immitis*. Vet Radiol Ultrasound 1995;36(1):23–9.

96. Supakorndej P, McCall JW, Jun JJ. Early migration and development of *Dirofilaria immitis* in the ferret, *Mustela putorius furo*. J Parasitol 1994;80(2): 237–44.

97. Fox JC, Wagner R, Crotty C. Development of a PCR test and an IFA test for Dirofilaria immitis in cats and their use along with an ELISA heartworm antigen test to determine the prevalence of infections in the Tulsa, Oklahoma area. Recent Advances in Heartworm Disease Symposium. Tampa (FL): 1998. p. 167–71.

98. Liu J, Song KH, Lee SE, et al. Serological and molecular survey of *Dirofilaria immitis* infection in stray cats in Gyunggi province, South Korea. Vet Parasitol 2005; 130(1–2):125–9.

99. Cottrell DK. Use of moxidectin (ProHeart 6) as a heartworm adulticide in four ferrets. Exotic DVM 2004;6:9–12.

100. Carlotti DN. Canine and feline demodex. Presented at the World Veterinary Congress. Vancouver, British Columbia, July 27–31, 2008.

101. Mencke N. Managing gastrointestinal helminth infections in small mammals. Proceedings of the North American Veterinary Conference. Orlando (FL): 2007. p. 1665–7.

102. McKenna PB, Cooke MM, Harper PR. Filaroides infections in wild ferrets (*Mustela putorius*) and stoats (*Mustela erminea*). N Z Vet J 1996;44(5):203.

103. Wisely SM, Howard J, Williams SA, et al. An unidentified filarial species and its impact on fitness in wild populations of the black-footed ferret (*Mustela nigripes*). J Wildl Dis 2008;44(1):53–64.

104. Jones A, Pybus MJ. Taeniasis and echinococcosis. In: Samuel WM, Pybus MJ, Kocan AA, editors. Parasitic diseases of wild mammals. 2nd edition. London: Manson Publishing, Ltd; 2001. p. 150–92.

105. Wenzel U, Heine J, Mengel H, et al. Efficacy of imidacloprid 10%/moxidectin 1% (Advocate/Advantage Multi) against fleas (*Ctenocephalides felis felis*) on ferrets (*Mustela putorius furo*). Parasitol Res 2008;103:231–4.

106. Lohse J, Rinder H, Gothe R, et al. Validity of species status of the parasitic mite *Otodectes cyanotis*. Med Vet Entomol 2002;16:133–8.

107. Miller DS, Eagle RP, Zabel S, et al. Efficacy and safety of selamectin in the treatment of *Otodectes cynotis* infestation in domestic ferrets. Vet Rec 2006;159(22): 748.

108. Noli C, van der Horst HHA, Willemse T. Demodicosis in ferrets (*Mustela putorius furo*). Vet Q 1996;18:28–31.

# Parasites of Captive Nonhuman Primates

Cathy A. Johnson-Delaney, DVM, Dipl ABVP-Avian*

KEYWORDS

• Nonhuman primate • Monkey • Endoparasite • Ectoparasite
• Protozoa • Zoonosis

Captive nonhuman primates include the prosimians (lemurs, bushbabies), new world primates (callitrichids: eg, marmosets, tamarins; cebids: eg, owl, squirrel, capuchin, spider monkeys), old world primates (cercopithecids: eg, vervets, guenons, macaques, baboons; colobids: eg, colobus, langurs), lesser apes (gibbons, siamangs) and great apes (bonobos, chimpanzees, orangutans, and gorillas) (see primate taxonomy in **Table 1**).[1] With the exception of wild-caught or feral-reared primates imported for laboratory animal use, most important in the United States are small numbers of zoologic species. The large numbers of colony/feral/wild-caught primates for laboratory use are primarily macaques (*Macaca* sp) collected from China or Southeast Asia. Smaller numbers of green monkeys (*Chlorocebus aethiops*) are imported from free-ranging island colonies in the Caribbean. A small number of marmosets, tamarins, and squirrel monkeys are imported for laboratory animal use from captive colonies in South America. These importations for use in laboratory animal medicine have parasite issues addressed within the federal quarantine program and often reflect conditions of exposure in the country of origin. Blood-borne parasites, such as *Plasmodium* sp, are more likely to be primate-host specific and should be identified and treated during or just after the federal quarantine period. Primate malaria does not seem to be maintained or amplified in outdoor captive primate facilities within North America, although if the appropriate vector was present, such infections could possibly occur. Continued surveillance and sentinel programs to monitor outdoor populations, particularly in tropical climates, should be established and promoted.

Zoo-dwelling nonhuman primates are regularly tested and treated and are unlikely to have disease associated with severe infections or infestations unlike those imported for laboratory animal use. Pet or privately owned individual monkeys with appropriate veterinary care rarely have intestinal or ectoparasites after initial examination and, if necessary, treatment. The exception to this is fleas or mites usually acquired in relation to other pets in the home.

Eastside Avian and Exotic Animal Medical Center, 13603 100th Avenue NE, Kirkland, WA 98034, USA
* Corresponding author.
E-mail address: cajddvm@hotmail.com

Vet Clin Exot Anim 12 (2009) 563–581
doi:10.1016/j.cvex.2009.07.002
1094-9194/09/$ – see front matter © 2009 Elsevier Inc. All rights reserved.

**Table 1**
**Taxonomy and common names of common captive nonhuman primates**

| Latin Name | Common Names |
| --- | --- |
| Prosimians | |
| *Galago senagalensis* | Lesser bush baby, northern bush baby |
| *Otolemur garnettii* | Greater bush baby, Garnett's greater bush baby |
| *Lemur catta (Eulemur catta)* | Ring-tailed lemur |
| *Varecia variegate* | Ruffed lemur |
| *Eulemur fulvus* | Brown lemur |
| New world monkeys | |
| *Callithrix jacchus* | Common marmoset, white-eared or white-tufted marmoset |
| *Callithrix penicillata* | Black tufted-eared marmoset |
| *Callithrix pygmaea* (previously *Cebuella pygmaeus*) | Pygmy marmoset |
| *Saguinus geoffroyi* | Geoffroy's tamarin, red-crested tamarin |
| *Saguinus labiatus* | Red-bellied tamarin |
| *Saguinus midas* | Golden-handed or red-handed tamarin |
| *Saguinus oedipus* | Cotton-top tamarin |
| *Leontopithecus rosalia* | Golden lion tamarin |
| *Aotus trivirgatus* | Gray-necked owl monkey, dourocouli |
| *Callicebus personatus* | Titi monkey, masked titi monkey |
| *Cebus albifrons* | White-fronted capuchin |
| *Cebus paella* | Tufted or brown capuchin |
| *Cebus cabucinus* | White-throated, white-faced capuchin |
| *Saimiri boliviensis* | Bolivian squirrel monkey |
| *Saimiri sciureus* | Common squirrel monkey |
| *Pithecia pithecia* | White-faced saki |
| *Alouatta* sp | Howler monkeys |
| *Ateles geoffroyi* | Black-handed spider monkey |
| Old world monkeys | |
| *Macaca arctoides* | Stump-tailed macaque |
| *Macaca fascicularis* | Long-tailed, crab-eating, cynomolgus, Java macaque |
| *Macaca fuscata* | Japanese or snow monkey, macaque |
| *Macaca mulatta* | Rhesus macaque |
| *Macaca nemestrina* | Pig-tailed macaque |
| *Macaca nigra* | Celebes, crested black macaque |
| *Macaca silenus* | Lion-tailed macaque, wanderoo |
| *Papio* sp | Baboons |
| *Mandrillus sphinx* | Mandrill |
| *Cercocebus torquatus atys* | Sooty mangabey |
| *Erythrocebus patas* | Patas monkey |
| *Chlorocebus aethiops* | Vervet, grivet, or green monkey |
| *Cercopithecus diana* | Diana monkey |
| *Cercopithecus neglectus* | De Brazza's monkey |

*(continued on next page)*

| Table 1 (continued) | |
| --- | --- |
| **Latin Name** | **Common Names** |
| Colobus guereza | Abysinnian, Guereza, or eastern black and white colobus |
| Semnopithecus entellus, Presbytis entellus | Hanuman langur |
| Pygathrix nemaeus | Douc langur, red-shanked douc |
| Lesser apes | |
| Hylobates lar | White-handed gibbon |
| Hylobates (Symphalangus) syndactylus | Siamang |
| Great apes | |
| Pongo sp | Orangutans |
| Gorilla gorilla | Lowland gorilla |
| Bonobo paniscus, Pan paniscus | Bonobo |
| Pan troglodytes | Chimpanzee |

Taxonomy is often under review and frequently disputed among primatologists.
*Data From* Hawkins JV, Clapp NK, Carson RL, et al. Diagnosis and treatment of Trichospirura leptosoma infection in common marmosets (Callithrix jacchus). Contemp Topics 1997;36:52–5.

Nonhuman primates are also susceptible to parasitic infections from other animals and humans, although they are not the primary host. These usually do cause disease and may be more difficult to diagnose and treat. Included in this group are toxoplasmosis, giardiasis, *Cryptosporidia* sp, *Sarcoptes* sp, *Baylisascaris procyonis*, *Ctenophalides felis*, pentastomiasis, dirofilariasis, and a wide variety of ticks and mites.

## SELECTED PARASITIC DISEASE OF PROSIMIANS

Practitioners are most likely to encounter gastrointestinal parasites. These include the protozoa: *Entamoeba* sp, *Trichomonas* sp, *Giardia* sp, and *Balantidium* sp. In large numbers, most of these cause clinical diarrhea. Detection is by means of direct fecal examination and common laboratory stains and test kits for *Giardia*. Gastrointestinal nematodes include *Strongylus*, *Strongyloides*, *Gongylonema*, *Physaloptera*, *Enterobius*, *Trichuris*, oxyurids, and ascarids. Ova are readily found in fecal flotation testing, with the exception of *Physaloptera*, which is only shed intermittently and may be difficult to find. Most respond well to common anthelminthics as listed in **Table 2**. Aberrant tapeworm larvae have caused hydatid disease and cysticercosis in lemurs and galagos. The primate consumes eggs from the canid tapeworm *Echinococcus granulosus* or *Taenia crassiceps*. Larvae develop into cysts in body cavities. Depending on the size and location of the cysts, drainage or surgical removal of the cysts may be necessary.

*Toxoplasma gondii* causes serious systemic disease, particularly in lemurs. Death is often peracute, with some cases following a 1- to 2-day course of nonspecific signs, such as depression and inappetence. Rarely, a more chronic neurologic form occurs, with signs that include ataxia, depression, head tilt, circling, anorexia, and paresis. Clinical pathologic findings may include elevations in liver and renal enzyme values and generalized stress and inflammation. Diagnosis can be made with paired serum samples or by histopathologic examination of many tissues demonstrating

**Table 2**
Prosimian parasite summary

| Disease | Agent | Location in Host | Transmission | Diagnosis | Treatment and Management |
|---|---|---|---|---|---|
| Stomach worms | *Physaloptera* | Stomach | Oral, intermediate host: cockroach | Fecal flotation, repeated | Levamisole, 2.5 mg/kg po q 24 h × 14 d<br>Fenbendazole, 50 mg/kg po q 24 h × 3 d<br>Vermin control |
| Hydatid disease | *Echinococcus*, *Taenia* | Muscle, organs, body cavities (aberrant host) | Canid host, ingestion ova from feces | Radiography, ultrasound, aspiration | Drain<br>Surgical removal<br>Prevent exposure to canid feces |
| Toxoplasmosis | *Toxoplasma gondii* | Systemic, multiple organs, nervous system | Ingestion ova from feline feces | Serology, cerebrospinal fluid tap, histopathologic examination | Sulfas<br>Supportive care<br>Prevent exposure to feline feces |
| Filariasis | *Dipetalonema* (presumed) | Peripheral blood | Bite from mosquito | Blood smear | Insect control<br>Protocols based on dogs or humans |
| Cerebral larval migrans | *Baylisascaris procyonis* | Brain, lemur aberrant host | Ingestion of ova from raccoon feces | Usually postmortem histologic examination of brain | Ivermectin has been tried at 0.2–0.4 mg/kg q 7 d<br>Supportive care<br>Prevent raccoon access to primate housing |

| | | | | |
|---|---|---|---|---|
| Intestinal nematodes | *Strongylus, Strongyloides, Gongylonema, Trichuris,* oxyurids, ascarids, *Enterobius* | Gastrointestinal tract | Ingestion ova (direct fecal-oral) | Fecal flotation | Ivermectin, 0.2–0.4 mg/kg sc, im, or po Thiabendazole, 50 mg/kg po Pyrantel, 5–10 mg/kg po q 24 h × 3 d Fenbendazole, 50 mg/kg po q 24 h × 8 d All treatments may need to be repeated at intervals |
| Protozoal infections | *Balantidium coli, Giardia* sp, *Entamoeba* sp, *Cryptosporidia* sp | Gastrointestinal tract | Ingestion, flora disruption, immunosuppression | Direct fecal cytology, trichrome staining, commercial *Giardia* test kits | Metronidazole, 25 mg/kg po q 24 h × 7 d Paromomycin, 15 mg/kg po q 12 h × 7 d No treatment directly for *Cryptosporidia* |

*Abbreviations:* d, days; h, hours; im, intramuscular; po, orally; q, every; sc, subcutaneous.

*Data from* Junge RE. Prosimians. In: Fowler ME, Miller RE, editors. Zoo and wild animal medicine. 5th edition. St. Louis (MO); 2003. p. 334–46; and Valverde CR. Primates. In: Carpenter JW, editor. Exotic animal formulary. 3rd edition. St. Louis (MO): Elsevier Saunders; 2005. p. 495–534.

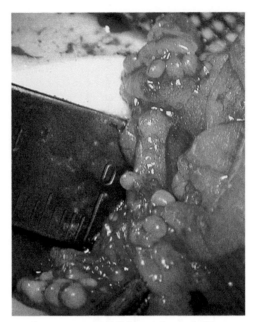

**Fig. 1.** Small cestode cysts from a macaque (*Macaca fascicularis*).

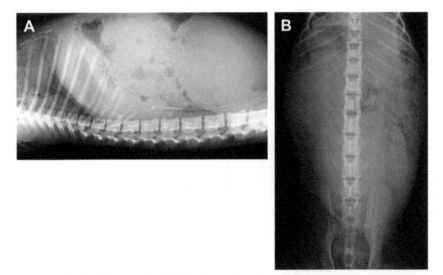

**Fig. 2.** Lateral (*A*) and ventrodorsal (*B*) radiographs of abdomen young female *Macaca fascicularis* with hydatid cysts. There is an increase in abdominal opacification and loss of normal visceral detail.

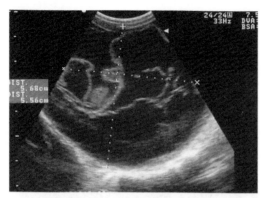

**Fig. 3.** Ultrasonography of abdomen of macaque with hydatid cysts. Thin-walled fluid-filled cysts may be seen.

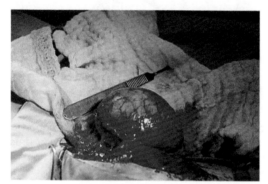

**Fig. 4.** Removal of hydatid cysts from young female macaque in **Fig. 3** at exploratory laparotomy.

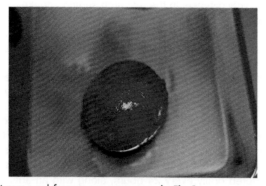

**Fig. 5.** Hydatid cyst removed from young macaque in **Fig. 3**.

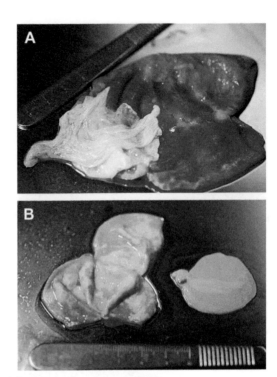

**Fig. 6.** Opened cyst from young macaque in **Fig. 3.**

tachyzoites. The disease is transmitted by ingestion of oocytes from infected cat feces. Treatment may be attempting using parenteral sulfa drugs and supportive care but is usually unsuccessful. Prevention is by excluding housecats from areas inhabited by the monkeys.

## MONKEYS AND APES

As mentioned previously, the parasite load of recently imported nonhuman primates is different than that of long-time captive residents. Because of sanitation, many parasites with direct life cycles can be eliminated over time with repeated treatments. Many cause little clinical disease. In the research setting, monkeys must be parasite-free; thus, even blood parasitic infections must be treated.

Pet nonhuman primates are frequently presented with fleas acquired through contact with household dogs and cats. The author has successfully used topical treatments as used in cats on several species. Human head lice have been transmitted from children in the household. Control is as with the infested children and household, using over-the-counter products. Use described on the label for application and frequency has been successful. Sarcoptes mites are not infrequently found and, again, are usually acquired from another member of the household. These cause intense pruritus and dermatitis. Treatment includes ivermectin at 0.2 to 0.4 mg/kg administered subcutaneously every 7 days along with an antihistamine, such as diphenhydramine at 2 to 5 mg/kg administered orally every 8 hours or meloxicam at 0.2 mg/kg administered orally every 24 hours, along with an antibiotic if secondary bacteria infection is present from self-inflicted wounds.

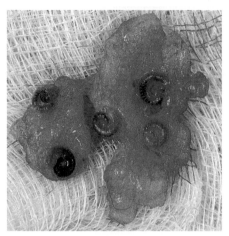

**Fig. 7.** Pentastomids from a macaque (*Macaca fascicularis*). Pentastomids were found throughout the mesentery. (*From* Johnson-Delaney CA. Reptile zoonoses and threats to public health. In: Mader DR, editor. Reptile medicine and surgery. 2nd edition. St. Louis (MO): Elsevier; 2006. p. 1017–30; with permission.)

Imported macaques for laboratory animal use have been found with a variety of parasites when placed into federally regulated Centers for Disease Control and Prevention quarantine. In the author's experience, those from Asia have been found with lice, *Sarcoptes* sp, pentastomids, acanthocephalids, various nematodes, cystocerciasis (hydatid disease), human liver flukes (*Gastrodiscoides hominis*), and cestodiasis (**Fig. 1**). Treatment within the mandated 31-day quarantine period included ivermectin at 0.4 mg/kg administered subcutaneously every 14 days and praziquantel at 40 mg/kg administered intramuscularly every 30 days (trematode dosage). Hydatid cysts would be drained (see **Fig. 1; Figs. 2** and **3**) or surgically removed (**Figs. 4–6**)

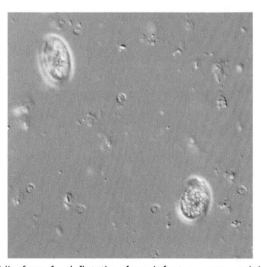

**Fig. 8.** Cryptosporidia from fecal flotation from infant macaque, original magnification ×1000.

**Table 3**
Nonhuman primate parasite disease summary

| Disease | Agent | Species Affected | Location in Host | Transmission | Diagnosis | Treatment and Management |
|---|---|---|---|---|---|---|
| Strongyloidiasis | *Strongyloides* sp. | Fatalities in patas, woolly monkeys | Intestinal tract | Eggs in feces, direct life cycle | FF | Sanitation Anthelminthics: thiabendazole, 50 mg/kg po q 24 h × 2 d, repeat in 21 d; ivermectin, 0.2–0.4 mg/kg po, repeat in 14–21 d; levamisole, 10 mg/kg po, repeat as needed |
| Pinworms | *Enterobius vermicularis* | Old world monkeys | Colon | Direct, ova spread air and dust, fecal/oral | FF, cellophane tape to perianal/perineal swabs | Ivermectin, 0.2–0.4 mg/kg po, repeat in 14–21 d; piperazine, 605 mg/kg po q 24 h × 10 d; pyrantel pamoate, 11 mg/kg po once, may repeat if needed |
| Trichuris | *Trichuris trichiura* | Old world monkeys | Gastrointestinal tract | Direct life cycle, fecal/oral | FF | Sanitation Levamisole, 10 mg/kg po, repeat as needed; ivermectin, 0.2–0.4 g/kg po, repeat in 14–21 d |

| Disease | Organism | Host | Location | Life cycle | Diagnosis | Treatment |
|---|---|---|---|---|---|---|
| Oesophagostomiasis | Oesophagostomum sp | Old world monkeys | Colon | Direct life cycle, larvae hatch in stool 48 hours, larvae are ingested and then penetrate colon wall | FF | Anthelminthics as above Sanitation |
| Trichospirura leptosoma | Trichospirura leptosoma | Callitrichids[3] | Pancreas | Indirect, cockroach | Formalin-ether sedimentation of stool, pancreatic biopsy | Fenbendazole, 50 mg/kg po q 24 h × 14 d Prevent cockroaches in habitat |
| Filariasis | Loa loa, Dipetalonema immitis, Onchocerca volvulus, etc. | Drills, baboons, mangabeys, vervets, Asian monkeys | Adult worms live outside digestive tract, female worms produce microfilaria | Indirect life cycle, blood-sucking insect vectors, microfilaria in peripheral blood and subcutaneous tissue | Blood spear, detection of microfilaria above buffy coat in spun hematocrit tube under microscope | Insect control Diethylcarbamazine, several regimens depending on species |
| Heartworm | Dirofilaria immitis | Pale-headed saki monkey[5] | Adult worm in heart | Dog/cat heartworm, mosquito larvae transmission | ELISA occult test, ultrasonography, radiographs | Prevent mosquito bites in endemic areas Ivermectin, 0.2 mg/kg po q 30 d, possibly preventive Continue to monitor if adult worms are detected |
| Anatrichosomiasis (nasal worm) | Anatrichosoma cutaneum, Anatrichosoma cynomolgi | Macaques, langurs, patas, talapoins, marmosets, mangabeys | Nasal mucosa, female worms migrate through skin depositing eggs | Direct contact | Nasal swabs, skin scrapings for eggs | Ivermectin Prevent contact between species Sanitation |

(continued on next page)

**Table 3**
*(continued)*

| Disease | Agent | Species Affected | Location in Host | Transmission | Diagnosis | Treatment and Management |
|---|---|---|---|---|---|---|
| Angiostrongylosis | *Angiostrongylus cantonensis* | *Alouatta caraya, Varecia variegata, Cercopithecus talapoin* (zoo species)[6] | Lungworm of rats; central nervous system signs, progressive, aberrant host | Ingestion of snails/slugs (intermediate host) | Histopathologic examination | Supportive care Possibly anthelminthics, anti-inflammatories Prevent ingestion of snails/slugs |
| Pterygodermitites nycticebi | *Pterygodermitites nycticebi* | Callitrichids | Adults in small intestine, anterior ends in submucosa | Roaches carry larvae, eaten by calltrichid | FF | Insect control Regular worming with fenbendazole or mebendazole Consult formulary |
| Gongylonema (tongue, oral worm) | *Gongylonema pulchrum* | Callitrichids[7,8] | Oral cavity, tongue, musculature | Direct | Scraping of tongue, oral mucosa for ova | Ivermectin, 0.3 mg/kg po q 7 d × 4 repeats; mebendazole, 70 mg/kg po q 24 h × three doses |
| | *Gongylonema macrogu-bernaculum* | *Macaca silenus, Cercopithecus buettikoferi*[9] | Oral cavity, tongue | Direct, squirrels are definitive host | Scraping of tongue, oral mucosa; histopathologic examination | As above |
| Acanthocephalus (thorny-headed worms) | *Acanthocephalus* sp | Tropical species | Usually free in abdominal cavity | | See at surgery | Can try mebendazole, 100 mg/kg po q 24 h for alternating weeks after surgical removal of worms in callitrichids |

| | | | | | | |
|---|---|---|---|---|---|---|
| Prosthenorchis | *Prosthenorchis elegans* | Marmosets | Intestinal mucosa, granulomatous inflammation, peritonitis | Indirect, cockroaches, beetles | Signs: cachexia, intussusception, rectal prolapse; biopsy | Surgical removal of parasite / Insect control / Anthelminthics / Supportive care |
| Hymenolepiasis (tapeworms) | *Hymenolepis nana* | Rhesus macaques, squirrel monkeys | Intestine | Direct autoinfect from eggs hatching in intestine or pass through beetle/flea | FF | Sanitation / Praziquantel, 15–20 mg/kg po or im, may need multiple treatments at 10-d intervals / Zoonotic |
| Hydatid disease | *Echinococcus* sp (see **Figs. 1–6**) | All | Cysts in abdomen, eyes, subcutis | Ingestion of canid feces | Ultrasonograph, radiograph, identification of scolices in aspirates | Ultrasound-guided drainage of large cysts / Surgical removal / Follow-up treatment with praziquantel, 30–40 mg/kg po or sc repeated at 2–3 weeks |
| Respiratory flukes *Dinobdella ferox* | | Macaques | Leech, upper respiratory tract | Indirect host, snails, adults are hermaphroditic, leeches are ingested | FF, visual examination | Prevent contact with snails / Praziquantel, 40 mg/kg po or im, may need to repeat |
| Liver flukes | *Gastrodiscoideus hominis* | Macaques | Human liver fluke, in liver, in abdominal cavity | Indirect, snail ingestion | Visual examination | Prevent contact with snails / Praziquantel, 40 mg/kg po or im, repeat in 14 d |

*(continued on next page)*

**Table 3**
*(continued)*

| Disease | Agent | Species Affected | Location in Host | Transmission | Diagnosis | Treatment and Management |
|---|---|---|---|---|---|---|
| Schistosomiasis | *Schistosoma mansoni*, etc. | Baboons | Inferior mesenteric veins, portal vein | Eggs accumulate in perivascular tissues and intestine, pass in stool. Eggs hatch, enter snail, are released from snail, penetrate primate skin, and migrate to vascular system | FF, direct smear | Prevent snail contact Anthelminthics Zoonotic |
| Malaria | *Plasmodium sp* | Many | Peripheral blood, blood cells, spleen | Indirect, sexual phase in mosquitos, asexual stage in human or nonhuman primates | Blood smear | Mosquito-proof enclosures Insect control Chloroquine, 10 mg/kg po or im once, Then 5 mg/kg 6 h later, then 5 mg/kg q 24 h × 2 days Concurrent treatment with primaquine, 0.3 mg/kg po q 24 h × 14 d; mefloquine, 25 mg/kg po once |
| Trypanosomiasis (Chagas' disease) | *Trypanosoma cruzi*, etc. | South American species | Blood, muscle cells, systemic | Transmitted by insects | Blood smear | Insect control Zoonotic |

| | | | | | |
|---|---|---|---|---|---|
| Entamoeba histolytica | *Entamoeba histolytica* | All species[10-12] | Mucosa: trophozoites invade, become abscesses in lung, liver, brain Langurs, colobus, proboscis monkey: gastric lesions | Ingestion of cysts, amoeba | Fecal direct smear, wet mount | Metronidazole, 17.5–25 mg/kg po q 12 h × 10 d; paromomycin, 10 mg/kg po q 8 h × 5–10 d in great apes; paromomycin, 12.5–15.0 mg/kg po q 12 h × 5–10 days for other species Zoonotic |
| Balantidium | *Balantidium coli* | All species | Usually asymptomatic, but large numbers in colitis | Direct ingestion | Fecal direct smear, wet mount | Doxycycline, 5 mg/kg po q 12 h once, then 2.5 mg/kg po q 24 h; diiodohydroxyquin, 12–16 mg/kg po q 8 h in great ape infants and juveniles; diiodohydroxy-quin, 20 mg/kg po q 12 h × 21 d for adults, use with metronidazole; diiodohydroxy-quin alone, 30–40 mg/kg po q 24 h × 3–21 d in great apes; metronidazole, 30–50mg/kg po q 12 h × 5–10 d; tetracycline in great ape adults: 500–1000 mg per animal po q 8 h × 10–14 d Zoonotic |

(continued on next page)

**Table 3**
*(continued)*

| Disease | Agent | Species Affected | Location in Host | Transmission | Diagnosis | Treatment and Management |
|---|---|---|---|---|---|---|
| Giardia | *Giardia lamblia* | All | Usually asymptomatic, self-limiting diarrhea, small intestine/jejunum | Direct ingestion | Fecal examination, trichrome stain, ELISA kits | Prevent fecal/oral ingestion Metronidazole, 25 mg/kg po q 12 h × 10 d; quinacrine, 2 mg/kg po q 8 h × 7 d in great apes (maximum: 300 mg/d) Zoonotic |
| Encephalitozoan | *Encephalitozoan cuniculi* | Squirrel monkeys | Microgranulomas in brain, kidney, lung, adrenal gland; cause stillbirths, abortions | Carried by rabbits, monkey is aberrant host | Possibly serology, histopathologic examination | Can try rabbit treatment of oxibendazole, 10 mg/kg po q 24 h for several weeks, unproved |
| Toxoplasmosis | *Toxoplasma gondii* | All new world monkeys, especially susceptible[13] | Retinal lesions, central nervous system signs, respiratory distress | Ingestion of food contaminated by cat feces, rodents may have eaten oocysts | Serology, histopathologic examination | Prevent access house cats, rodents Can try sulfadiazine, 50 mg/kg po q 6 h; combine with pyrimethamine, 2 mg/kg q 24 h × 3 d, then 1 mg/kg q 24 h × 28 d (great apes) |
| Cryptosporidium | *Cryptosporidia* sp (**Fig. 8**) | All species, particularly infants, immuno-suppressed | Intestinal mucosa causing diarrhea | Direct ingestion of cysts, frequently from contaminated water supplies | | In nonimmuno-suppressed animals, it is usually self-limiting Treatment: supportive only, may try treatments used in humans (usually ineffective) Zoonotic |

| Scabies | Sarcoptes scabei | Macaques, all | Adults in skin, dermatitis, pruritic | Direct contact, transmissible to other species and humans | Skin scraping | Ivermectin, 0.2–0.4 mg/kg sc or po with repeated treatments<br>Medicated bath to soothe, supportive care for itching, secondary bacterial dermatitis<br>Zoonotic |
|---|---|---|---|---|---|---|
| Psorergates | Psorergates pitheci | Guenons, baboons | Adults in skin, dermatitis, some pruritus | Direct contact | Skin scraping | Ivermectin, 0.2–0.4 mg/kg sc or po with repeated treatments<br>Medicated bath to soothe, supportive care for itching, secondary bacterial dermatitis |
| Respiratory mites | Pneumonyssoides, Pneumonyssus simicola, Rhinophaga sp | Macaques, baboons asymptomatic carriers; langurs, proboscis monkeys clinical disease | Mites in lungs | Nasal discharge by means of direct contact with mucus | Tracheal wash, cytology of discharge, fluid cysts in lungs, radiographs for lung pathologic findings | Ivermectin, 0.2–0.4 mg/kg sc, repeat as needed |
| Fleas | Ctenophalides felis, etc. | All | Pruritic dermatitis, flea dirt | From environment and other animals | Visualization, flea dirt seen | Fipronil or imidocloprid at feline doses<br>Environmental control<br>Zoonotic |

Abbreviations: d, days; FF, fecal flotation; h, hours; im, intramuscular; po, orally; sc, subcutaneously.

after quarantine, with histopathologic examination confirming no live cestode. There is no treatment for pentastomids (**Figs. 7** and **8**) or Acanthocephala, which were only apparent during abdominal surgery or at necropsy. Rarely would *Plasmodium* spp be found on blood smears, with no obvious clinical signs. Asymptomatic baboons in research facilities are not infrequently diagnosed with *Babesia* sp in blood smears. These baboons would be excluded from transplant studies and as blood donors, although treatment with oral doxycycline at 30 mg/kg administered orally every 12 hours for 14 days would eliminate the parasite from peripheral blood.

Captive marmosets and tamarins have been diagnosed with the pancreatic worm, *Trichospirura leptosoma*. The nematode has been associated with wasting and increased mortality in marmoset colonies the United States, Europe, and the United Kingdom. It causes a lymphocytic, verminous, fibrosing chronic pancreatitis. The life cycle is 14 to 15 weeks, with 5 to 6 weeks within the cockroach. The marmoset ingests the cockroach. The prepatent period is 8 to 9 weeks, and eggs and larvae may be found by the formalin-ether sedimentation technique of feces for up to 2 years. After that, worms contain embryonated eggs within the pancreas. As few as three worms per pancreas may cause slow destruction of the pancreas. Clinical chemistries of an ill marmoset may show markedly elevated aspartate aminotransferase and pancreatic amylase. Most show moderate anemias with hematocrits less than 30% (N = 39–53). Treatment consists of fenbendazole at 50 mg/kg administered orally every 24 hours for 14 days along with supportive care, including replacement of pancreatic enzymes.[2–4] The presence of this parasite should be considered in the differential list for any case of marmoset or tamarin wasting disease (**Table 3**).

## CONTROL AND PREVENTION

All facilities should establish a program for regular surveillance and rotating anthelminthic and ectoparasite control programs based on the species of nonhuman primate. This includes changing substrates and bedding at regular intervals and sanitary practices that remove feces frequently. A vermin (insects, mollusks, rodents) control program can prevent many parasites from completing their life cycle and continually infecting a colony. Because so many parasite problems have direct fecal-oral life cycles, keeping monkeys parasite-free can be a challenge.

## SUMMARY

Captive nonhuman primates can be infected with a variety of parasites, many of which could be considered zoonotic. Practitioners may work with nonhuman primates in zoos, in laboratory animal facilities, in sanctuaries, or as pets. Captive-born animals have a different parasite potential than those wild-caught or imported from outdoor breeding facilities in Asia, Africa, or the Caribbean. Parasite loads of animals housed indoors, particularly individuals or those in laboratory cages, are usually far less and easier to control than those of animals housed outdoors, particularly on soil. Regular surveillance and treatment programs should be established for each situation. This also includes prevention of access from vermin, mollusks, and insects that may serve as intermediate hosts or vectors for some parasites.

## ACKNOWLEDGMENTS

The author thanks the Washington National Primate Research Center, University of Washington (Seattle, WA) and SNBL USA, Ltd. (Everett, WA).

**REFERENCES**

1. Rowe N. The pictorial guide to the living primates. Charlestown (RI): Pogonias Press; 1996.
2. Joslin JO. Other primates excluding great apes. In: Fowler ME, Miller RE, editors. Zoo and wild animal medicine. 5th edition. St. Louis (MO): Sanders Elsevier. p. 346–81.
3. Hawkins JV, Clapp NK, Carson RL, et al. Diagnosis and treatment of Trichospirura leptosoma infection in common marmosets (*Callithrix jacchus*). Contemp Topics Lab Anim Sci 1997;36:52–5.
4. Loomis MR. Great apes. In: Fowler ME, Miller RE, editors. Zoo and wild animal medicine. 5th edition. St. Louis (MO). p. 391–7.
5. Gamble KC, Fried JJ, Rubin GJ. Presumptive dirofilariasis in a pale-headed saki monkey (*Pithecia pithecia*). J Zoo Wildl Med 1998;29:50–4.
6. Aguilar RF, Topham K, Healtey JJ, et al. Neural angiostrongylosis in nonhuman primates: diagnosis, treatment and control of an outbreak in southern Louisiana. In: Proceedings of the American Association of Zoo Veterinarians 1999:272–6.
7. Adkesson MJ, Langan JN, Paul A. Evaluation of control and treatment of Gongylonema spp. infections in callitrichids. J Zoo Wildl Med 2007;38:27–31.
8. Duncan M, Tell L, Gardiner CH, et al. Lingual gongylonemiasis and pasteurellosis in Goeldi's monkeys (*Callimico goeldii*). J Zoo Wildl Med 1995;26:102–8.
9. Craig LE, Kinsella JM, Lodwick LJ, et al. Gongylonema macrogubernaculum in captive African squirrels (*Funisciurus substriatus* and *Xerus erythropus*) and lion-tailed macaques (Macaca silenus). J Zoo Wildl Med 1998;29:331–7.
10. Pang VF, Chang CC, Chang WF. Concurrent gastric and hepatic amoebiasis in a dusky leaf monkey (*Presbytis obscurus*). J Zoo Wildl Med 1993;24:204–7.
11. Suzuki J, Kobayashi S, Murata R, et al. Profiles of a pathogenic Entamoeba histolytica-like variant with variations in the nucleotide sequence of the small subunit ribosomal RNA isolated from a primate (De Brazza's guenon). J Zoo Wildl Med 2007;38:471–4.
12. Suzuki J, Kobayashi S, Murata R, et al. A survey of amoebic infections and differentiation of an entamoeba histolytica-like variant (JSK2004) in nonhuman primates by a multiplex polymerase chain reaction. J Zoo Wildl Med 2008;39:370–9.
13. Gyimesi ZS, Lappin MR, Dubey JP. Application of assays for the diagnosis of toxoplasmosis in a colony of woolly monkeys (*Lagothrix lagotricha*). J Zoo Wildl Med 2006;37:276–80.

# Selected Infectious Diseases of Reptiles

Sathya K. Chinnadurai, DVM, MS[a,b,*],
Ryan S. DeVoe, DVM, DACZM, DABVP–Avian[b]

**KEYWORDS**

• Bacterial • Fungal • Infectious disease • Parasitic • Reptile

Bacterial, fungal and parasitic diseases in reptiles are occasionally caused by primary pathogens but often are the result of an immunocompromising condition, such as inappropriate temperatures, humidity, or enclosure hygiene.[1] Treating bacterial and fungal diseases usually requires addressing the predisposing husbandry deficiency. Although the focus of this article is on bacterial and parasitic diseases, several important fungal diseases are mentioned as important to keep in mind as differentials. Although viral diseases are not discussed in this article, the importance of viruses as predisposing factors for other infectious diseases has been well described.[2,3]

Recent comprehensive publications list many reported bacterial, fungal, and parasitic pathogens. This article does not repeat existing material; instead it discusses general methods for diagnosing and treating infectious diseases and discusses certain diseases in relation to body system. Special attention is placed on recently reported diseases.

## THE IMPORTANCE OF NORMAL FLORA

A myriad of organisms can be cultured from captive reptiles and their environment. The increasing standard of care in reptile medicine has allowed clinicians to develop treatment plans based on microbiologic culture and antimicrobial sensitivity results. Although culture and sensitivity testing greatly increases the chances of treatment success by identifying appropriate antimicrobials, there is the potential for isolating nonpathogenic and commensal microorganisms from the animal. There has thus been a recent increase in studies that identify bacterial and fungal organisms colonizing the skin and gastrointestinal tract of apparently healthy reptiles.[1,4–10] When interpreting microbiologic cultures in clinically affected animals, it is important to differentiate pathogenic and commensal bacteria. All animals carry commensal

[a] Department of Clinical Sciences at North Carolina State University, College of Veterinary Medicine, 4700 Hillsborough Street, Raleigh, NC 27606, USA
[b] The North Carolina Zoological Park, 4401 Zoo Parkway, Asheboro, NC 27203, USA
* Corresponding author. North Carolina Zoological Park, 4401 Zoo Parkway, Asheboro, NC 27205.
*E-mail address:* sathya_chinnadurai@ncsu.edu (S.K. Chinnadurai).

Vet Clin Exot Anim 12 (2009) 583–596
doi:10.1016/j.cvex.2009.06.008
1094-9194/09/$ – see front matter © 2009 Elsevier Inc. All rights reserved.

vetexotic.theclinics.com

bacteria and fungi that are usually nonpathogenic and can protect the body from colonization by pathogenic organisms.

Many fungal diseases are caused by ubiquitous organisms, which take hold in animals that are compromised. Modes of transmission include airborne, fomite, and waterborne dissemination. One study determined that up to 13 different genera of fungi are found on the skin of healthy squamates.[4] Potential opportunistic fungi include species from the genera *Aspergillus*, *Mucor*, *Candida*, *Penicillium*, and *Geotrichum*.

Various nonpathogenic protozoa and nematodes make their homes in reptiles, causing limited inflammation and disease. Ciliates, such as *Balantidium*, *Paramecium*, and *Nyctotherus* spp are considered normal intestinal flora in healthy lizards.[11] In separate recent surveys of captive sea kraits (*Laticauda colubrina*) and tokay geckos (*Gekko gecko*), numerous nematodes, trematodes, cestodes, arthropods, and protozoa were identified in the intestines and lungs of dead animals.[12,13] None of the parasites found in the sea kraits were determined to be the cause of death and most existed without histologic evidence of inflammation. The parasite density in the affected animals may have been increased because of systemic immunosuppression associated with captivity stress or concurrent diseases.

In many cases, commensal organisms may provide the host with resistance to potentially pathogenic invaders. Even commensal organisms have the potential to reproduce unchecked in animals with a compromised immune system and could cause disease.

## DIAGNOSTICS

The vast numbers of normally occurring, nonpathogenic organisms can cloud the interpretation of culture results, making biopsy and histopathology an important tool. A definitive diagnosis of bacterial or mycotic disease often requires both histopathology and culture. Although a culture can provide a name of an organism, only histopathology can characterize the host reaction to the organism and the extent of tissue damage. Conversely, a biopsy can identify inflammation and deep invasion of a fungus or bacteria, but culture is required to identify the offending microorganism and determine the best antimicrobial treatment.

Samples collected in and around the primary site of infection often provide the most diagnostic specimens. Tracheal washes, endoscopy, and skin or shell biopsies can provide material for culture and sensitivity, histopathology, and cytology. Many infected lesions are covered with thick exudate and necrotic material, preventing uncontaminated sample collection. In these cases, it is important to collect deep samples and potentially collect samples after aggressive surgical débridement.

Infectious material must be collected into and grown on appropriate media. Appropriate time and temperature for sample growth is essential. For many reptile pathogens, incubation of samples at 37°C is inappropriate because the organisms may be optimized for growth at lower reptilian body temperatures.[1,14] Some organisms may take weeks to months to produce a diagnostic sample; this is especially true for *Mycobacterium* and *Mycoplasma* spp. Thick granulomatous material, slow-growing bacteria, and sample contamination can lead to false-negative culture results and failure to identify a true pathogen.

Cytology of lesions can provide a good deal of information quickly without considerable expense. Simply identifying the type of inflammation and presence of etiologic agents can narrow down the list of potential causes.[15] Impressions smears stained with a Gram stain can guide treatment of bacterial diseases while cultures are pending. Yeast and hyphae can be readily identified on standard stains, such as Wright-Geimsa. For further conformation of fungal hyphae, lactophenol cotton blue stain can be used. Acid-fast organisms (*Mycobacterium*, *Nocardia* spp) are potentially missed with standard stains and require an acid-fast stain.[16]

Molecular diagnostics, such as polymerase chain reaction (PCR), are rapid and useful supplemental diagnostic tests. Although fungal cultures may take weeks to months to produce an identifiable isolate, PCR can be used to identify DNA sequences unique to certain groups of bacteria and fungi and may allow speciation. Parasite speciation relies heavily on the expertise of parasitologists to visually identify organisms. Molecular tools, including PCR, have been used to identify reptile parasites, such as *Cryptosporidium* spp.[17–19]

## GENERAL GUIDELINES FOR THERAPY

A treatment plan begins with identifying and addressing the predisposing cause, if possible. Pharmacologic treatment of infectious diseases requires physiologic stabilization of the patient before or during administration of drugs. Administering antimicrobials and antiparasitics to hypothermic, dehydrated, or otherwise debilitated reptiles increases the potential for toxicosis and may decrease the metabolism and distribution of the drug. Supportive care consisting of temperature maintenance and fluid and nutritional support is essential to survival of systemically ill reptiles.

In the absence of culture and sensitivity, the systemic antibiotic regimen should include a gram-negative spectrum. Reasons for treatment failure include problems of drug penetration into abscessed tissue and inadequate duration of therapy. Many bacterial infections in reptiles require months of antimicrobial therapy. One report of shell phaeohyphomycosis in an Aldabra tortoise (*Geochelone gigantea*) required more than 1 year of oral and topical antifungal therapy.[20] Local wound treatment often consists of deep débridement, lavage, and topical antibacterial and antifungal therapy. In addition to patient treatment, many diseases also require habitat disinfection, including enclosure cleaning and sterilizing or discarding bedding material.

## DISEASE CONDITIONS
### Pneumonia

Pneumonia in reptiles is typically a chronic disease at the time of diagnosis and can be attributable to suboptimal husbandry. Although viruses are often primary pathogens, bacteria can cause severe pneumonia in all reptile taxa.[14,21] Reptiles presenting for lethargy, anorexia, or open-mouth breathing should be evaluated for pneumonia. For aquatic chelonians, pneumonia may result in abnormal buoyancy.

Bacterial pneumonia is often due to gram-negative pathogens, including *Klebsiella*, *Pseudomonas*, *Aeromonas*, *Escherichia coli*, *Salmonella*, and *Proteus* spp. *Mycoplasma* spp can cause rhinitis and pneumonia in chelonians and has been linked to disease outbreaks in wild tortoises and alligators.[22–28] Although uncommon in squamates, fungal pneumonia can be common in chelonian patients and can involve *Aspergillus*, *Fusarium*, and *Candida*.[29] Fungal pneumonia can be secondary to prolonged antibiotic therapy, high humidity, moldy bedding, and inadequate ventilation. Parasitic pneumonia is reported in squamates often due to lungworms (*Rhabdias*) or pentastomid arthropods (*Armillifer*). Intranuclear coccidian infections in tortoises cause disseminated infections and can present as pneumonia.[30]

For animals that have pneumonia, radiographs may be indicated. Radiographs of snakes that have pneumonia are of limited value because lesions may only be evident with advanced disease, if at all. A recent study highlights the usefulness of CT for diagnosing pneumonia in Indian pythons.[31] In chelonian patients, three-view radiographs are essential.[29] Unilateral disease is common in chelonians (**Fig. 1**) and may be missed by a lateral radiograph. In all reptiles, bronchoscopy provides a valuable tool for visualization of lesions and sample collection (**Fig. 2**). Because reptiles lack true alveoli, a true bronchoalveolar lavage is not possible.[32] A lung wash and fluid collection for culture and cytology is possible in most reptiles. If bronchoscopy equipment is not available, clinicians can perform a transtracheal wash.

Physiologic and anatomic differences between reptiles and mammals can make treatment and resolution of infectious diseases difficult. The structure of the reptile lung differs greatly by taxa; lung types include unicameral, paucicameral, and multicameral forms.[33] In most reptile species, the lung structure has relatively low surface area and high dead space. This structure provides a small area of perfused tissue for drug delivery to the lung. Reptiles lack a diaphragm and cannot efficiently cough; this inability coupled with high pulmonary dead space provides ample area for pooling of inflammatory exudates.[31]

### Dermatitis

Skin diseases are the maladies most easily recognized by reptile owners and keeper staff, leading to increased veterinary attention to dermatitis. In squamates, dermatitis can present with increased frequency of shedding or abnormal patterns of shedding (dysecdysis). In chelonians, cutaneous lesions over the shell often penetrate through the keratin layer into the bone and are commonly termed septicemic cutaneous ulcerative disease (SCUD). *Citrobacter freundii* is the most commonly reported cause of SCUD in chelonians.[6] Because dermatitis is often an indicator of inappropriate husbandry and immune compromise, chronic skin lesions can be expected to progress to systemic and occasionally fatal disease.[1,6]

Sources of secondary bacterial infections include bites from live prey items and poor cage maintenance. *Dermatophilus* is a frequent cutaneous bacterial infection of reptiles, especially animals kept in damp environments. *Dermatophilus* is considered a cause of brown spot disease in crocodilians raised for leather in the United States and Australia.[34] A filamentous bacterium distinct from *Dermatophilus congolensis* was isolated from turtles and named *D chelonae*.[35] This new species is

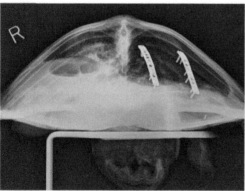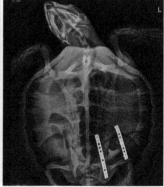

**Fig. 1.** Anteroposterior and dorsoventral radiographs of a Kemp's Ridley sea turtle (*Lepidochelys kempi*) that had unilateral bacterial pneumonia. Radiopaque strips are orthopedic plates from a previous carapacial fracture repair. The animal developed abnormal buoyancy 2 months after stranding.

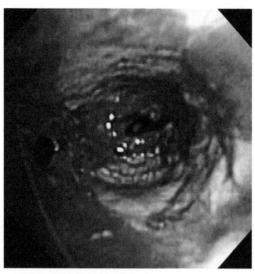

**Fig. 2.** Bronchoscopy of the same Kemp's Ridley sea turtle (*Lepidochelys kempi*) showing severe pneumonia with granulomatous exudate.

apparently adapted to ectothermic animals and has caused cutaneous and visceral infections in chelonians and snakes.[35,36]

Fungal dermatitis is the most common fungal disease in snakes and lizards. Typical keratinophilic dermatophytes, such as *Microsporum* and *Trichophyton*, are rare. Many cases are opportunistic infections by organisms such as *Candida* spp and *Fusarium* spp. One organism that has been described as primary pathogen and is rarely isolated from normal skin is the *Chrysosporium* anamorph of *Nannizziopsis vriesii* (CANV).[4,37–39]

Mites and ticks are the most common cause of parasitic skin disease in squamates. The common snake mite (*Ophionyssus* spp) is frequently found on snakes, lizards, and in one report, chelonians.[40] Both hard (ixodid) and soft (argasid) ticks can infest reptile patients. These parasites can be transmitted from newly imported animals to naïve hosts. Mites are typically identified in the interscalar skin and oral commissures of squamates. Acariform parasites can potentially transmit blood-borne disease but the cutaneous disease is often limited to inflammation at the site of attachment. In marine turtles, barnacles (*Balanus* spp and *Chelonibia* spp) and leeches (*Ozobranchus* spp) can be part of the normal epibiota but can overwhelm an already debilitated animal (**Fig. 3**).[41]

Cytology can provide a rapid, noninvasive diagnostic test. Cytology can be performed on skin scrapings or pieces of shed skin (exuvium). Care should be taken when collecting full-thickness biopsies of skin lesions because inflamed, infected skin may be prone to dehiscence and biopsy sites may need to be managed as open wounds. For chelonian shell lesions, aggressive curettage of living, sensitive bone may be necessary to collect representative samples (**Fig. 4**).[20,42] When débriding shell lesions for diagnosis and treatment, appropriate anesthesia and posttreatment analgesia are necessary. Identifying ticks and mites relies on visualizing the parasite in the interscalar skin or at the oral commissure (**Fig. 5**). Patients can be wiped with a wet white paper towel to remove mites for identification. Many owners notice the mites in a water bowl where the affected reptile soaks to alleviate a heavy infestation.

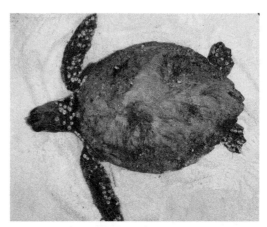

**Fig. 3.** Cold-stunned green sea turtle (*Chelonia mydas*) with numerous epibionts, including barnacles, leeches, and algae. In healthy turtles, these organisms typically exist in low numbers, but they can proliferate unregulated in debilitated animals.

For skin diseases, a combination of systemic and topical therapies and patience is needed for success. Topical therapy often consists of diligent débridement and treatment with antibacterial and antifungal rinses, flushes, and ointments. Topical wipes with water, mineral oil, or ivermectin have been used to treat mite infestations, although close attention is necessary to not overdose a patient with topical medications.

### Gastroenteritis and Colitis

Diagnosis and treatment of gastroenteritis can be challenging in reptile patients. Many captive reptiles are fed infrequently, and therefore signs associated with dysfunction of the gastrointestinal (GI) tract may not be noted for some time. For instance, a snake that has clinical cryptosporidiosis and is only fed once a month may only regurgitate or vomit once a month and otherwise appear in good health. For these reasons, it is

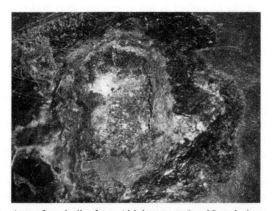

**Fig. 4.** Fungal infection of a shell of an Aldabra tortoise (*Geochelone gigantea*). Image shows the lesions after aggressive surgical débridement. (*Courtesy of* Elizabeth Stringer, Indianapolis, IN.)

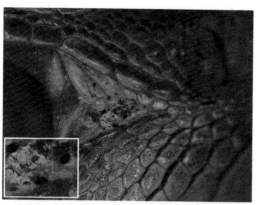

**Fig. 5.** Mites imbedded in the oral commissure of a green iguana (*Iguana iguana*). See inset box for closer magnification.

critical that a thorough history is taken and analyzed with a working knowledge of the natural history and husbandry requirements of the species in question.

Assessment of the fecal consistency can be difficult for the novice. There are some species of reptile, such as snakes, that eat primarily fish or other snakes, which normally have loose, messy stool. On the opposite end of the spectrum are the grassland tortoises that tend to have dry feces with a large amount of undigested fiber passed intact. Evaluation is made more difficult when an animal has historically received an inappropriate diet and what the owner or keeper perceives as normal is actually representative of an abnormal state. For a good example of this phenomenon, we look again at the grassland tortoises. Many leopard and sulcata tortoises that are purchased by well-meaning but ignorant owners are fed diets that are much too heavy in fruits and leafy green vegetable matter and too low in fiber. As a consequence their feces are always moist and sticky and resemble the stool one might see from a rodent-eating snake.

There are several microorganisms that can infect the gastrointestinal tract of reptiles. Some of these organisms are primary pathogens and are transmitted between animals, but others are opportunistic and only cause infections in animals that are otherwise compromised. To further complicate things, there are several organisms that are host adapted and are harbored by some species without causing disease. When these organisms are passed to a novel species it is difficult to predict how the naïve animal will respond. Although various microorganisms can be responsible for causing dysfunction of the GI tract, the same basic approach can be taken to diagnose most infections. A thorough history, physical examination, complete blood count, and chemistry panel should constitute the initial database for a reptile patient that has GI disease. Great effort should be taken to carefully palpate the organs of the coelom, especially the stomach and colon. In many cases of chronic gastroenteritis the affected area of the GI tract is palpably thickened or irregular.

Plain and contrast radiographs can be helpful in ruling out foreign bodies, outflow obstructions, perforations, or mass effects that are affecting the GI tract. A standard technique for GI contrast studies has been published for green iguanas.[43] For contrast radiographs the authors typically use iohexol or barium sulfate delivered by gavage. Barium sulfate usually gives better detail but iohexol is less of a concern if a perforation exists. Both iohexol and barium are given at a dose of 1% of body weight by volume. Ultrasonographic evaluation can be useful, especially in patients that are of sufficient size and possess anatomy that is amenable to imaging. Clinicians can use ultrasound to diagnose ascites and liver disease in reptiles and to aid in sample collection.

Gastric lavage can be used to detect infectious agents in the stomach. The technique is simple: an appropriately sized lubricated flexible tube is placed orally into the stomach and sterile saline (3% of bodyweight is a good starting point) is infused. The stomach is gently massaged externally and the contents are aspirated by way of the tube. Typically, a small fraction of the volume infused is recovered on aspiration. Cloacal or colonic lavage can be performed using the same technique, except the tube is placed through the vent instead of the mouth. The material recovered can be submitted for culture and sensitivity and PCR for a specific organism, such as *Cryptosporidium serpentis* or *C saurophilum*. The fluid should also be used for stained and wet-mount cytology. When *Cryptosporidium* is suspected, an acid-fast stain for the regurgitant, feces, or gastric lavage fluid should be performed. Identification of an acid-fast protozoan can indicate *Cryptosporidium* and should be confirmed with gastric biopsy or PCR. Diagnosis of *Entamoeba* can be made by identifying the organism or cyst on a fecal float or by direct fecal exam. PCR testing has been developed for *Entamoeba* also.

Endoscopy is the authors' favored method for evaluating the GI tract in reptiles. Endoscopy allows for the direct visualization of the esophageal, gastric, and colonic mucosa and evaluation of the contents of the lumen. In small animals most GI endoscopy can be performed with a rigid scope. Larger animals may require some of the longer, flexible endoscopes to perform a thorough examination. In addition to directly visualizing the mucosal surfaces of the GI tract by endoscopy, one can also obtain biopsies with instruments passed through the operating ports of the endoscope.

Cloacal or fecal cultures are often performed on ill reptiles, but the results can be somewhat difficult to interpret. The normal flora of the reptilian gastrointestinal tract can vary between species and even individuals. Bacteria such as *Salmonella*, *Shigella*, and *Campylobacter* spp, which are considered pathogenic in mammalian and avian species, are often harbored by reptiles with no ill effect. Bacterial enteritis does occur in reptiles, but it is usually a secondary process and the result of a predisposing condition. For instance, when reptiles develop severe hemorrhagic enteritis from amoebiasis, there is usually a bacterial component because isolates that are normal flora infiltrate tissues and cause damage. If an ill reptile has diarrhea, culture of feces in conjunction with cytology and fecal sedimentation and flotation is warranted.

Gram-negative bacteria cause most reptilian bacterial infections. Gram-positive infections do occur in reptiles, but at a much lower rate. In some cases, clinical disease is caused by bacterial toxemia.[44] Recently, *Chlamydophila pneumoniae* has been implicated in an outbreak of repeated regurgitation and death in emerald tree boas.[45,46] A myriad of parasites can result in gastrointestinal disease; of special concern are the protozoal pathogens, *Cryptosporidium* and *Entamoeba*. *Entamoeba* and *Cryptosporidium* are transmitted directly by the fecal–oral route and can cause severe morbidity and mortality within captive populations of susceptible reptiles.[11] Multiple protozoa in the genus *Entamoeba* can cause amoebiasis. *E invadens* is the species most frequently blamed for clinical disease, although in most cases little to no effort is made to definitively identify the organism. Cryptosporidiosis causes hypertrophic gastritis in snakes and gastritis and enteritis in lizards. In severely affected snakes and lizards the thickened colon (amoebiasis) or thickened stomach (cryptosporidiosis) is easily palpated in the coelomic cavity.

Treatment of any type of gastroenteritis consists of supportive care, especially fluid support, elevated ambient temperature, and antibiotics and antiprotozoals as appropriate. Even primary parasitic and viral gastroenteritis can involve a secondary bacterial infection. Of paramount importance is nutritional support with an easily digested diet at proper environmental conditions. Disease and inadequate husbandry can lead to alterations in GI transit time, resulting in putrefaction of ingesta instead of proper digestion.

### Disseminated Infections and Osteomyelitis

Prolonged primary infections of the skin, respiratory, and gastrointestinal systems can lead to systemic infections. Septicemia can also result in bacterial seeding of the liver, bone, and central nervous system, especially during immune compromise from environmental stressors. Sepsis should be a differential for unexplained neurologic disease and considered as a likely sequela to chronic infections, including pneumonia and dermatitis.

Aeromonas hydrophila is a frequently cultured bacterium from septicemic American alligators (Alligator mississippiensis), although it has also been cultured from the oral cavities and viscera of apparently healthy alligators.[6,47,48] Mycoplasmosis was associated with an outbreak of pneumonia, neurologic disease, and polyserositis in farmed alligators.[26,49] Corynebacterium, Clostridium, Mycobacterium, and Stenotrophomonas have been isolated from blood, bone, and tissues of septicemic squamates.[5,44,50–52]

Likely differentials for infectious osteomyelitis lesions in reptiles include Salmonella, Mycobacterium, Mycoplasma, and various fungal organisms.[6] Mycobacterial species that have been isolated from osteomyelitis lesions in reptiles include Mycobacterium chelonae in sea turtles,[53] Mycobacterium terrae in Eastern box turtles (Terrapene carolina carolina), and an unidentified atypical Mycobacterium in a bearded dragon (Pogona vitticeps).[54] Mycoplasma iguanae has been associated with vertebral disease in feral iguanas (Iguana iguana) in Florida.[55] Special attention should be paid to Salmonella as a pathogen in reptiles. Most reports of Salmonella in reptiles relate to the zoonotic potential, but there are multiple reports of Salmonella causing disease in the reptile host. In a recent report, Salmonella arizonae was isolated from spinal osteomyelitis lesions in a collection of rattlesnakes.[56,57] Clostridium sepsis has been associated with proliferative, nonlytic, spinal lesions causing hind-limb paralysis in monitors.[44]

Cutaneous fungal infections have often progressed to systemic disease by the time of diagnosis. Fatal disseminated cases of fungal disease have been reported in Fly River turtles (Carettochelys insculpta) and a Galapagos tortoise.[58,59] The CANV has been reported to cause systemic mycosis in tentacled snakes after progressing from severe dermatitis.[60] Intranuclear coccidiosis has been documented to cause disseminated parasitic infections with lesions noted in the brain, lungs, and liver. Entamoeba is another example of a gastrointestinal parasite that causes systemic disease. It is generally accepted that chelonians, aquatic lizards, and snake-eating snakes carry Entamoeba asymptomatically. When introduced to a susceptible species, the organism begins by invading the colon. Subsequently, the amoebae enter the bloodstream and can spread to the liver and nervous system or disseminate throughout the body. A severe hemorrhagic diarrhea usually develops, followed by symptoms related to the specific organ system infected.

In systemically ill animals, complete blood count and plasma biochemistry are indicated to determine extent of systemic compromise. Aseptic blood collection can provide vital samples for aerobic and anaerobic blood culture. Blood culture is often indicated for cases of osteomyelitis and encephalitis when sampling of the target organ is not feasible.

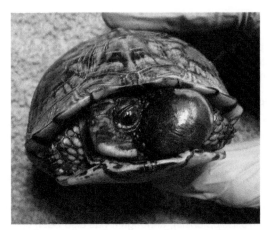

**Fig. 6.** Unilateral bacterial aural abscess is an Eastern box turtle (*Terrapene carolina carolina*). This lesion resolved with surgical débridement, repeated saline flushing, and systemic antibiotic therapy.

## Newly Recognized Infectious Diseases in Reptiles

### Aural abscesses in turtles

Aural abscesses are problem commonly reported in eastern box turtles and other species (**Fig. 6**).[61–63] The condition may be linked to environmental organochlorine exposure and alteration in body stores of vitamin A. Recent literature suggests that the cause of this disease may be more complex.[64,65] The condition typically responds to surgical débridement and systemic and topical antimicrobial therapy. The incidence of recurrence is unknown.

### Bartonella and Cowdria

Until recently, *Bartonella* was believed to be an invertebrate-borne pathogen of terrestrial mammals. Recently, *B henselae* DNA has been identified by PCR in the blood of sea turtles.[66] The transmission and significance of this organism is unknown. Another potentially vector-borne disease recently reported in reptiles is *Cowdria* isolated from African vipers. In the past decade, *Cowdria* (*Ehrlichia*) *ruminantium* was isolated from *Amblyomma sparsum* ticks on tortoises imported into the United States.[67,68] Although the tortoises in the original report did not show disease associated with *Cowdria* infection, an unrelated report described pulmonary hemorrhage, vomiting, diarrhea, and death in *Cowdria*-infected African vipers.[69]

## SUMMARY

We have described the common clinical signs, diagnostic plan, and therapeutic options for several reptile infectious diseases. The breadth of this article prevents us from providing detailed descriptions of different causes; instead we have highlighted the similarities found in common reptile diseases presented by organ systems.

## REFERENCES

1. Pare JA, Sigler L, Rosenthal KL, et al. Microbiology: fungal and bacterial diseases of reptiles. In: Mader D, editor. Reptile medicine and surgery. 2nd edition. Philadelphia: WB Saunders; 2006. p. 217–38.

2. Wellehan JF, Johnson AJ. Reptile virology. Vet Clin North Am Exot Anim Pract 2005;8:27–52.
3. Jacobson ER. Viruses and viral diseases of reptiles. In: Jacobson ER, editor. Infectious diseases and pathology of reptiles. Boca Raton (FL): CRC Press; 2007. p. 409–12.
4. Pare JA, Sigler L, Rypien K, et al. Cutaneous mycobiota of captive squamate reptiles with notes on the scarcity of the Chysosporium anamorph of Nannizziopsis vriesii. J Herp Med Surg 2003;13(4):10–5.
5. Hejnar P, Bardon J, Sauer P, et al. Stenotrophomonas maltophilia as a part of normal oral bacterial flora in captive snakes and its susceptibility to antibiotics. Vet Microbiol 2007;121:357–62.
6. Jacobson ER. Bacterial diseases of reptiles. In: Jacobson ER, editor. Infectious diseases and pathology of reptiles. Boca Raton (FL): CRC Press; 2007. p. 461–526.
7. Maria R, Ramer J, Reichard T, et al. Biochemical reference intervals and intestinal microflora of free-ranging Ricord's iguanas (Cyclura ricordii). J Zoo Wildl Med 2007;38:414–9.
8. Saelinger CA, Lewbart GA, Christian LS, et al. Prevalence of Salmonella spp in cloacal, fecal, and gastrointestinal mucosal samples from wild North American turtles. J Am Vet Med Assoc 2006;229:266–8.
9. Salb A, Mitchell MA, Riggs S, et al. Characteristics of intestinal microflora of captive green iguanas (Iguana iguana). J Herp Med Surg 2007;17(1):12–5.
10. Santoro M, Hernandez G, Caballero M. Aerobic bacterial flora of nesting green turtles (Chelonia mydas) from Tortuguero National Park, Costa Rica. J Zoo Wildl Med 2006;37:549–52.
11. Jacobson ER. Parasites and parasitic diseases of reptiles. In: Jacobson ER, editor. Infectious diseases and pathology of reptiles. Boca Raton (FL): CRC Press; 2007. p. 572–97.
12. Chinnadurai SK, Brown DL, Van Wettere A, et al. Mortalities associated with sepsis, parasitism, and disseminated round cell neoplasia in yellow-lipped sea kraits (Laticauda colubrina). J Zoo Wildl Med 2008;39:626–30.
13. Reese DJ, Kinsella M, Zdziarski JM, et al. Parasites in 30 captive tokay geckos, (Gekko gecko). J Herp Med Surg 2004;14(2):21–5.
14. Pees M, Schmidt V, Schlomer J, et al. Significance of the sampling points and the aerobic microbiological culture for the diagnosis of respiratory infections in reptiles. Dtsch Tierarztl Wochenschr 2007;114:388–93.
15. Jacobson ER. Host responses to infectious agents and identification of pathogens in tissue section. In: Jacobson ER, editor. Infectious diseases and pathology of reptiles. Boca Raton (FL): CRC Press; 2007. p. 261–2.
16. Campbell TW. Clinical pathology of reptiles. In: Mader D, editor. Reptile medicine and surgery. 2nd edition. Philadelphia: WB Saunders; 2006. p. 453–70.
17. Xiao L, Ryan UM, Graczyk TK, et al. Genetic diversity of Cryptosporidium spp. in captive reptiles. Appl Environ Microbiol 2004;70:891–9.
18. Plutzer J, Karanis P. Molecular identification of a Cryptosporidium saurophilum from corn snake (Elaphe guttata guttata). Parasitol Res 2007;101:1141–5.
19. Pedraza-Diaz S, Ortega-Mora LM, Carrion BA, et al. Molecular characterization of Cryptosporidium isolates from pet reptiles. Vet Parasitol 2009;160:204–10.
20. Stringer EM, Garner MM, Proudfoot JS, et al. Phaeohyphomycosis of the carapace in an Aldabra tortoise (Geochelone gigantea). J Zoo Wildl Med 2009;40:160–7.
21. Coke RL. Respiratory biology and diseases of captive lizards (sauria). Vet Clin North Am Exot Anim Pract 2000;3:531–6.

22. Feldman SH, Wimsatt J, Marchang RE, et al. A novel Mycoplasma detected in association with upper respiratory disease syndrome in free-ranging eastern box turtles (Terrapene carolina carolina) in Virginia. J Wildl Dis 2006;42: 279–89.

23. Dickinson VM, Schumacher IM, Jarchow JL, et al. Mycoplasmosis in free-ranging desert tortoises in Utah and Arizona. J Wildl Dis 2005;41:839–42.

24. Brown DR, Zacher LA, Carbonneau DA. Seroprevalence of Mycoplasma alligatoris among free-ranging alligators (Alligator mississippiensis) in Florida-2003. J Zoo Wildl Med 2005;36:340–1.

25. Brown DR, Merritt JL, Jacobson ER, et al. Mycoplasma testudineum sp. nov., from a desert tortoise (Gopherus agassizii) with upper respiratory tract disease. Int J Syst Evol Microbiol 2004;54:1527–9.

26. Brown DR, Farley JM, Zacher LA, et al. Mycoplasma alligatoris sp. nov., from American alligators. Int J Syst Evol Microbiol 2001;51:419–24.

27. Brown MB, McLaughlin GS, Klein PA, et al. Upper respiratory tract disease in the gopher tortoise is caused by Mycoplasma agassizii. J Clin Microbiol 1999;37: 2262–9.

28. Penner JD, Jacobson ER, Brown DR, et al. A novel Mycoplasma sp. associated with proliferative tracheitis and pneumonia in a Burmese python (Python molurus bivittatus. J Comp Pathol 1997;117:283–8.

29. Origgi FC, Jacobson ER. Diseases of the respiratory tract of chelonians. Vet Clin North Am Exot Anim Pract. 2000;3:537–49.

30. Garner MM, Gardiner CH, Wellehan JF, et al. Intranuclear coccidiosis in tortoises: nine cases. Vet Pathol 2006;43:311–20.

31. Pees MC, Kiefer I, Ludewig EW, et al. Computed tomography of the lungs of Indian pythons (Python molurus). Am J Vet Res 2007;68:428–34.

32. Lafortune M, Gobel T, Jacobson E, et al. Respiratory bronchoscopy of subadult American alligators (Alligator mississippiensis) and tracheal wash evaluation. J Zoo Wildl Med 2005;36:12–20.

33. O'Malley B. Reptiles. In: O'Malley B, editor. Clinical anatomy and physiology of exotic species. Edinburgh: Elsevier Saunders; 2005. p. 17–39.

34. Buenviaje GN, Ladds PW, Martin Y. Pathology of skin diseases in crocodiles. Aust Vet J 1998;76:357–63.

35. Bemis DA, Patton CS, Ramsay EC. Dermatophilosis in captive tortoises. J Vet Diagn Invest 1999;11:553–7.

36. Wellehan JF, Turenne C, Heard DJ, et al. Dermatophilus chelonae in a king cobra (Ophiophagus hannah). J Zoo Wildl Med 2004;35:553–6.

37. Bowman MR, Pare JA, Sigler L, et al. Deep fungal dermatitis in three inland bearded dragons (Pogona vitticeps) caused by the Chrysosporium anamorph of Nannizziopsis vriesii. Med Mycol 2007;45:371–6.

38. Pare A, Coyle KA, Sigler L, et al. Pathogenicity of the Chrysosporium anamorph of Nannizziopsis vriesii for veiled chameleons (Chamaeleo calyptratus). Med Mycol 2006;44:25–31.

39. Abarca ML, Martorell J, Castella G, et al. Cutaneous hyalohyphomycosis caused by a Chrysosporium species related to Nannizziopsis vriesii in two green iguanas (Iguana iguana). Med Mycol 2008;46:349–54.

40. Wiechert JM. Infection of Hermann's tortoises, Testudo hermanni boettgeri, with the common snake mite, Ophionyssus natricis. J Herp Med Surg 2007;17(2): 53–5.

41. Greiner EC, Mader D. Parasitology. In: Mader D, editor. Reptile medicine and surgery. 2nd edition. Philadelphia: WB Saunders; 2006. p. 343–64.

42. Li XL, Zhang CL, Fang WH, et al. White-spot disease of Chinese soft-shelled turtles (Trionyx sinens) caused by Paecilomyces lilacinus. J Zhejiang Univ Sci B 2008;9:578–81.
43. Smith D, Dobson H, Spence E. Gastrointestinal studies in the green iguana: technique and reference values. Vet Radiol Ultrasound 2001;42(6):515–20.
44. Bertelsen MF, Weese JS. Fatal clostridial enterotoxemia (Clostridium glycolicum) in an ornate Nile monitor (Varanus ornatus). J Zoo Wildl Med 2006;37:53–4.
45. Jacobson ER, Heard D, Andersen A. Identification of Chlamydophila pneumoniae in an emerald tree boa, Corallus caninus. J Vet Diagn Invest 2004;16:153–4.
46. Lock B, Heard D, Detrisac C, et al. An epizootic of chronic regurgitation associated with chlamydophilosis in recently imported emerald tree boas (Corallus caninus). J Zoo Wildl Med 2003;34:385–93.
47. Novak SS, Seigel RA. Gram-negative septicemia in American alligators (Alligator mississippiensis). J Wildl Dis 1986;22:484–7.
48. Gorden RW, Hazen TC, Esch GW, et al. Isolation of Aeromonas hydrophila from the American alligator, Alligator mississippiensis. J Wildl Dis 1979;15:239–43.
49. Clippinger TL, Bennett RA, Johnson CM, et al. Morbidity and mortality associated with a new Mycoplasma species from captive American alligators (Alligator mississippiensis). J Zoo Wildl Med 2000;31:303–14.
50. Martinez J, Segura P, Garcia D, et al. Septicemia secondary to infection by Corynebacterium macginleyi in an Indian python (Python molurus). Vet J 2006;172:382–5.
51. Girling SJ, Fraser MA. Systemic mycobacteriosis in an inland bearded dragon (Pogona vitticeps). Vet Rec 2007;160:526–8.
52. Hernandez-Divers SJ, Shearer D. Pulmonary mycobacteriosis caused by Mycobacterium haemophilum and M. marinum in a royal python. J Am Vet Med Assoc 2002;220:1661–3, 1650.
53. Greer LL, Strandberg JD, Whitaker BR. Mycobacterium chelonae osteoarthritis in a Kemp's Ridley sea turtle (Lepidochelys kempii). J Wildl Dis 2003;39:736–41.
54. Kramer MH. Granulomatous osteomyelitis associated with atypical mycobacteriosis in a bearded dragon (Pogona vitticeps). Vet Clin North Am Exot Anim Pract 2006;9:563–8.
55. Brown DR, Demcovitz DL, Plourde DR, et al. Mycoplasma iguanae sp. nov., from a green iguana (Iguana iguana) with vertebral disease. Int J Syst Evol Microbiol 2006;56:761–4.
56. Ramsay EC, Daniel GB, Tryon BW, et al. Osteomyelitis associated with Salmonella enterica SS arizonae in a colony of ridgenose rattlesnakes (Crotalus willardi). J Zoo Wildl Med 2002;33:301–10.
57. Grupka LM, Ramsay EC, Bemis DA. Salmonella surveillance in a collection of rattlesnakes (Crotalus spp.). J Zoo Wildl Med 2006;37:306–12.
58. Lafortune M, Wellehan JF, Terrell SP, et al. Shell and systemic hyalohyphomycosis in Fly River turtles, Carettochelys insculpta, caused by Paecilomyces lilacinus. J Herp Med Surg 2005;15(2):15–9.
59. Manharth A, Lemberger K, Mylniczenko N, et al. Disseminated phaeohyphomycosis due to an Exophiala species in a Galapagos tortoise, Geochelone nigra. J Herp Med Surg 2005;15:20–6.
60. Bertelsen MF, Crawshaw GJ, Sigler L, et al. Fatal cutaneous mycosis in tentacled snakes (Erpeton tentaculatum) caused by the Chrysosporium anamorph of Nannizziopsis vriesii. J Zoo Wildl Med 2005;36:82–7.
61. Brown JD, Richards JM, Robertson J, et al. Pathology of aural abscesses in free-living eastern box turtles (Terrapene carolina carolina). J Wildl Dis 2004;40:704–12.

62. Brown JD, Sleeman JM, Elvinger F. Epidemiologic determinants of aural abscessation in free-living eastern box turtles (Terrapene carolina) in Virginia. J Wildl Dis 2003;39:918–21.
63. Joyner PH, Brown JD, Holladay S, et al. Characterization of the bacterial microflora of the tympanic cavity of eastern box turtles with and without aural abscesses. J Wildl Dis 2006;42:859–64.
64. Kroenlein KR, Sleeman JM, Holladay SD, et al. Inability to induce tympanic squamous metaplasia using organochlorine compounds in vitamin A-deficient red-eared sliders (Trachemys scripta elegans). J Wildl Dis 2008;44:664–9.
65. Sleeman JM, Brown J, Steffen D, et al. Relationships among aural abscesses, organochlorine compounds, and vitamin A in free-ranging eastern box turtles (Terrapene carolina carolina). J Wildl Dis 2008;44:922–9.
66. Valentine KH, Harms CA, Cadenas MB, et al. Bartonella DNA in loggerhead sea turtles. Emerg Infect Dis 2007;13:949–50.
67. Burridge MJ, Simmons LA, Simbi BH, et al. Evidence of Cowdria ruminantium infection (heartwater) in Amblyomma sparsum ticks found on tortoises imported into Florida. J Parasitol 2000;86:1135–6.
68. Peter TF, Mahan SM, Burridge MJ. Resistance of leopard tortoises and helmeted guineafowl to Cowdria ruminantium infection (heartwater). Vet Parasitol 2001;98:299–307.
69. Kiel JL, Alarcon RM, Parker JE, et al. Emerging tick-borne disease in African vipers caused by a Cowdria-like organism. Ann N Y Acad Sci 2006;1081:434–42.

# Bacterial and Parasitic Diseases of Amphibians

Eric Klaphake, DVM, DACZM, DABVP–Avian[a,b,*]

**KEYWORDS**

- Bacteria • Parasite • Amphibian • Frog • Salamander • Toad

Whether in private practice or in a zoologic setting, veterinarians of the exotic animal persuasion are asked to work on amphibians. As with most nondomestic species, many health issues in amphibians are traced back to problems with husbandry or nutrition. Because these areas are more adequately addressed in zoos, and even by hobbyists and pet stores, veterinarians are able to evaluate more thoroughly for true medical issues, with infectious diseases at the forefront. Until quite recently, many infectious diseases were unknown or even misdiagnosed as being caused by opportunistic secondary organisms. The challenge of convincing a client or even a curator to invest in diagnostic testing is often formidable. Likewise, amphibians can be a challenge to collect samples from in useful quantities for such testing. Amphibians have been proposed as environmental sentinels, but the dearth of research on infectious amphibian diseases is remarkable in opposing our support of that statement. Many times, the diagnosis comes from a necropsy, histopathologic examination, or various DNA polymerase chain reaction (PCR) test results that do not obviously help that individual animal but can be critical for managing and preventing the disease in the rest of the collection. One of the best current resources for amphibian diseases of all kinds and current updates is Rick Speare's (James Cook University, Townsville, Queensland, Australia).[1] This Web site served as a reference for many of the topics discussed in this article.

## BRIEF MENTION OF RANAVIRUS AND *BATRACHOCHYTRIUM DENDROBATES*

Although this article is focused on bacteria and parasites, one must recognize that more and more research is coming to light indicating that underlying or concurrent viral and fungal infections play roles in bacterial and fungal infections.[2] A late 2008 review of journal articles in required reading for individuals studying to become a diplomate of the American College of Zoologic Medicine found that since 2004, 25% of all articles published on infectious diseases in amphibians were on viruses and 56% were

[a] Animal Medical Center, 216 8th Avenue, Bozeman, MT 59715, USA
[b] ZooMontana, 2100 South Shiloh Road, Billings, MT 59106, USA
* Corresponding author. Animal Medical Center, 216 8th Avenue, Bozeman, MT 59715.
*E-mail address:* dreklaphake@msn.com

Vet Clin Exot Anim 12 (2009) 597–608
doi:10.1016/j.cvex.2009.06.005
1094-9194/09/$ – see front matter © 2009 Elsevier Inc. All rights reserved.

on fungal diseases. A brief summary of the two most devastating viral and fungal diseases is included in this article.

Ranavirus is a genus of iridovirus. Iridoviruses are the new viruses on the block, although most of the "new" is actually in reference to their recognition in reptiles. Some have implicated amphibians as the reservoir of reptile infection. Previously, iridoviruses had been noted only in fish and amphibians, with lymphocystis in fish being the classic example. Ranaviruses have been implicated in frog and tiger salamander die-offs. Ranavirus type III is the cause of tadpole edema syndrome, because adults are subclinical carriers. As implied, the clinical signs in tadpoles are edema and subcutaneous hemorrhage. Iridoviruses are large double-stranded DNA viruses identified by an eosinophilic intranuclear inclusion in red blood cells or a basophilic intracytoplasmic inclusion in stomach gland cells.[1,3–6] DNA PCR testing is currently available for zoologic collections through the San Diego Zoo's Institute for Conservation Research. Frozen tissue (eg, liver, kidney, skin), buffy coat, pharyngeal or cloacal swab, and skin biopsy may be used (Allan Pessier, personal communication, 2009). For private practitioners, the author is currently unaware of antemortem testing options but recommends consulting with your exotic or zoologic pathologist for options. At this time, treatment tends to consist of supportive care, isolation, and culling. Although no antiviral agents have been tested against ranaviruses, the chances of obtaining cure of chronically affected or carrier amphibians is small. Glutaraldehyde, bleach, and artificially generated ultraviolet light are effective disinfectants.[1]

Most fungal infections are opportunistic as a result of suppressed immune systems from other infections or improper husbandry and diet. *Batrachochytrium dendrobates* (Bd) is the most important infectious disease of amphibians to understand as a clinician, however. Named after the first species it was identified in—the poison dart frog species (*Dendrobates azureus* and *D auratus*) and White's tree frog *(Litoria caerulea)*, the species' affected range has expanded to almost every anuran, some urodelian, and even caecilian species.[7] Infections are so severe in the wild that many species have gone extinct as a result of exposure to Bd. Research suggests that *Xenopus laevis* use for detection of human pregnancy throughout the world in the middle of the twentieth century contributed to its worldwide spread. Other species, such as the marine toad (*Bufo marinus*) and American bullfrog (*Rana catesbeiana*), have been implicated as subclinical carriers and spreaders of Bd. Clinical signs include acute death, general malaise, skin shed, ventral edema or petechi, and toe-tip lesions in adults. Best samples to collect are toe tips or drink patch area. This disease generally does not seem to affect tadpoles clinically, although keratin beak deformities are noted.[1,6] At this time, PCR-based testing is the diagnostic method recommended because it has shown greater sensitivity than histopathologic examination or wet mount slides. DNA PCR testing is currently available for zoologic collections through the San Diego Zoo's Institute for Conservation Research using a skin swab (Allan Pessier, personal communication, 2009). The company Zoologix, Inc. (Chatsworth, California) offers testing for private practitioners (identified on the Web site as chytrid fungus[8];). Treatment generally consists of itraconazole or miconazole baths, isolation, and culling.[9] Raising environmental temperatures (not always the best thing to do for amphibians) seems to help the amphibians to avoid or resist Bd infections. Disposable gloves can act as a fomite; thus, new gloves or, less preferably, bare hands are recommended with each animal.[10] At this time, Bd is viewed as an amphibian-only disease. Typically, the organism functions poorly at temperatures approaching mammal body temperature; thus, zoonotic concerns are currently considered unwarranted.

## BACTERIA
### Normal Microflora

Amphibian skin is used for respiration and a barrier against disease. An important part of this barrier is the natural microflora found in the skin and also the microflora found in the gastrointestinal tract. When evaluating for bacterial infection, simply growing bacteria in culture does not equate to disease. Information on the normal flora is important for such evaluation. Unfortunately, there are few studies that have evaluated this; one must be careful with too much interspecies extrapolation, and regional, seasonal, gender, age, and other factors may also affect what the normal microflora is. In one study, the natural bacterial flora found on the skin of apparently healthy adult eastern newts (*Notophthalamus viridescens*), larval bullfrogs (*R catesbieana*), and red-backed salamanders (*Plethodon cinereus*) living in natural field sites in Virginia included five bacterial species from the newts, three bacterial species from the bull-frogs, and four bacterial species and one yeast from red-backed salamanders. It has also been found that only a subset of bacteria in the environment is able to colonize amphibian skin successfully.[11] In evaluating gastrointestinal normal microflora, researchers found in southern toads *(B terrestris)* and spring peepers *(Pseudacris crucifer)* that higher levels of enteric gram-negative bacteria were observed during metamorphosis in the intestines of each species. Gut content had no effect on bacterial levels in *B terrestris*. Much higher bacterial levels were recorded in smaller metamorphs. The results suggested that enteric microflora may play an ecologic role in anuran development and metamorphosis in these species.[12] As previously mentioned, defining "normal" microflora can be a challenging task.

### Antimicrobial Effects of Natural Microflora

In fact, several recent studies have shown that normal microflora and its byproducts actually protect against viral, fungal, other bacterial, and parasitic infection. A species of anti-Bd skin bacteria was added to skins of red-backed salamanders *(P cinereus)* and reduced the severity of Bd symptoms in experimentally infected individuals. This could slow or halt epidemic outbreaks and allow successful reintroduction of amphibian species that have become locally or globally extinct in the wild.[13] Skin peptides collected from tiger salamander (*Ambystoma tigrinum*) larvae and adults and tested against Bd and the *A tigrinum* virus (ATV), in addition to bacteria isolated from *A tigrinum*, inhibited growth of Bd, *Staphylococcus aureus*, and *Klebsiella* sp, but activity against ATV was unpredictable. Environmental temperature and skin pH were major factors in effectiveness.[14]

With widespread resistance of bacteria to current antibiotics, naturally occurring antimicrobial peptides (AMPs) from amphibian skin are considered promising candidates for future therapeutic use. In vitro bactericidal activities of five AMPs from three different species of anurans against multidrug-resistant clinical isolates belonging to species often involved in nosocomial infections (*S aureus*, *Enterococcus faecium*, *Pseudomonas aeruginosa*, *Stenotrophomonas maltophilia*, and *Acinetobacter baumannii*) were assessed. The peptides tested were temporins A, B, and G from the European common frog (*R temporaria*), the fragment from positions 1 to 18 of esculetin 1b [Esc(1–18)] from the edible frog (*R esculenta),* and bombinin H2 from the yellow-bellied toad *(Bombina variegate).* When tested in buffer, all the peptides were bactericidal against all bacterial species tested (three strains of each species), with only a few exceptions. The temporins were more active against gram-positive bacteria, especially in human serum; Esc(1–18) showed fast and strong bactericidal activity, within 2 to 20 minutes, especially against gram-negative species; and bombinin H2 displayed similar bactericidal activity toward all isolates. Interestingly, although the activities of the temporins and bombinin H2 were almost completely inhibited in the presence of 20% human serum, the activity of Esc(1–18) against the gram-negative species was partially preserved in the presence of 40% serum.[15] Thus, obviously, these peptides are even more effective in their natural environment of the frog skin.

### Gram-Negative Pathogenic Bacteria

The classic frog infection was always referred to as "red leg," although there are several caveats that need to be considered with this terminology. First, many frog species are naturally red on the ventrum of the legs, and it can be a secondary gender characteristic in some males or an indication of stress. When it was believed to be a clinical sign of disease, the cause had been relegated to a bacterial infection, most likely attributable to gram-negative rods—usually *Aeromonas* sp. In retrospect, many of these infections involving die-offs may have had primary viral or fungal components, as mentioned previously, that were overlooked because of lack of diagnostics or funds. As the immune system was overwhelmed by the primary infection, the secondary gram-negative rod infection took advantage of the opportunity. There can be primary bacterial infections, most attributable to poor husbandry and water quality. These infections cause erythema as a result of rupture and dilation of capillaries from disseminated septic thrombi—the red leg. Hydrops and hydrocoelom often follow. *Flavorbacter* sp and *Aeromonas* sp have high epizootic potential. It is important to treat for secondary bacterial infections with any viral or fungal infection for this reason.[2,5,6,16]

### Chlamydophilosis and Chlamydiosis

*Chlamydophila* sp is a common organism of concern in birds and, more recently, in reptiles. In amphibians, it was reported as causing red leg in *Xenopus* sp and Solomon Island eyelash frogs (*Ceratobatrachus guentheri*). The diagnosis was attributable to no bacterial growth plus intracytoplasmic inclusions of elementary bodies (the infectious form) and reticular bodies.[1,6,16,17] Generally, if present, other etiologies may be indicated by a granulomatous response, and thus rule out *Mycobacteria* spp and certain systemic fungal diseases. Some isolated strains from amphibians have been identified as *Chlamydia pneumoniae*. Whether these strains of *C pneumoniae* are still capable of infecting humans or crossed the host barrier some time ago remains to be determined but may provide further insights into the relation of this common respiratory infection to its human host.[18] Diagnosis can be performed by DNA PCR; however, as evidenced in the retrospective study by Blumer and colleagues,[17] its presence may be subclinical and of no clinical consequence, with histopathologic examination necessary to pathological significance. Treatment is doxycycline, although other tetracyclines have been used.[6]

### Mycobacteriosis

*Mycobacterium* spp identified in amphibians include *M marinum*, *M xenopi*, and *M ranae*. As with *Chlamydophila* spp, however, *Mycobacteria* spp are likely to undergo significant reclassification in the years ahead as DNA PCR technology continues to progress and be refined. Most are believed to be from a water or soil source, with the clinical sign being weight loss despite good appetite. Mycobacterial infection of amphibians has been reported only in captivity and occurs mainly in immunocompromised animals. Mortality is usually low. Natural resistance to mycobacteria, which are ubiquitous in aquatic environments, is higher in ectotherms versus homeotherms. Infections may primarily involve the skin, respiratory tract, or intestines. Frogs have been found with single large tumor-like masses or with disseminated nodules throughout internal organs. Such organs as the liver, spleen, kidney, or testes may become almost completely destroyed by the infection before the animal dies, usually with cachexia. Early granulomas are composed of mostly epithelioid macrophages, which may progress to form encapsulated foci with dry caseous centers. Granulomas typically contain large numbers of acid-fast bacilli.[1] Identification of the organism is as standard for *Mycobacteria* spp. Zoonotic potential is assumed but ultimately unknown. There is no recommended treatment beyond isolation of exposed amphibians, culling of clinical animals, and environmental control.

### Bacterial Zoonoses

Amphibians may carry pathogenic *Salmonella* sp but are rarely clinically affected; however, zoonotic concerns need to be considered. Prevalence from clinically normal amphibians is 10% to 60%. Amphibians may be good reservoirs of *Salmonella* spp, with a high potential to contaminate the environment.[1]

A series of papers reported that marine toads (*B marinus)* and coqui frogs *(Eleutherodactylus johnstonei)* in Barbados could be reservoirs for zoonotic *Leptospira* spp, and other species of unknown zoonotic potential were found. The prevalence of *Leptospira* spp isolated was approximately 4%, but serologic evidence of past infection was much higher (>21%).[1]

### PARASITES

The final group of potential infectious organisms in amphibians is parasites. It is important to remember that most parasites have evolved to be a minimal drain on their host so as to avoid "killing the goose with the golden egg." There are a lot of articles on normal parasites found in amphibians, but in this article, the author focuses on those causing disease. Many parasites can actually be commensal, and treatment of those may cause more harm than good.

### Pathogenic Protozoa

Amphibians have a large range of protozoa, many of which seem to be commensals in the gastrointestinal tract. Only the potentially pathogenic protozoa are mentioned in this section. Most research has been done on the taxonomy of the protozoa, with little research on pathogenicity and biology.

Amoebiasis has been reported in amphibians, with *Entamoeba ranarum* reported in anurans. The anuran ingests the infective cyst in a direct life cycle, which, like many amoeboid cysts, is durable in environment. Once infected, trophozoites mature in the colon to the cyst form. A renal form in *B marinum* occurs as an ascending infection; hepatic abscessation has also been reported. Clinically, most infected amphibians have general illness signs, some with gastrointestinal manifestation, and possible edema and coelomic fluid. Some amphibians may have commensal amoebas, which can be difficult to differentiate from pathogenic ones, but if large numbers of amoeba and clinical signs are seen, pathogenic disease should be highly suspected. Treatment usually involves metronidazole, even as a bath.[6]

Ciliated protozoa are classified in the category of possible commensal status with uncertain pathogenicity, in the gastrointestinal tract and urinary bladder (for amphibians with those). Consider treatment if they are subjectively found in a high density of organisms, with inflammation or with clinical signs. For aquatic species, external pathogenic ciliates can cause cloudy skin patches or gills, and ulcers. This actually often indicates a water filtration problem rather than a ciliate problem.[6]

Hemoprotozoa are being more thoroughly evaluated in terms of their role in disease. Diagnostically, it is important to differentiate these parasites from viral or chlamydophilic inclusions. More than 60 species of trypanosomes have been reported in anurans, but the taxonomy is confusing. Most are nonpathogenic; however, *Trypanosoma inopinatum* is lethal to European green frogs *(Hyla arborea)* and causes hemorrhage, swollen lymph glands, anemia, and death, whereas *T rotatorium* can be pathogenic in tadpoles or in heavy infections, with trypanosomes accumulating in the kidneys. *T pipientis* causes spleen enlargement but rarely causes death.[1] In Oregon spotted frogs *(R. pretiosa),* a *Lankesterella* sp and a *Trypanosoma* sp were detected in 31% and 35%, respectively. Parasite loads were generally light, with *Lankesterella* sporozoites in 1% to 2% of erythrocytes and extracellular trypanosomes at one parasite per 200 fields of view at a ×1000 magnification.[19] In captivity, these are introduced into the amphibian by feeder fish or other live foods. Preventative recommendations include dipping food items in a hypertonic bath for approximately 5 minutes and then rinsing.[6]

Other internal parasites of pathologic interest include microsporidia causing septicemia and ulcerative dermatitis in South American tree frogs (*Phyllomedusa* sp). Recommended treatment is chloramphenicol.[1,6]

The microsporidian, *Pleistophora myotrophica*, causes high mortality in captive common toads *(B bufo).* This parasite infects all striated muscles, resulting in atrophy and emaciation. White streaks between muscle fibers are obvious grossly, and, microscopically, spaces in the muscle fibers are packed with microsporidian spores. Muscle regeneration occurred with long chains of sarcoblasts adjacent to damaged muscle. Tadpoles were not infected experimentally, but their development was arrested. Only 1 of 12 experimental common frogs *(R temporaria)* became infected and had spores in the tongue, whereas 100% of *B bufo* were infected.[1]

Fatal renal myxosporean infection was reported in a collection of Asian horned frogs (*Megophrys nasuta*) and identified as *Chloromyxum* sp. Histologic changes in the kidneys included varying degrees of renal tubular dilation and necrosis and mild to severe nonsuppurative tubulointerstitial nephritis associated with vegetative stages of the myxosporidian. This is the second known identification of *Chloromyxum* sp in amphibian kidneys and the first report of death attributable primarily to the parasite.[20]

*Myxidium immersum* was introduced to Australia with the marine toad (*B marinus*). It has a low host specificity and has spread into native frog species, including 12 species of *Litoria*; 4 species of *Limnodynastes*; and 1 species each of *Mixophyes*, *Ranidella*, and *Uperoleia*. The large immobile trophozoites (1–5 mm) are found freely floating in bile in the gallbladder.[1]

*Myxobolus hylae* was found in the reproductive organs of *L aurea*. Infected frogs appeared sickly and emaciated. The testes and vasa deferentia were infected in male frogs, and the oviducts were infected in female frogs. In cases of heavy infection, the whole testis was swollen and covered with white cysts up to 2 to 3 mm composed of myriads of spores.[1]

A proliferous, polycystic, and sometimes fatal kidney disease attributable to an infection with *Myxosporidia* was reported in hyperohid frogs (*Afrixalus dorsalis*, *Hyperolius concolor*, and *Hyperolius* sp) from Nigeria, Ghana, and Tanzania. The disease was described as "frog kidney enlargement disease" and was caused by *Hoferellus anurae*. Myxosporidian plasmodia, different developmental stages, and spores occurred in the kidney, ureter, urinary bladder, and intestines.[21]

Myositis associated with infection by *Ichthyophonus*-like organisms was reported in wild amphibians collected in Quebec, Canada, from 1959 to 1964 and from 1992 to

1999. Infection was diagnosed in six species (frogs [*R clamitans*, *R sylvatica*, *R catesbeiana*, *R palustris*, and *Pseudacris crucifer*] and newts [*Notophthalmus viridescens*]). Spores of the organisms invaded striated muscle fibers and were associated with variable degrees of granulomatous and eosinophilic inflammation. Infection was considered fatal in two green frogs, one wood frog, and one red-spotted newt. It was considered potentially significant in three additional green frogs in which up to 100% of the fibers of some muscles were replaced by spores associated with a severe granulomatous reaction. This report shows that ichthyophonosis is enzootic in amphibians from Quebec.[1] The amphibian leech (*Placobdella picta*) has been implicated in *Ichthyophonus* sp transmission, by acquiring infection when inserting its proboscis into the muscles beneath the skin of infected newts and transmitting the infection in subsequent feeding bouts. Anthropogenic eutrophication might lead to more frequent or severe outbreaks of *Ichthyophonus* sp infection in amphibians.[22]

A mesomycetozoan (fungus-like protists), *Amphibiocystidium ranae*, infects several European amphibian species and was associated with a recent decline of frogs in Italy. In the Eastern red-spotted newt (*N viridescens*), a new species—*A viridescens* in the order Dermocystida—with evidence of mortality attributable to infection has been reported.[23]

### Pathogenic Nematodes

Nematodes are another parasitic group in which the question becomes how many is too many? Disease is common in captivity, but none has been reported to cause epidemics in the wild. Amphibians have helminth fauna with low diversity and low infection levels compared with other vertebrates. This may be attributable to host specificity of the parasites or to aspects of host biology.[1]

*Rhabdia* spp are the most common lungworms in anurans. In a direct life cycle, the larvae penetrate the anuran skin, molt, and travel to the lungs, with larvae moving up the airway to be swallowed and shed in feces. A heavy infection can cause pathologic change.[6] Experimental transmission of *Rhabdias bufonis* to *B bufo* resulted in a dose-dependent decrease in growth rates, fitness, and survival. *B marinus* exposed to infective larvae of *R sphaerocephala* died overnight, with hundreds of larvae found in internal organs, including the heart muscle, liver, and eye. Larvae may reach the lungs indirectly by way of the blood stream or by direct migration to the lungs, although some may encyst in other organs, inciting granuloma formation.[1] Wood frogs (*R sylvatica*) were assessed for susceptibility to lung nematodes (*R ranae*), with variations in susceptibility to lung nematodes being influenced by host gender and gender-specific relations to the developmental rate. Further, male hosts might prove to be a more important source of infective stages of worms than female hosts.[24] Juvenile leopard frogs (*R pipiens*) exposed to six pesticides (atrazine, metribuzin, aldicarb, endosulfane, lindane, and dieldrin) and challenged with *R ranae* had a higher prevalence of lung infection by *R ranae*, suggesting that agricultural pesticides alter the immune response of frogs and affect their ability to deal with parasitic infection.[25] Recommended treatment and management include isolating infected animals and ivermectin or levamisole baths.[6]

*Strongyloides* spp also have a direct life cycle and have been reported to cause gastrointestinal lesions. *Foleyella* spp can cause death as a result of heavy infections with microfilaria or adult worms. Infections may occur at a high prevalence in a population and seem asymptomatic.[1] *Pseudocapillaroides xenopi* is a capillarioid nematode that burrows in the epidermis. Infection resulted in deaths in captive *X laevis*. Bacterial and fungal opportunists contributed to the pathogenesis. Clinical signs developed over 4 months and included ulcers, sloughing of the epidermis, erythema, and weight loss.[1]

### Pathogenic Cestodes and Trematodes

Most trematodes and cestodes are usually larval forms in anurans that serve as intermediate hosts, causing minimal clinical signs and focal pathologic change once encysted but clinically relevant pathologic change and disease during migration through tissues. Adult trematodes can be found in the lungs, urinary bladder, kidney, gastrointestinal tract, and skin. Recent concern and research have centered on *Ribeiroia* sp and a relation to the formation of supernumerary limbs in the boreal toad (*B boreas*).

Spargana are the intermediate stage of cestodes (Order Pseudophyllidea) and occur in frogs worldwide. They are potentially pathogenic, but their effects in frogs have not been well studied. The adult *Spirometra erinacei* inhabits the small intestine of carnivores, whereas the procercoid stage occurs in copepods, and the plerocercoid stage (spargana) is found in tadpoles and adult frogs that ingest infected copepods.[1] In Australian amphibians, spargana have been reported in wild adults of *B marinus* (3.7% with light infections, 59% of spargana found in thighs, spargana had a marked local inflammatory response, and more than half of the spargana were dead), *L aurea*, *L caerulea* (25% of one population), *L nasuta*, and *L rubella*, and experimental infections were produced in adults of *L latopalmata* and *Limnodynastes tasmaniensis* and tadpoles of *L latopalmata*, *L caerulea*, and *L tasmaniensis*. In a survey of Malaysian frogs, 11.8% were found infected with spargana, 57% with bleeding or swelling at infection sites.[1]

Metacercariae of various trematode species occur in tadpoles and frogs. The definitive host may be snakes, frogs, birds, or mammals. Usually, encysted larvae are not pathogenic, although infections have been found in vital organs, such as the eyes, heart, liver, lungs, and central nervous system. Metacercariae of the *Neascus* group encysted in the dermis along the lateral line system of captive adults of *X laevis*, leading to paralysis and death. *Diplostomulum xenopi* infected the pericardial cavity of *X laevis*, causing pericarditis, respiratory distress, and death. Heavy experimental infections with *Cercaria ranae* caused bloat in tadpoles.[1]

Many pesticides and other chemicals to which amphibians can be exposed have been shown to increase problems with many trematodes. Embryonic exposure to the organophosphate Malathion in pickerel frog (*R palustris*) tadpoles on susceptibility to the trematode parasite *Echinostoma trivolvis* found increased parasite encystment rates. Other side effects were decreased hatching success and viability rates and increased incidence of malformations (ventralization and axial shortening).[26] The use of the herbicide atrazine was the best predictor of the abundance of larval trematodes in *R pipiens* and was consistent across trematode taxa. The combination of atrazine and phosphate-principal agrochemicals in global corn and sorghum production accounted for 74% of the variation in the abundance of these often debilitating larval trematodes (atrazine alone accounted for 51%). Both agrochemicals increase exposure and susceptibility to larval trematodes by augmenting snail intermediate hosts and suppressing amphibian immunity.[27] *R sylvatica* tadpoles exposed to atrazine had a significantly higher intensity of parasitism than did larval frogs not exposed or exposed to lower levels.[28]

*Ribeiroia ondatrae*, a trematode that causes limb deformities in amphibians, had 80% to 90% of offered cercariae ingested within 10 minutes by *Hydra* sp, damselfly larvae, dragonfly larvae, and copepods. This suggested that conservation of the biodiversity and numbers of aquatic predators may limit adverse impacts of trematode infections in vertebrate hosts.[29] The trematode parasite *R ondatrae* sequentially infects birds, snails, and amphibian larvae, frequently causing severe amphibian limb deformities and mortality. Mechanistically, eutrophication (excessive plant growth and decay) promotes amphibian disease through two distinctive pathways: by increasing the density of infected snail hosts and by enhancing per snail production of infectious parasites.[30] Larval amphibians under crowded conditions experience increased susceptibility to trematode establishment in nature but only if they metamorphose within the time period when cercariae are still available.[31] Tadpoles treated with exogenous corticosterone developed higher parasite loads, which may explain apparent increases in the numbers of trematode-induced deformities in amphibian populations during recent decades.[32]

The author was recently contacted by a researcher studying the cardiopulmonary system in wild caught leopard frogs (*R pipiens*). *Rhabdia* sp and a hemoflagellate had been noted but were considered subclinical; however, a *Haematoloechus* sp was thought to be affecting the study (M. Flood, personal communication, 2009). *Haematoloechus medioplexus* infects the lungs of amphibians, particularly frogs. Eggs are released by the adult worm and pass up the respiratory tract, are swallowed, pass through the digestive tract, and are released in the feces. The eggs are ingested by an aquatic snail, and the miracidium hatches, moves to the hepatic gland, and become a sporocyst. The sporocyst produces cercariae, which are released and can live and swim for up to 30 hours. The cercariae search for a dragonfly nymph to be the second intermediate host. The cercaria penetrates the gills of the nymph and encysts as a metacercaria. When the dragonfly transforms to the adult, the metacercaria is retained. When the adult dragonfly leaves the water and is eaten by a frog, the metacercaria is digested out and migrates up the esophagus to the bronchi, where it enters the lungs and develops to the adult stage.[33] With the complexity of the life cycle, successful removal of adult worms should eliminate that parasite. Levamisole had been reported by other researchers as an effective treatment; however, with the difficulty in getting levamisole in the United States, oral praziquantel was recommended instead. Success of treatment was unknown at time of this article's publication.

### Acanthocephala

The spines of Acanthocephala inhabiting the stomach and intestine of frogs can cause perforation, coelomitis, and death. *Acanthocephalus ranae* is a common species in Europe. It does require an arthropod intermediate host; thus, it is usually self-limiting in captivity.[1,6]

### External Parasites

Most leeches are ectoparasites, although one species has been reported to get into the lymphatics of anurans. They can also transmit an *Ichthyophonus* sp-like organism, as previously discussed.[23] Recommended treatment for external leeches is a hypertonic saline bath.[6] Likewise, external copepods are treated with salt baths.[6]

With trombiculid mites, remember that larvae are the only problem; all other life stages of "chiggers" live in the environment. Reptiles and amphibians are the natural hosts of these larvae, which can lead to blood depletion and erythematous vesicles on those hosts (As an aside, in humans, the larvae feeds and then realizes you are not the natural food source, regurgitates the tissue/blood/digestive juices back into the wound, and then leaves. The itchiness you feel is the reaction to the vomit, but the parasite is long gone). Treatment options include ivermectin and hypertonic salt baths. For infested exhibits, soil can be heated in the oven to kill the other life stages.[6]

*Amblyomma* ticks occur on *B marinus* in Central and South America. They occur on all areas of the body and cause transient focal congestion and hemorrhage. Ticks have not been found on *B marinus* in Australia or on native amphibians.[1]

Larvae of the fly families Sarcophagidae, Calliphoridae, and Chloropidae can develop within amphibians. The "toad fly," *Bufolucilia bufonivora*, lays eggs in the nostrils of toads, and the larvae destroy the epithelium and penetrate deeper into the orbit or brain, which kills most toads. Larvae of *Notochaeta bufonivora* parasitized wild Costa Rican variable harlequin toads (*Atelopus varius*) and farmed *R catesbiana*. *A. varius* in early stages of myiasis had a single small wound on the posterior surface of one thigh, and all hosts died within 4 days after they were found. Female frogs were parasitized more often. Larvae occurred in the mouth and caused necrotic perforations associated with a range of aerobic and anaerobic bacteria, including *Clostridium* spp in the farmed *R catesbiana*. In Australia, *Batrachomyia* spp have been found in 11 frog species, inhabiting the dorsal lymph sac with their posterior spiracles in or close to a hole in the frog's skin. They leave the frog and drop to the ground to pupate. The number of maggots[2-6] is much less than that seen with *B bufonivora*, suggesting that the eggs are not laid directly on frog skin but are picked up from the soil. Frogs are reported to have survived this infection and had little obvious tissue damage, although death can result at the time of larval emergence. A *Pseudophryne bibronii* (Bibron's toadlet) was found with perforation of the peritoneal wall, and the rostral end of the maggot lay within the peritoneal cavity. An *L caerulea* infected with a larva of *B mertensis* was in poor body condition and did not eat well until the larva was surgically removed.[1]

## SUMMARY

In summary, although Bd and viral diseases are in the forefront of research for amphibians, parasitic and bacterial diseases often present secondarily and, occasionally, even as the primary cause. Full diagnostic workups, when possible, can be critical in determining all the factors involved in morbidity and mortality issues in amphibians.

## REFERENCES

1. Speare R, Berger L. Available at: http://www.jcu.edu.au/school/phtm/PHTM/frogs/ampdis.htm. Accessed May 1, 2009.
2. Miller DL, Rajeev S, Brookins M, et al. Concurrent infection with ranavirus, Batrachochytrium dendrobatidis, and Aeromonas in a captive anuran colony. J Zoo Wildl Med 2008;39:445–9.
3. Schock DM, Bollinger TK, Chinchar VG, et al. Experimental evidence that amphibian ranaviruses are multi-host pathogens. Copeia 2008;133–43.
4. Duffus ALJ, Pauli BD, Wozney K, et al. Frog virus 3-like infections in aquatic amphibian communities. J Wildl Dis 2008;44:109–20.
5. Green DE. Pathology of amphibia. In: Wright KM, Whitaker BR, editors. Amphibian medicine and captive husbandry. Malabar (FL): Krieger Publishing Company; 2001. p. 401–85.
6. Wright KM. Overview of amphibian medicine. In: Mader DR, editor. Reptile medicine and surgery. 2nd edition. St. Louis (MO): Saunders-Elsevier; 2006. p. 941–71.
7. Longcore JE, Pessier AP, Nichols DK. Batrachochytrium dendrobatidis gen. et sp. nov., a chytrid pathogenic to amphibians. Mycologia 1999;91:219–27.
8. Available at: http://www.zoologix.com/zoo/Datasheets/ChytridFungus.htm. Accessed July 24, 2009.

9. Forzán MJ, Gunn H, Scott P. Chytridiomycosis in an aquarium collection of frogs: diagnosis, treatment, and control. J Zoo Wildl Med 2008;39:406–11.

10. Mendez D, Webb R, Berger L, et al. Survival of the amphibian chytrid fungus Batrachochytrium dendrobatidis on bare hands and gloves: hygiene implications for amphibian handling. Dis Aquat Org 2008;82:97–104.

11. Culp CE, Falkinham JO, Belden LK. Identification of the natural bacterial microflora on the skin of eastern newts, bullfrog tadpoles and redback salamanders. Herpetologica 2007;63:66–71.

12. Fedewa LA. Fluctuating gram-negative microflora in developing anurans. J Herpetol 2006;40:131–5.

13. Harris RN, Lauer A, Simon MA, et al. Addition of antifungal skin bacteria to salamanders ameliorates the effects of chytridiomycosis. Dis Aquat Org 2009;83: 11–6.

14. Sheafor B, Davidson EW, Parr L, et al. Antimicrobial peptide defenses in the salamander, Ambystoma tigrinum, against emerging amphibian pathogens. J Wildl Dis 2008;44:226–36.

15. Mangoni ML, Maisetta G, Di Luca M, et al. Comparative analysis of the bactericidal activities of amphibian peptide analogues against multidrug-resistant nosocomial bacterial strains. Antimicrobial Agents Chemother 2008;52:85–91.

16. Taylor SK, Green DE, Wright KM, et al. Bacterial diseases. In: Wright KM, Whitaker BR, editors. Amphibian medicine and captive husbandry. Malabar (FL): Krieger Publishing Company; 2001. p. 159–79.

17. Blumer C, Zimmermann DR, Weilenmann R, et al. Chlamydiae in free-ranging and captive frogs in Switzerland. Vet Pathol 2007;44:144–50.

18. Bodetti TJ, Jacobson E, Wan C, et al. Molecular evidence to support the expansion of the host range of Chlamydophila pneumoniae to include reptiles as well as humans, horses, koalas and amphibians. Syst Appl Microbiol 2002;25:146–52.

19. Stenberg PL, Bowerman WJ. Hemoparasites in Oregon spotted frogs (Rana pretiosa) from central Oregon, USA. J Wildl Dis 2008;44:464–8.

20. Duncan AE, Garner MM, Bartholomew JL, et al. Renal myxosporidiasis in Asian horned frogs (Megophrys nasuta). J Zoo Wildl Med 2004;35:381–6.

21. Mutschmann F. Pathological changes in African hyperoliid frogs due to a myxosporidian infection with a new species of Hoferellus (Myxozoa). Dis Aquat Org 2004;60:215–22.

22. Raffel TR, Dillard JR, Hudson PJ. Field evidence for leech-borne transmission of amphibian Ichthyophonus sp. J Parasitol 2006;92:1256–64.

23. Raffel TR, Bommarito T, Barry DS, et al. Widespread infection of the Eastern red-spotted newt (Notophthalmus viridescens) by Amphibiocystidium, a genus of a new species of fungus-like mesomycetozoan parasites not previously reported in North America. Parasite 2008;135:203–15.

24. Dare OK, Forbes MR. Rates of development in male and female wood frogs and patterns of parasitism by lung nematodes. Parasite 2008;135:385–93.

25. Christin MS, Gendron AD, Brousseau P, et al. Effects of agricultural pesticides on the immune system of Rana pipiens and on its resistance to parasitic infection. Environ Toxicol Chem 2003;22:1127–33.

26. Budischak SA, Belden LK, Hopkins WA. Effects of Malathion on embryonic development and latent susceptibility to trematode parasites in ranid tadpoles. Environ Toxicol Chem 2008;27:2496–500.

27. Rohr JR, Schotthoefer AM, Raffel TR, et al. Agrochemicals increase trematode infections in a declining amphibian species. Nature 2008;455:1235–9.

28. Koprivnikar J, Forbes MR, Baker RL. Contaminant effects on host-parasite inter-actions: atrazine, frogs, and trematodes. Environ Toxicol Chem 2007;26:2166–70.

29. Schotthoefer AM, Labak KM, Beasley VR. Ribeiroia ondatrae cercariae are consumed by aquatic invertebrate predators. J Parasitol 2007;93:1240–3.

30. Johnson PTJ, Chase JM, Dosch KL, et al. Aquatic eutrophication promotes path-ogenic infection in amphibians. Proc Natl Acad Sci U S A 2007;104:15781–6.

31. Dare OK, Rutherford PL, Forbes MR. Rearing density and susceptibility of R. pipiens metamorphs to cercariae of a digenetic trematode. J Parasitol 2006; 92:543–7.

32. Belden LK, Kiesecker JM. Glucocorticosteroid hormone treatment of larval tree-frogs increases infection by Alaria sp trematode cercariae. J Parasitol 2005;91: 686–8.

33. Dick TA, Graham TC. Available at: http://www.umanitoba.ca/faculties/science/zoology/faculty/dick/z346/haematohome.html. Accessed May 1, 2009.

# Bacterial and Parasitic Diseases of Pet Fish

Helen E. Roberts, DVM[a],*, Brian Palmeiro, VMD, DACVD[b,c],
E. Scott Weber III, VMD, MSc[d]

**KEYWORDS**

- Pet fish • *Aeromonas* • *Ichthyophthirius*
- Wet-mount cytology • Ornamental fish

## BACTERIAL DISEASE IN PET FISH

Bacterial disease is extremely common in ornamental fish and is most frequently associated with bacteria that are ubiquitous in the aquatic environment acting as opportunistic pathogens secondary to stress. Less commonly, bacterial disease is caused by primary or obligate pathogens. Most bacterial infections of fish are caused by gram-negative organisms and include the genera *Aeromonas*, *Citrobacter*, *Edwardsiella*, *Flavobacterium*, *Pseudomonas*, and *Vibrio*.[1–3] Bacterial disease in fish is complex and involves the interplay of various factors including the environment, the host (immune system function, host susceptibility, etc.), and pathogen-specific factors such as virulence. Stress can result in immune suppression and is critical in the pathogenesis of bacterial disease in fish with poor environmental conditions as the most common stressor involved in precipitation of bacterial disease. Water quality should routinely be assessed when investigating any disease outbreaks in aquatic organisms. Major bacterial pathogens in fish can be divided into the following four major groups[1] and one minor newly emerging group of pathogens:

Ulcer forming or systemic, gram-negative bacteria. This group includes bacteria in the genera Aeromonas, Vibrio, Edwardsiella, Pseudomonas, Flavobacterium, and others. This is the most common group of bacterial pathogens that affect fish.

External, gram-negative bacteria. This group of bacteria most commonly causes external infections. Some of these bacteria may also cause systemic infections.

[a] Aquatic Veterinary Services of WNY, PC, 5 Corners Animal Hospital, 2799 Southwestern Blvd., Suite 100, Orchard Park, NY 14127, USA
[b] Pet Fish Doctor, 645 Pennsylvania Ave, Prospect Park, PA 19076, USA
[c] Veterinary Referral Center, Malvern, PA 19355, USA
[d] Companion Avian and Exotic Animal Service, Department of Aquatic Animal Health, University of California, Medicine and Epidemiology, 2108 Tupper Hall, Davis, CA 95616, USA
* Corresponding author.
*E-mail address:* nyfishdoc@aol.com (H.E. Roberts).

Vet Clin Exot Anim 12 (2009) 609–638
doi:10.1016/j.cvex.2009.06.010
1094-9194/09/$ – see front matter © 2009 Elsevier Inc. All rights reserved.

Included in this group are Flavobacterium columnarae, Flexibacter maritimus, yellow-pigmented bacteria, Cytophaga spp, and others.

Systemic, gram-positive, rapidly growing bacteria. These bacteria generally cause systemic infections and include Streptococcus spp and related species.

Slow-growing, acid-fast bacteria. These bacterial pathogens cause systemic, chronic, granulomatous disease. The most common pathogens in this group are Mycobacterium spp.

Newly emerging intracellular rickettsial pathogens.

Clinical signs of bacterial disease may be peracute (mortality without gross evidence of disease), acute, or chronic and varies with the particular pathogen and various host related factors. With misuse of antibiotics, antibiotic resistance is becoming more important in treating bacterial diseases in fish. This article discusses specific bacterial diseases in fish including clinical presentation, diagnostics, and treatments.

## ULCER-FORMING AND SYSTEMIC INFECTIONS CAUSED BY GRAM-NEGATIVE BACTERIA

This is the most common group of bacterial pathogens that affect fish and includes bacteria in the genera *Aeromonas*, *Vibrio*, *Edwardsiella*, *Pseudomonas*, *Flavobacterium*, and others. Clinical signs of ulcer-forming and systemic infections caused by gram-negative bacteria include lethargy, anorexia, abnormal swimming patterns or spinning, hemorrhagic lesions on the skin, ulcerative skin lesions, abdominal distension, ascites, abnormal position in the water column, exophthalmia ("pop-eye"), skin darkening, gill necrosis, and mortality.[1–3] With gill involvement, respiratory signs such as increased opercular rate, piping (gasping for air at the water surface) and respiratory distress may be seen.

### Motile Aeromonad Septicemia

Motile aeromonads are the most common bacterial pathogens of fish and may result in a syndrome called motile aeromonad septicemia (MAS). MAS is most commonly caused by ubiquitous aquatic bacteria of the *Aeromonas hydrophila* complex, including *A hydrophila*, *A sobria*, and *A caviae*. *A hydrophila* is the most common isolate and is more commonly isolated from freshwater than marine fish. MAS is almost always secondary to an underlying stressor and is most commonly found in conjunction with eutrophic water quality conditions. In fishponds, this aeromonad is commonly isolated from clinically ill fish in the warmer months of the year. Common clinical signs include cutaneous hemorrhages and ulcers that can be deep through the dermis to connective tissue and muscle, visceral hemorrhages, edema, dropsy or ascites, and exophthalmia.[1–3]

### Ulcerative Dermatitis in Koi (Cyprinus carpio)

Ulcerative dermatitis (UD) is a multifactorial syndrome seen in koi (*Cyprinus carpio*) and related cyprinids such as goldfish (*Carassius auratus*) that results in ulcerative skin lesions. Clinical signs include raised or erythematous and missing scales, and ulcers that extend from the skin into the underlying musculature; in severe cases, bone may be exposed or penetration into the coelomic cavity may occur. Progression to septicemia can also occur resulting in clinical signs such as those seen with MAS. Osmotic distress due to loss of epidermal integrity may result in fluid retention, exophthalmos, and dropsy. **Fig. 1** exhibits the typical ulcers in a koi with UD. Various bacterial pathogens have been isolated from these cases including *A salmonicida* and *A hydrophila*.[1,2,4] *A salmonicida* can be difficult to culture as it is fastidious and quickly overgrown by other rapidly growing bacteria such as motile aeromonads.[1] In a recent

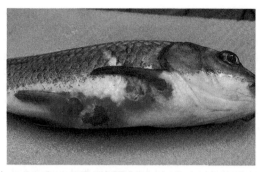

**Fig. 1.** A koi with ulcerative dermatitis exhibiting typical cutaneous ulcers. Note exposure of underlying musculature and peripheral annular rims of hemorrhage surrounding the ulcers.

abstract, *A salmonicida* DNA was detected by way of polymerase chain reaction (PCR) in 77% of koi with ulcerative skin lesions.[5] Although not always the case, UD lesions caused by *A salmonicida* have been diagnosed by one of the authors (ESW) more in autumn and winter, when water temperatures are cooler. Numerous pathogens have been isolated from these cutaneous lesions by way of sterile-swab and sterile-tissue cultures including *Aeromonas* spp, *Pseudomonas* spp, *Citrobacter* spp, *Chryseobacterium* spp, *Delfia* spp, and *Shewanella putrefaciens*.[6]

Causes of UD in koi can be divided into predisposing, primary, secondary, and perpetuating factors (**Table 1**).[7]

| Table 1 | | | |
|---|---|---|---|
| **Predisposing, primary, secondary, and perpetuating causes of ulcerative dermatitis in koi** | | | |
| **Predisposing** | **Primary** | **Secondary** | **Perpetuating** |
| Chemical stressors: poor water quality or other undesirable environmental conditions | Ectoparasites | Secondary bacterial invaders—motile aeromonads, *Pseudomonas*, *Flavobacterium*, *Citrobacter*, etc | Fibrosis and scarring, granulation tissue, tissue weakening |
| Physical stressors: shipping, overcrowding, aggression, etc | *Aeromonas hydrophila* complex | *Saprolegnia* | Recruitment of inflammatory cells and enzymatic tissue degradation |
| Poor husbandry: filtration, tank or pond design, nutrition, etc | *Aeromonas salmonicida* | Parasites that invade damaged epidermis—nematodes, flukes, *Trichodina*, *Ichthyobodo*, etc | Osmotic stresses due to lack of epidermal integrity |
| — | Trauma | — | Septicemia |
| — | Koi Herpes Virus | — | — |
| Physiologic stresses | — | — | — |
| Genetic factors | — | — | — |
| — | — | Algae | — |

*From* Palmeiro BS. Bacterial Diseases. In: Roberts HR, editor. Fundamentals of ornamental fish health. Wiley-Blackwell. In Press; with permission.

In most cases, many of these factors interact together to result in clinical disease, emphasizing the need for a thorough diagnostic evaluation. Systemic antibiotics are often used in the treatment of this condition. Prolonged bath immersion treatment with salt at 0.1% to 0.3% is typically used to decrease osmotic stresses. In some cases, debridement of the ulcer and removal of necrotic tissue or scales may be necessary. Various topical treatments such as silver sulfadiazine can also be helpful. No treatment should be initiated without assessing and addressing water quality concerns. More information on treatment can be found under treatment of systemic or ulcer gram-negative infections below.

### Aeromonas salmonicida

*A salmonicida* is a nonmotile species of *Aeromonas* that causes a chronic-to-subacute bacterial infection resulting in cutaneous ulcerations of the skin. There are three reported subspecies of *A salmonicida* including *salmonicida*, *achromogenes*, and *masoucida*.[3] The subspecies *salmonicida* is usually associated with systemic infections and is the causative agent of furunculosis in salmonids.[3] The atypical subspecies *achromogenes* is more commonly associated with ulcerative skin lesions in nonsalmonid species such as goldfish, common carp, and eels. It is also the causative agent of carp erythrodermatitis and has been implicated as the causative agent of UD in koi. *A salmonicida* is considered an obligate pathogen of fish, but carrier fish can occur.[3]

### Pseudomonas *spp*

Most Pseudomonal-associated septicemia cases in ornamental species are due to *P fluorescens*.[2] Infections are more common in warmer water temperatures and are typically secondary to environmental stressors,[2] although one author (ESW) has diagnosed an infection in a cold marine Atlantic cod. There is still disagreement among fish health specialists if *Pseudomonas* represents a primary or secondary pathogen or a nonpathogenic environmental contaminant.

### Vibriosis

Bacteria of the genus *Vibrio* are ubiquitous in the marine and estuarine environment and most commonly cause disease in marine fish. In a survey of 129 cases from tropical marine fish, nearly 50% had either *Aeromonas* or *Vibrio* infections.[8] Species that have been shown to cause disease in fish include *V anguillarum* (most common), *V salmonicida*, *V ordalii*, *V alginolyticus*, *V parahaemolyticus*, *V vulnificus*, and *Photobacterium damselae* subspecies *piscicida*. *V anguillarum* and *V ordalii* are the two most commonly identified from marine ornamentals.[2] Clinically, vibriosis is very similar to motile aeromonad septicemia and results in hemorrhagic septicemia with cutaneous hemorrhages and ulcers.[2] As with other bacterial infections, underlying environmental stressors are often present.

### Photobacterium damselae *subspecies* piscicida

One common species recently classified in the *Vibrio* family causing pathology in marine tropical fish is *Photobacterium damselae* subspecies *piscicida*. It is found in a variety of freshwater and marine tropical and temperate species. It can manifest in an acute outbreak with varying mortality, or the disease can be marked by an insidious chronic form with pseudotubercle formation in the kidney and spleen with internal necrosis.[9] This disease was formerly known as piscine pasteurellosis. Outbreaks are associated with high temperatures and can cause catastrophic losses in several species of marine fish. This disease has been treated using various oral antibiotics.

### Edwardsiella tarda

*Edwardsiella tarda* is a gram-negative rod associated with septicemia with or without ulceration in a wide variety of freshwater and marine species.[10] Disease associated with *E tarda* often occurs during the summer in ponds. Reports of disease in ornamental fish have been reported in coral reef grunts and squirrelfish, and a keyhole angelfish.[8] This bacterium can infect all poikilothermic vertebrates and is zoonotic. In disease outbreaks, antibiotics are commonly added to feed.

### DIAGNOSIS OF GRAM-NEGATIVE ULCER FORMING OR SYSTEMIC INFECTIONS

Diagnosis is based on history, clinical signs, and bacterial culture or sensitivity. Samples should be submitted to laboratories that are familiar with culturing aquatic pathogens. Most fish pathogens are best cultured at room temperature (22–25°C), not 37°C, which is the common protocol in mammalian microbiology laboratories. A nonselective agar such as blood agar is a good medium for the growth of most fish pathogens.[3] In marine fish, a medium with 1% to 2% sodium chloride may be needed. In some cases, selective specialized media can be used to enhance the growth and isolation of certain pathogens.

The organ of choice for bacterial culture (**Fig. 2**) in systemic infections is the posterior kidney.[1–3] Dorsal and ventral approaches to the posterior kidney have been described.[2] Other organs that may be cultured include the brain (especially when neurologic signs are present), liver, spleen, and anterior kidney. Blood culture has been described as a nonlethal test in cases of systemic bacterial infections. A recent report described good correlation between blood culture results and posterior kidney tissue cultures in a small population of fish.[11] Blood cultures were obtained aseptically from the caudal vein; samples were incubated in brain heart infusion broth and then transferred to blood agar plates.[11] When culturing cutaneous ulcers, tissue cultures obtained aseptically are preferred to superficial swabs as secondary pathogens commonly invade ulcerative lesions. When culturing, samples should be obtained from the leading edge of the ulcerative lesion. Taking a small biopsy for histology or cytologic staining is also recommended to help support microbiologic findings. *A salmonicida* can be very difficult to culture as it is quickly overgrown by less fastidious secondary pathogens. Molecular techniques (such as PCR, ELISA, and immunostaining) can be used to illustrate the presence of *A salmonicida* or other pathogens in ulcerative skin lesions or various tissue samples.[5]

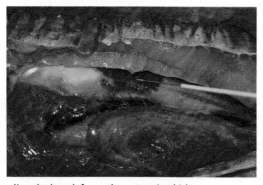

**Fig. 2.** Bacterial sampling (culture) from the posterior kidney.

## TREATMENT OF GRAM-NEGATIVE ULCER FORMING OR SYSTEMIC INFECTIONS

Treatment of gram-negative ulcer forming and systemic infections in fish should always involve a thorough analysis of the environment, and improvement of any poor environmental or husbandry-related problems or other related stressors. The mainstay of treatment for gram-negative systemic or ulcerative disease in fish is antimicrobials. Antimicrobials can be administered parenterally, orally, or as a bath treatment. Parenteral administration of antibiotics is the most effective method to achieve therapeutic blood levels that exceed the minimum inhibitory concentration for aquatic pathogens. Ideally, antimicrobials are selected based on culture and antibiotic susceptibility tests (disk diffusion, automated-broth microdilution techniques) as antimicrobial resistance is common in aquatic bacterial pathogens. Empiric first choice antibiotic should be effective against gram-negative bacteria. Few antimicrobials have been studied pharmacokinetically in ornamental fish. The antibiotics studied in ornamental fish include enrofloxacin, florfenicol, and oxytetracycline. **Table 2** lists common antimicrobials used in pet fish, including dosing information when applicable.

Injectable antibiotics are typically given as intramuscular or intracoelomic injections. Intramuscular injections are most commonly given in the dorsal epaxial musculature. Intracoelomic injections can be given in the scaleless region at the base of the pelvic fin. **Fig. 3** illustrates an intracoelomic injection in a koi.

Oral antibiotics are most commonly used when treating large numbers of fish and when injections are not practical. Antibiotics are either mixed with the feed or top-dressed on the feed using a binding agent such as canola oil. Gel-based diets (such as those by Mazuri Purina Mills, Grey Summit, Missouri) offer the practitioner a convenient and palatable diet in which oral antibiotics can easily be mixed. Oral antibiotics can also be administered by way of oral gavage tube.

Administration of antibiotics in the water is commonplace in the aquarium industry and numerous antibiotics are available over the counter to fish hobbyists. Problems associated with use of bath antibiotics include limited absorption or insufficient dose, damage to the biofilter and development of bacterial resistance.[1] Pharmacokinetic data for bath antibiotics is generally lacking in ornamental fish; absorption is likely greater in marine fish because of increased water consumption. Bath antibiotics should be limited to cases of external infections (such as columnaris disease and "fin rot") and in fish that are anorexic.

## EXTERNAL GRAM-NEGATIVE BACTERIAL INFECTIONS

Bacterial diseases caused by gram-negative bacteria that are typically more limited to the skin include columnaris disease and fin rot. Columnaris disease is caused by *Flavobacterium columnare* and results in cottony proliferative lesions on the skin and fins.[1] Common locations for the lesions include perioral, periocular, fins, dorsum, and tail regions. The synonym "cotton-wool" disease describes the fluffy white cotton-like masses, patches, or plaques often seen with *F columnare*. Given this clinical appearance, columnaris disease is often misdiagnosed as fungal disease in aquarium fish; wet-mount examination of affected areas can be used to differentiate between these two conditions and rule out parasitic infestations (**Fig. 4**). *F columnare* may also affect the gills resulting in respiratory signs. A large number of other similar gram-negative rods including *Cytophaga* spp, *Flexibacter* spp, *Flavobacterium* spp, *Sporocytophaga* spp, and *Myxobacterium* spp have been isolated from fish with similar lesions.[2] All these gram-negative bacteria form yellow to orange pigmented colonies and are occasionally collectively referred to as yellow-pigmented bacteria.[5] Columnaris-type infections caused by *F maritimus* have been reported to cause a marine form of columnaris disease with similar clinical signs to the freshwater counterpart.[2,3]

Wet-mount examination of the skin reveals characteristic long, thin rods with gliding or flexing motion; "hay stack" protrusions of rod-shaped bacteria may also be noted.[1–3] Columnaris disease is common in live bearers such as guppies, platies, mollies, and swordtails. Treatment of columnaris disease can be achieved with antibiotic bath treatment with oxytetracycline (see **Table 2** for dosing) repeated daily for 10 days. Other treatment options include potassium permanganate as a prolonged bath, copper sulfate, and diquat herbicide (Reward Syngenta, Greensboro, North Carolina) dosed at 2 to 18 mg/L for four-hour bath immersions.[1] Treatment should be repeated daily for three to four treatments with large water changes after each bath treatment. Systemic antimicrobials may be needed in more severe infections. A recent study found that a single hydrogen peroxide ($H_2O_2$) treatment of 3.1 mg/L or more for one hour effectively eliminated external bacteria in the green swordtail *Xiphophorus helleri*.[12]

Fin-rot refers to a characteristic necrosis of the fins resulting in an irregular notched to ragged appearance to the fins. Fin rot is usually secondary to underlying stressors and poor husbandry. Several different species of bacteria can be isolated from these lesions in ornamental fish including *Flavobacterium columnare*, *Flexibacter maritimus*, and *Cytophaga* spp.[2] Treatment of this condition involves searching and removing underlying stressors and using antimicrobials as for columnaris disease.

## SYSTEMIC, GRAM-POSITIVE, RAPIDLY GROWING BACTERIA

The most common bacteria in this group that cause disease in fish are *Streptococcus* spp; other gram-positive genera that are closely related to *Streptococcus* and cause disease in fish include *Lactococcus*, *Enterococcus*, and *Vagococcus*. Clinical signs are similar to those involving systemic gram-negative infections such as skin discolorations, exophthalmos, ascites, skin ulcerations, and hemorrhages.[2,13] Neurologic signs are extremely common in fish with streptococcal infections; abnormal swimming behavior such as spiraling or spinning is often reported.[13] High mortality may also occur. On gross necropsy, *Streptococcus* can cause granulomas in the kidney, spleen, or liver. Diagnosis is confirmed by culturing *Streptococcus* and related bacteria. In acute outbreaks of streptococcus, kidney cultures are routinely taken. As many cases invade the central nervous system, culturing the brain in suspected cases is critical when neurologic signs are observed. Antibiotics that may be effective against *Streptococcus* and related species include erythromycin (1.5g/lb of food fed for 10–14 days), amoxicillin or ampicillin, and florfenicol.[13] Immunostimulants added to the feed, such as beta-glucans and nucleotides, have been shown to increase survival for *Streptococcus*-infected redtail black shark populations.[14] In addition to being a human pathogen, *S iniae* causes disease in cultured marine and freshwater fish and is difficult to eradicate from hatcheries and grow-out facilities.

## SLOW-GROWING, ACID-FAST BACTERIA: MYCOBACTERIOSIS

Mycobacteriosis in fish is caused by nontubercle-forming *Mycobacterium* species that are ubiquitous in the aquatic environment. The two most common species associated with ornamental fish disease are *M marinum* and *M fortuitum*.[2,15,16] *M chelonae* also causes disease in fish (typically cold-water salmonids) but is less commonly reported.[3] Mycobacteriosis is zoonotic and can cause "fish tank granuloma" in people. A recent study in zebrafish illustrated that the primary route of infection is

**Table 2**
Dosage information for common antimicrobials in pet and ornamental fish

| Drug | Parenteral Administration | Oral Administration | Bath | Notes |
|---|---|---|---|---|
| Amikacin | 5 mg/kg IM q 12 h[a] | — | — | Not studied pharmacokinetically in pet fish Used commonly by koi hobbyists |
| Aztreonam | 100 mg/kg IM, ICe q 48 h[a] | — | — | Not studied pharmacokinetically in pet fish Used commonly by koi hobbyists |
| Ceftazidime | 20 mg/kg IM q 72h[b] | — | — | Not studied pharmacokinetically in pet fish Used commonly by fish veterinarians |
| Enrofloxacin | 5–10 mg/kg IM, ICe q 48–72 h (koi)[c] 5 mg/kg IM q 48 h (red pacu)[d] | 5 mg/kg PO every 24–48 hr (red pacu)[d] | 2.5 mg/L × 5 h every 24–48 h (red pacu)[d] | Only studied pharmacokinetically in koi[c] and pacu,[d] but used commonly by fish veterinarians in many species |
| Florfenicol | Red pacu: 20–30 mg/kg IM q 24 h[e] Koi: 25 mg/kg q 24–48 h; shorter half-life in three-spot Gourami may necessitate more frequent dosing[f] | 50 mg/kg po q 24 h in koi; shorter half-life in gourami may necessitate q 12 h dosing[f] | Minimal absorption as bath treatment in koi[f] | Studied pharmacokinetically in red pacu,[e] koi,[f] and three-spot gourami[d] |
| Kanamycin | — | 300 mg/lb food/d × 10d[g] 50 mg/kg/d in feed[a] | 50–100 mg/L × 5 hr, repeat every 3 d for 3 treatments[a,g] | Not studied pharmacokinetically in pet fish May cause renal damage |
| Oxolinic acid | — | 150 mg/lb food/d for 10 d[g] | 38 mg/10 gallons for 24 h, repeat as needed[g] 95 mg/gallon for 15 min, repeat twice daily for 3 d[g] | Not studied pharmacokinetically in pet fish May cause lethargy when used as bath treatment, inhibited by hard water |

| | | | | |
|---|---|---|---|---|
| Oxytetracycline | Red pacu: 7 mg/kg IM q 24 h[h] | 1.12 g/lb food/d for 10 d[g] | 750–3,780 mg/10 gallons for 6–12 h, repeat daily for 10 d (dose will depend on hardness of water)[g] 50%–75% water changes between treatments | Studied pharmacokinetically in red pau[h] Increased Ca and Mg inactivate, not useful in marine systems as bath treatment |
| Nitrofurazone | — | 1.12 g/lb food/d for 10 d[g] | 189–756 mg/10 gallons for 1 h, repeat daily for 10 d[g] 378 mg/10 gallons for 6–12 h, repeat daily for 10 d[g] | Not studied pharmacokinetically in pet fish Systemic absorption from bath treatment questionable, best reserved for external infections Carcinogenic Inactivated in bright light |
| Sulfadimethoxine/ ormethoprim (Romet B Hoffman-LaRoche) | — | 50 mg/kg/d for 5 d[a] | Not useful as bath treatment | Not studied pharmacokinetically in pet fish |
| Trimethoprim sulfa | — | 30 mg/kg PO q 24 hr × 10–14 d[a] | 20 mg/L × 5 h q 24 h × 5–7d[a] | Not studied pharmacokinetically in pet fish |

*Abbreviations:* ICe, intracoelomic; IM, intramuscular.

[a] Mashima T, Lewbart GA. Pet fish formulary. VCNA Exotic Animal Practice 2000;3(1):117–30.

[b] Palmeiro B and Roberts H. Bacterial disease in fish. In: Mayer J, editor. Clinical Veterinary Advisor: Exotic Medicine. 2009. In Press.

[c] Lewbart GA, Butkus D, Papich M, et al. Evaluation of a method of intracoelomic catheterization in koi. JAVMA 2005;226:784–8.

[d] Lewbart GA, Vaden S, Deen J et al. Pharmacokinetics of enrofloxacin in the red pacu (*Colossoma brachypomum*) after intramuscular, oral and bath adminis-tration. J Vet Pharmacol Therap 1997;20:124–8.

[e] Lewbart GA, Papich MG, Whitt-Smith D. Pharmacokinets of florfenicol in the red pacu (*Paractus brachypomus*) after single dose intramuscular administration. J Vet Pharacol Therap. 2005;28:317–9.

[f] Yanong RPE, Curtis EW, Simmons R et al. Pharmacokinetic studies of florfenicol in koi carp and threespot gourami *Trichogaster trichopterus* after oral and intramuscular treatment. Journal of Aquatic Animal Health 2005;17:129–37.

[g] Yanong R. Use of antibiotics in ornamental fish aquaculture. VM-84. Florida Cooperative Extension Service, UF-IFAS. 2006. Available at: http://edis.ifas.ufl.edu. Accessed June 15, 2009.

[h] Doi AM, Stoskopf MK, Lewbart GA. Pharmacokinetics of oxytetracycline in the red pacu following different routes of administration. J Vet Phamacol Therap 1998;21:364–8.

*From* Palmeiro BS. Bacterial Diseases. In: Roberts HR edition. Fundamentals of Ornamental Fish Health. Wiley-Blackwell. In Press; with permission.

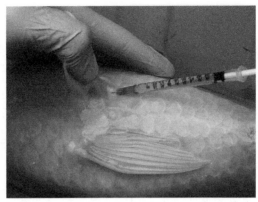

**Fig. 3.** Intracoelomic injection in a koi. The injection is administered in the scaleless region at the base of the pelvic fin.

through the intestinal tract.[17] Fish can be infected by consuming contaminated feed, by way of cannibalism of infected fish and carcasses or aquatic detritus.[3,15,16]

*Mycobacterium* spp are ubiquitous in the aquatic environment; a recent report found 75% of water samples from decorative aquaria to be positive for *Mycobacterium* spp.[18] Environmental factors that favor growth of mycobacterium include low dissolved oxygen, low salinity, low pH, warmer water, and high organic loads.[15]

Although mycobacteriosis has been reported in greater than 150 species of freshwater, brackish, and marine species, tropical aquarium fish are most commonly affected.[16] Members of the freshwater families *Anabantidae* (bettas and gouramis),

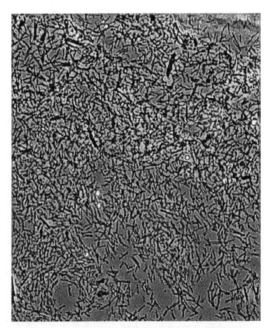

**Fig. 4.** A wet-mount preparation showing *Flavobacterium columnare*, the etiologic agent of columnaris disease.

*Characidae* (tetras and piranhas), and *Cyprinidae* (danios and barbs) appear to be particularly susceptible.[16] Also, marine sygnathids are regularly diagnosed with mycobacteriosis on necropsy and histopathology. In cultured and wild finfish, striped bass (*Morone saxatilis*) are commonly affected with the disease, now endemic in the Chesapeake Bay.

Clinical signs of mycobacteriosis are usually nonspecific and can include ulcerative skin lesions, reduced appetite, emaciation, lethargy, exophthalmia ("pop-eye"), swollen abdomen, anorexia, fin or tail rot, and skeletal abnormalities.[1,2] This disease is usually chronic, slowly progressive, and causes low-to-moderate mortalities. Mycobacteriosis is the most commonly diagnosed chronic wasting disease of aquarium fish. **Fig. 5** illustrates a goldfish with dropsy (generalized edema) secondary to systemic mycobacteriosis. On internal examination, granulomas will develop in the liver, kidney, spleen, heart, muscle, gill, and other tissues. Granulomas are typically pale gray to tan but are only visible to the naked eye in more advanced cases.

Diagnosis is based on clinical signs, the presence of granulomas, and the demonstration of acid-fast bacterial rods in tissues. Typical granulomas can be found on light microscopy of internal organ wet mounts (most commonly kidney, spleen, and liver). Granulomas can also be found in skin wet mounts, and less commonly, gill biopsies. **Fig. 6** illustrates the typical appearance of granulomas on light microscopy, with a dark-brown center and surrounding capsule.

When granulomas are found, an acid-fast stain should be performed. Acid-fast stains can be performed on cytologic preparations or histopathological sections. A positive acid-fast stain reveals red-to-pink, rod-shaped bacteria against a light green background. Culture of *Mycobacterium* for definitive species identification can be lengthy and difficult but is best performed on mycobacterial selective media such as Lowenstein-Jensen agar. *M marinum* is classified as a slow-growing mycobacterium, whereas *M fortuitum* and *M chelonae* are classified as rapidly growing.[16] Molecular diagnostics such as PCR are also useful in species identification. Because *Mycobacteria* sp are so ubiquitous in the environment, the gold standard for diagnosis is a positive culture supported by histopathology and PCR identification.

There is no effective cure for mycobacteriosis in fish. In aquaculture, retail, and wholesale situations, depopulation and disinfection is often recommended. Treatment is often different in public aquaria or zoos and private collections, and mycobacteriosis is often managed differently at these institutions and locations. Various antibiotics such as rifampin, erythromycin, streptomycin, kanamycin, doxycycline and minocycline have been suggested as possible treatments, but a clinical cure is unlikely.[1,2,15] Mycobacteria are resistant to many commonly used bactericidal agents at standard

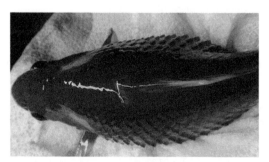

**Fig. 5.** Dropsy (generalized edema) in a goldfish (*Carassius auratus*) with systemic mycobacteriosis. Note protruding scales and abdominal distension ("pine cone disease"). Also, note exophthalmos.

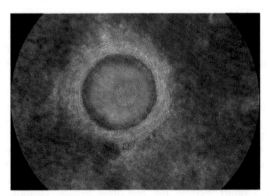

**Fig. 6.** Granulomas found on internal wet-mount examination of the spleen in a fish with mycobacteriosis. Note dark-brown center with surrounding lighter capsule.

dosage rates, including chlorine bleach and quaternary ammonium compounds.[15] As much as 10,000 parts per million chlorine has been reported necessary to kill mycobacteria.[15] In a recent study comparing efficacy of common disinfectants against *M marinum*, ethyl alcohol (50% and 70%), benzyl-4-chlorophenol/phenylphenol (Lysol) (1%), and sodium chlorite (mixed as 1:5:1 or 1:18:1 [base:water:activator]) were the most effective disinfectants with elimination or reduction of *M marinum* within one minute of contact.[19] Sodium hypochlorite (50,000 mg/L) was moderately effective but required a minimum contact time of 10 minutes to reduce bacterial counts.[19] Disinfectants that were ineffective after sixty minutes of contact time included ethyl alcohol (30%), N-alkyl dimethyl benzyl ammonium chloride (1:256), and potassium peroxymonosulfate-sodium chloride (1%).[19]

## OTHER ORGANISMS: *RICKETTSIA*

Intracellular rickettsial organisms are an emerging disease problem in several species of tropical and temperate freshwater fish species.[20] In mortalities of blue-eyed plecostomus catfish, *Panaque suttoni*, shipped from Columbia, Khoo and colleagues[21] identified rickettsial-like organisms from moribund specimens on transport. The most commonly described rickettsial pathology and infection, called piscirickettsiosis, is caused by *Piscirickettsia salmonis* in Chinook salmon. Fish may or may not exhibit clinical signs, and mortality can be as high as 95%.[20] Current antibiotic treatment has not been successful in treating for piscirickettsiosis, necessitating changes in management to control outbreaks and prevent infection.

## PARASITIC DISEASES OF FISH

Parasitic diseases are the most common infectious disease seen in pet fish. Fish parasites are a very diverse group and include protozoans, trematodes, turbellarians, nematodes, cestodes, leeches, acanthocephalans, monogeneans, pentastomes, copepods, and crustaceans.[22] Life cycles range from simple and direct, requiring no intermediate host, to complex and indirect, requiring one or more intermediate hosts. Fish may serve as final, paratenic, or intermediate hosts in a parasite life cycle.[22–24] Understanding the life cycles of any diagnosed parasites is critical for effective and successful treatment.[22,23] For example, only the free-swimming life stage (theront) of the common, external, ciliated parasite *Ichthyophthirius multifiliis* are susceptible to chemical treatments.

### Introduction of Parasites

Parasites are most often introduced into a naïve, closed population by failing to quarantine and treat infected animals. Other methods of parasite introduction include the addition of live plants without prior disinfection, through fomites (nets, and other commonly shared equipment), by the use of contaminated source water, from wild birds, frogs, and turtles in outdoor ponds, and by way of aerosol droplet transmission between aquaria.[25–28] Standard biosecurity practices including quarantine protocols can reduce the potential for exposure of established populations and allow for treatment of animals in quarantine systems before introduction.

### Diagnosis of Parasites in Fish

All sick fish should be evaluated using a standard minimum database that includes a detailed history from the owner, water quality testing, observation for any apparent clinical signs, physical examination, microscopic examination of wet-mount cytology of skin scrapes, gill biopsies, and fecal samples. There are no specific pathognomonic clinical signs for parasitic diseases in fish, although a group of clinical signs can be suggestive. These include: flashing (rubbing on the bottom of the tank or pond, indicative of pruritus); lethargy; cutaneous lesions including scale loss, ulcerations, and increased mucus production; rapid, opercular movements (increased "gilling"); gasping or piping; weight loss; "yawning"; osmoregulatory disruption, and deaths.[29]

Most external parasites can be readily identified on direct observation, and wet-mount skin and gill cytology preparations of sedated or anesthetized fish.[22–24,28,29] Internal parasite infections may be identified by wet-mount preparation of fresh fecal samples, gross visualization of the parasite at the vent (eg *Camallanus* sp), evaluation of blood smears, organ squash preparations, histopathology, and necropsy examination.[22–24,28,29] These two procedures are described below.

Skin scraping procedure (**Fig. 7**)

a. Place a drop of water from the tank or pond on a prepared glass slide.
b. A glass or plastic cover slip is gently scraped at a 45-degree angle in a cranial-to-caudal direction in small areas of the body.
c. If lesional skin is present, these areas should be sampled. In fish with no obvious lesions, two to three sites should be sampled. Commonly sampled locations that may yield a high number of ectoparasites are areas that are least hydrodynamic so parasites can best adhere to the skin or gills, including the skin behind the fins, on the caudal peduncle or tail, under the chin and on the ventrum.

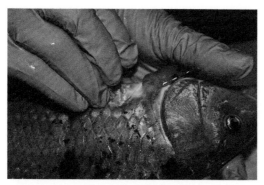

**Fig. 7.** A skin scrape taken from a koi (*Cyprinus carpio*).

d. Place the cover slip with mucus sample on a slide prepared with a drop of the fish's own water.
e. Starting with the lowest power objective, examine under the microscope for parasites. Identification of parasites is based on observation of their characteristic movements and size. During microscopy, the condenser should be down to improve contrast.
f. The slide is not stained and must be examined immediately. Slides may dry when examined outdoors or in warm or drafty environments. Parasites will become less active and die when left on a slide for a prolonged time, although they may need a few seconds to warm under the microscope's light source in cold temperatures to begin moving for identification.
g. If available, use both light and dark fields to scan the slide.

Gill biopsy procedure (**Fig. 8**)

1. Using gloved hands, the operculum of the sedated or anesthetized fish is gently lifted to reveal the gills.
2. With fine scissors such as iris tenotomy or suture removal scissors, snip a tiny section from the distal end of a few primary lamellae.
3. Place the gill tissue on a slide prepared with a drop of water from the 'fish's own environment.
4. As mentioned above, the slide is not stained and must be examined immediately for evidence of parasites.
5. The sample can also be examined for gill architecture. Gill pathology such as hyperplasia, hypertrophy, necrosis, lamellar fusion, and telangiectasia may be found.
6. In extremely large fish, one may only be able to scrape the gills. Gill rakers should be examined carefully during the physical examination as many larger parasites will lodge in these areas.

Parasites of clinical importance in fish can be divided into seven major groups and will be discussed in detail below.

### Protozoan Parasites of Clinical Importance

### Ciliated protozoans
*Ichthyophthirius multifiliis*, "whitespot disease" or "ich," is the most common parasitic disease affecting freshwater fish worldwide.[22,27,30] The parasite can survive in a wide range of temperatures and host susceptibility varies among species with scaleless

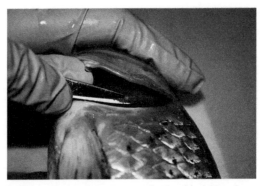

**Fig. 8.** A gill biopsy being performed on an anesthetized koi (*Cyprinus carpio*).

fish, such as catfish, being particularly vulnerable.[30] Overcrowded systems and poor water quality, which lead to increased stress and reduced immune function in fish, can result in increased morbidity and mortality.[31] Disease caused by *I multifiliis* can present acutely and result in up to 100% mortality.[30,31] The marine counterpart is *Cryptocaryon irritans.* Both have nearly identical pathology and clinical signs. The life cycle of both parasites is direct with a free-swimming infective stage (theront) that is the only stage susceptible to treatment. Trophonts are the encysted feeding stage seen on the host as white nodules. Trophonts break through the epithelium to become encysted tomonts with sticky external capsules that attach to inanimate substrate materials in the environment, including gravel, nets, plants, and so forth.[22,24,27–30,32] These tomonts divide, producing tomites that break through the nodule wall to releasing motile, infective theronts. At 25°C (77°F), infective theronts have 48 hours to find a new host or perish.[24,28,30,32] Upon finding a host, the theront penetrates the epithelium and develops into the ciliated trophont. *Ichthyophthirius* can be transmitted by aerosol dispersion of the infective stage.[26] The life cycle of ich is temperature dependent. It lasts 3 to 6 days at 25°C (77°F), and 10 days at 15°C (59°F). Outbreaks are most common at 15 to 25°C (59–77°F). One difference between marine and freshwater ich is duration of the life cycle. *Cryptocaryon* has a longer life cycle so treatment duration will need to be extended (up to 1 month) when compared with *Ichthyophthirius.*

Clinical signs include white, raised nodules up to 1 mm (0.5 mm for *Cryptocaryon*) on the skin and gills, flashing, increased mucus production, lethargy, dyspnea, secondary bacterial or fungal infections, and osmoregulatory compromise due to the epithelial and gill damage caused by the parasite.[24,27–30,32] Microscopic evaluation of the gills can show hyperplasia, necrosis, excess mucus, and necrosis.[30,32–35] Diagnosis is made by examination of a wet-mount cytology preparation of the skin or gills. Ich is a large parasite, entirely covered in cilia, moves in a characteristic slow-rolling motion, and has a C- or horseshoe-shaped nucleus (**Figs. 9–11**). The nucleus of *Cryptocaryon* differs from *Ichthyophthirius*; it is lobulated with four bead-like segments.[30]

*Trichodina* and *Trichodinella* spp are other common ciliated parasites found on both freshwater and marine pet fish. There are many species of these parasites, most with a predilection for skin and gill epithelium, but some will parasitize the urinary bladder or oviduct. These parasites are often associated with high levels of organic debris in the

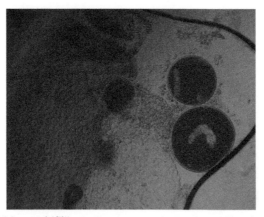

**Fig. 9.** *Ichthyophthirius multifiliis* as seen on a wet-mount examination of a skin scrape (40× magnification).

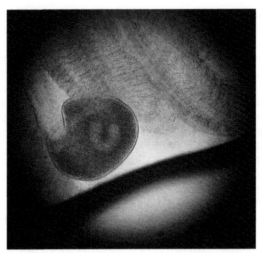

**Fig. 10.** *Ichthyophthirius multifiliis* on gill prep from a goldfish (*Carassius auratus*). Note the characteristic horseshoe-shaped nucleus (40× magnification).

water, poor nutrition, overcrowding, and subsequent poor water quality.[27,28,36] It is not uncommon to find these parasites on pond fish such as goldfish and koi that exist in ponds with high levels of detritus or organic debris. As with many other protozoan parasites, there is a direct life cycle and reproduction occurs by binary fission. Trichodinids can be introduced by fomites and live plants added to ponds and tanks.

Clinical signs of heavy infestations include flashing, increased mucus production giving a cloudy appearance to the skin, cutaneous hemorrhages, frayed fins and tail, lethargy, and chronic low level mortalities; with severe branchial infestations, respiratory signs may be present.[24,27,29,30,36] Secondary bacterial and fungal infections may occur because of extensive tissue damage. Observation of the circular, ciliated parasite with a prominent internal denticular ring on a wet-mount examination of gills or skin is diagnostic (**Fig. 12**). The parasite has been described as a flying saucer or "scrubbing bubble"[36] (E.L. Johnson, DVM, personal communication, February

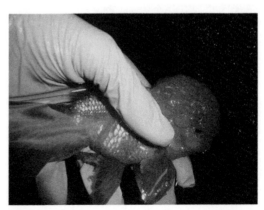

**Fig. 11.** An oranda affected by *Ichthyophthirius*. Small pinpoint white nodules may be seen on the wen (ornate head growth).

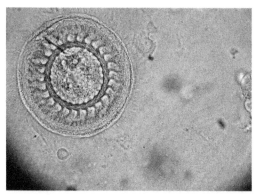

**Fig. 12.** Trichodina sp on a wet-mount prep from a skin scrape performed on a koi (*Cyprinus carpio*). This koi was being held in poor water conditions at 2°C (36°F).

2009). The motion of this parasite has been described as rotating,[28] scooting,[30] erratic, whirling, and hyperactive.

*Chilodonella* sp is a ciliated parasite shaped like a heart or an onion, with a flattened appearance. Cilia are located longitudinally on the parasite and may be seen as visible striations. *Chilodonella* can survive a wide variety of temperature ranges, is found worldwide, and can survive in brackish water.[27,30,32] *Brooklynella hostilis* is the marine counterpart named after its discovery at the Brooklyn aquarium. Both parasites are highly pathogenic and severe tissue damage can occur before any gross pathology is visible.[27,30] Clinical signs include respiratory distress (gasping, piping, opercular flaring, increased gilling), clamped fins, a ragged appearance to the skin, excess mucus production, secondary cutaneous ulcers, pathologic gill changes including hyperplasia and fusion of the lamellae, depression, and mortalities.[27–30,32] Diagnosis is based on observation of the parasite on wet mount examinations of skin and gills. *Chilodonella* moves in a gliding motion or circular motion on wet-mount preparation.

*Tetrahymena* sp (freshwater) and *Uronema* sp (marine) are ciliated parasites that cause external (skin and gill) lesions and internal, systemic infections. *Uronema* infects a wide variety of marine species and over a wide temperature range (8–28°C). External signs include small, white patches on the skin, skin hemorrhages, sloughing, and necrosis, and gill aneurysms.[28,30,32,36] Fish with systemic infections may show nonspecific signs such as anorexia and lethargy. Death can occur rapidly once infection is established. *Tetrahymena*, also known as "guppy disease" or "guppy killer," is found most often in guppies, other livebearers, tetras, and cichlids.[28,30] This organism can also be found colonizing organic debris in the water. Poor water quality, bacterial infections, and other stressors may predispose fish to *Tetrahymena* infections.[28,30,32] Clinical signs are similar to *Uronema*. Muscle swelling and periocular lesions can also be seen with *Tetrahymena* infections. Keratitis can also occur with this protozoan and other parasites (*Cryptocaryon, Ichthyophthirius, Henneguya,* and *Glugea*) due to the close connection of the skin and cornea.[37] Deep or systemic infections carry a poor prognosis. Diagnosis is made with wet-mount examination or histopathology of skin and gill tissue. Deep or systemic infections will require histopathology of the affected organ or tissue.

Sedentary or sessile ciliates are most commonly seen on pond-reared fish (koi, catfish, and goldfish) in water with high levels of organic debris and high levels of suspended solids.[28,30] They also occur as secondary invaders on cutaneous ulcers and other causes of epithelial damage in other pet fish species. Species most often encountered include *Epistylis* (also known as *Heteropolaria*), *Capriniana piscium* (previously known as *Trichophyra*), *Apiosoma* (**Fig. 13**) (previously known as *Glossatella*), and *Ambiphyra* (previously known as *Scyphidia*).[29,30,32] *Epistylis* produces white, fluffy lesions on fins and tail margins, opercular margins, and oral cavity.[30] These lesions can easily be mistaken for fungal lesions or columnaris disease owing to their similar appearance. *Capriniana* has a predilection for gill tissue and can cause severe respiratory distress by mechanically blocking gill tissue in infected fish.[30] Wet-mount cytology (**Fig. 14**) and histopathology of affected tissues are methods used to diagnose sessile ciliate infestations.

### Flagellated Protozoans of Clinical Importance

Parasitic dinoflagellates can be found in both marine (*Amyloodinium ocellatum*) and freshwater (*Piscioodinium* sp) tropical fish. Both parasites share characteristic morphology, are temperature sensitive, and have similar life cycles to *Ichthyophthirius*. Only the free-living dinospore is susceptible to treatment. *A ocellatum* can parasitize both elasmobranchs and teleosts.[30] Similar to *Ichthyophthirius*, *A ocellatum* has also been shown to be transmissible by aerosol dispersion of water droplets, up to three meters in dynamic airflow systems.[25] For both parasites, the gills and skin are the preferential site of infestation and heavy infestation can result in edematous changes, hyperplasia, inflammation, hemorrhage, osmoregulatory compromise, and necrosis of the gill filaments.[27–30,32] Mortalities, in as little as 12 hours, result from hypoxia, secondary bacterial infections, and osmoregulatory compromise.[27,28,36] In addition to respiratory distress, another clinical sign that may be seen is a dusty, gold appearance to the skin, hence the names "velvet disease," "gold dust disease," and "rust disease." Diagnosis is made by wet-mount cytology or histopathology of the skin and gills. In addition to the introduction of infected fish to a system, fomites and the introduction of "infected" water may play a role in transmission.[27]

*Ichthyobodo*, previously known as *Costia*, is a very small, flagellated parasite (about the size of a red blood cell) of freshwater fish found in a wide variety of species with a global distribution. The parasite can survive a wide temperature range (2–30°C) and has been occasionally on marine fish.[27,30,32] The life cycle is direct and transmission occurs from fish to fish. Mortalities are higher in fry, young fish, and stressed,

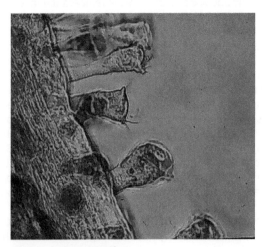

**Fig. 13.** *Apiosoma* sp Wet-mount preparation.

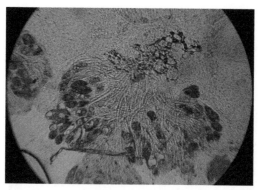

**Fig. 14.** Sessile ciliate infestation on a wet-mount preparation.

debilitated adult fish. Clinical signs include severe respiratory distress, lethargy, depression, flashing, anorexia, epithelial irritation, heavy mucus production, and deaths. Deaths may occur before any clinical signs. Diagnosis is based on wet-mount cytology. The organism's movement has been described as a "flickering" candle, or erratic spiraling. Other flagellates of clinical importance include *Hexamita* sp, *Spironucleus* sp, and *Cryptobia* sp. These parasites are found primarily in the gastrointestinal tract of freshwater fish although there are some species that can be found externally on fish. Of the seven species of *Cryptobia* that have been associated with the gastrointestinal tract of fish, only *C iubilans* is reported to be pathogenic and parasitic. *C branchialis* and *C agitans* typically parasitize gill tissue.[30,32] *Spironucleus* has been isolated from lesions characteristic of "hole-in-the-head-disease" in discus (*Symphysodon* sp) and angelfish (*Pterophyllum* sp) but the role it plays in this multifactorial syndrome is unknown.[29,36] These flagellates are most commonly found to cause clinical disease in freshwater angelfish, cichlids, and anabantids. Clinical signs of gastrointestinal infections include: severe weight loss, anorexia, lethargy, abdominal distension, mucoid enteritis, mucoid or pale feces, exophthalmos, darkening of the skin, buoyancy disorders, redness at the vent, and deaths (**Fig. 15**).[27–29,30,38,39] Concurrent infections with other parasites, poor water quality and other stressors such as overcrowding are not uncommon and increase morbidity. *C iubilans* induces granulomatous disease, primarily seen in the stomach of affected fish (**Fig. 16**).[40]

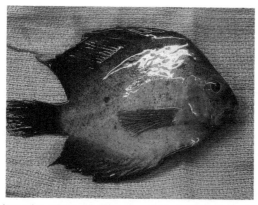

**Fig. 15.** Thin discus (*Symphysodon* sp) *with a Cryptobia iubilans infection.*

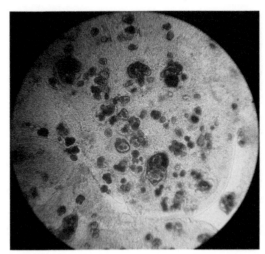

**Fig. 16.** Wet-mount squash preparation of the stomach wall in a discus with *Cryptobia iubilans*. Note the severe granulomatous gastritis effacing the normal stomach architecture.

Diagnosis of intestinal flagellates can be made by wet-mount fecal examination although an intestinal squash prep or histopathology is more likely to yield a diagnosis. For *Spironucleus* or *Hexamita*, trophozoites are small (12.5–20 μm in length), flagellated, actively motile, with an ellipsoid to pear shape. Trophozoites of *Spironucleus* or *Hexamita* are often localized in the anterior intestinal lumen and therefore may not be present on fecal examination. They have six anterior and two posterior flagella. Species identification and differentiation between *Hexamita* and *Spironucleus* requires electron microscopy. *Cryptobia* is most commonly detected by identifying granulomas in squash preparation wet mounts of the stomach. An acid-fast stain should be performed to rule out mycobacteriosis (another common cause of granulomas in ornamental fish). Motile trophozoites are not commonly seen on wet mounts. When present, flagellated trophozoites are elongate (acute infection) to oval or teardrop shape (chronic infection) with a characteristic slow, undulating movement. The organism has two flagella. Species identification requires electron microscopy.

### Microsporidians, Coccidia, Cryptosporidium, and Myxozoans

Microsporidians are intracellular parasites with a direct life cycle and several species have been reported in pet fish. *Pleistophora* is the etiologic agent of "neon tetra disease," causing white cysts (xenomas) to develop in the muscle and other tissues.[28–30] These cysts may be visible below the skin.[32] The xenomas can cause severe deformity of the tissues. Rupture of the xenoma releases spores that are released and ingested by new hosts.[28–30,32] *Pleistophora* also affects angelfish, rasboras, barbs, and tetras. Clinical signs include muscle wasting, erratic swimming behavior, color loss, lethargy, secondary bacterial infections at the site of cyst rupture, and deaths. Diagnosis is made by wet-mount examination of the lesions, squash prep of affected organs, and histopathology. Other Microsporidians occasionally encountered in pet fish species include *Glugea* sp and *Heterosporis* sp. There are no reported effective treatments for Microsporidians; however, toltrazuril (Baycox Bayer Animal Health) has shown some efficacy in experimental conditions.[39]

Coccidia are another group of intracellular parasites that can infect a variety of species of fish. Most species show a predilection for the gastrointestinal system causing emaciation, chronic enteritis, anorexia, mucoid stool, and deaths.[27–30,32] Goldfish are the most common pet species presented with infections in a pet fish-practice setting. Immune suppression due to poor water quality and other environmental disorders may predispose the fish to infection. Other organs that may be affected include the reproductive organs, swim bladder, liver, spleen, and kidney. Diagnosis of intestinal infection can be made by wet-mount examination of a fresh fecal sample or cloacal wash. Histopathology and squash preps of affected organs may also be used.

A few species of *Cryptosporidium* have been identified in teleost fish.[28,40,41] Clinically affected fish may show anorexia, food regurgitation, undigested food passed in the feces, weight loss, and deaths.[28] Much is still unknown with regards to the distribution, pathogenesis, and transmission of this parasite.

Myxozoans are spore producing parasites with complex life cycles and a worldwide distribution that infect a wide variety of cultured and wild fish. Species vary from nonpathogenic to highly pathogenic. Clinical signs will depend on the affected area or organ. Species of clinical importance include *Henneguya* (marine and freshwater), *Hoferellus* (freshwater, polycystic kidney disease in koi and goldfish), *Kudoa* (marine, muscle necrosis), and *Myxobolus* sp. Lesions can range from small, white focal areas on skin to granulomatous masses in the affected tissues. Wet-mount preps, organ-squash preps, histopathology, and special staining may be all required for diagnosis. There is no effective treatment for Myxozoans infections although fumagillin (used to treat a Microsporidean disease caused by *Nosema apis* in honeybees) and malachite green have been tried.[27,39]

**Table 3** lists the treatments for the most common protozoans encountered in pet fish medicine.

### Monogeneans (flukes) of Clinical Importance

Flukes, or parasitic flatworms, are very common in marine and freshwater pet fish. Most species are found on the skin and gills of affected fish, but a few species can be found on the eye (*Neobenedinia* sp, a marine fluke), body cavity, rectal cavity, ureters, and blood vascular system.[28,30,37] In freshwater fish, the primary species seen are *Dactylogyrus* (the "gill" fluke) and *Gyrodactylus* (the "skin" fluke). Either can be located on the skin and gills. There is no species specificity seen by either fluke type. Dactylogyrids are egg layers and are often found on imported fancy goldfish, angelfish, and discus. *Gyrodactylus* is a live-bearing fluke. Oviparous monogeneans (Dactylogyridae) release eggs into the water, which hatch into a free-swimming stage (oncomiracidium) that seeks out a fish host. Viviparous monogeneans (Gyrodactylidae) release live larvae that are immediately parasitic.

Clinical signs include flashing, rubbing, gasping, lethargy, "yawning," clamped fins, excess mucus production, secondary cutaneous ulcerations, scale loss, and deaths in severe infestations.[27–30,32] Flukes can predispose fish to secondary ulcers, bacterial diseases, and eventual osmoregulatory compromise due to epithelial damage created by their attachment and feeding behavior.[4] Wet-mount cytology of the gills or skin is used to diagnose monogenean infestations. *Dactylogyrus* can be recognized by the prominent two to four anterior eyespots and a four-pointed anterior end. Gyrodactylids (**Fig. 17**) have no eyespots, and often an embryo is visible inside the fluke. On gill tissue or mucus, either species can be seen anchored and appear to be "bobbing" or stretching and compressing its body. Marine species (referred to as capsalids) of clinical importance include *Neobenedenia* sp, *Benedenia* sp, and *Dermophthirius*.[30,32]

**Table 3**
**Antiprotozoal treatments**

| | | | |
|---|---|---|---|
| 2-amino-5-nitrothiazol | 4.4 mg/gm of food oral treatment | Cryptobia iubilans | Not 100% effective, may only reduce infestation[40] |
| Amprolium | 0.63 mL/L of a 9.6% solution given over 2 d in water | Coccidiosis | [27] |
| Chloroquine | 10 mg/L prolonged immersion | Dinoflagellates | — |
| Copper | 0.2 mg/L free copper ion prolonged immersion 100 mg/L bath | Protozoan ectoparasites and dinoflagellates in marine fish | Not recommended for freshwater systems<br>Bound to inorganic compounds<br>Toxic to invertebrates<br>Elasmobranchs may react adversely<br>Copper levels should be monitored daily<br>Solubility affected by pH and alkalinity<br>Immunosuppressive and toxic to gill tissue |
| Dimetridazole | 20 mg/gm of food Oral treatment | Cryptobia iubilans | Not 100% effective, may only reduce infestation[40] |
| Formalin (37% formaldehyde) | 0.125–0.25 mL/L Bath q 24h × 2–3 d for up to 60 minutes 0.015–0.025 mL/L (15–25ppm) prolonged immersion, every 2–3 d Change 50% water on nontreatment days | Protozoan parasites, crustacean ectoparasites | Carcinogenic<br>Depletes oxygen, additional aeration required<br>Some fish very sensitive<br>Not for use in stressed fish<br>Do not use if white precipitate forms<br>Contraindicated >27°C<br>Toxic to invertebrates |
| Freshwater | Used as a dip | Marine protozoan ectoparasites and some monogenean infestations | Not effective against all protozoans<br>A common quarantine procedure |

| Metronidazole | 7–15 mg/L q 24-48h × 5–10 d Prolonged immersion Change 50% water between treatments 25–50 mg/kg (0.25% in food fed at 1% bodyweight/d) for 3 d | Some protozoal flagellates including *Hexamita* and *Spironucleus* | Not very water soluble One oral treatment may be as effective as three water treatments |
|---|---|---|---|
| Monensin | 100 mg/kg bodyweight/ | Coccidiosis | Experimentally effective[27,30] |
| Potassium permanganate | 2 mg/L prolonged immersion 5–20 mg/L 1 h bath | External infections ectoparasites (protozoan, monogenean trematodes) | Inactivated by organic compounds in water Caustic Toxic in high pH water Stains Can be toxic in some fish species Can cause blindness (powder) Watch for signs of stress with use Safer products are available |
| Sodium chloride | 3–6 gm/L prolonged immersion 10–30 gm/L Dip (minutes or until fish is stressed) | Protozoan parasites Protozoan parasites | Dip is often used in quarantine protocols |
| Toltrazuril (Baycox, Bayer Animal Health) | 7–10 mg/kg orally q 24 h × 5 d | coccidiosis | Caution with some species |

*From* Roberts H. Freshwater Ornamental Fish. In: Johnson-Delaney C, editor. British Small Animal Veterinary Association Manual of Exotic Pets. 5th edition. BSAVA. In Press; with permission.

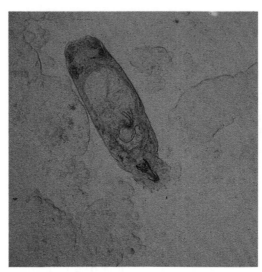

**Fig. 17.** Wet-mount prep showing a *Gyrodactylus* sp monogenean trematode. An embryo is visible inside the fluke.

*Neobenedenia* and *Benedenia* are large, and are typified by a large circular opisthohaptor on the posterior end and two smaller suckers on the anterior end. *Benedenia* has two pairs of tightly apposed, curved anchors, whereas *Neobenedenia* has three pairs. These two parasites adhere to the skin, gills, and eyes of susceptible fish, causing significant mechanical damage in large numbers.[42] Treatment methods include the use of praziquantel as a bath or prolonged immersion treatment (2–10 mg/L). The eggs of *Dactylogyrus* sp and marine capsalids are not susceptible to treatment and multiple treatments are required. In addition the eggs of the marine capsalids can be long and have attachments that can adhere to anything in the tank, making treatment and management of these parasites difficult (**Fig. 18**).[42] Other treatment options include organophosphates (to which some fish species are very sensitive), mebendazole, formalin, and potassium permanganate. An ovine anthelmintic, Supaverm (Janssen Animal Health), (closantel 5 mg/mL and mebendazole 75 mg/L) has

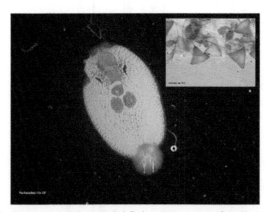

**Fig. 18.** *Neobenedenia* sp, a marine capsalid fluke, 200× magnification. Inset picture shows eggs with long sticky strands that attach to many surfaces.

been used to treat monogeneans in koi *(Cyprinus carpio)*.[43] The dose used anecdotally is 1 mL/400 L. This product has been shown to be uniformly toxic to goldfish *(Carassius auratus)* and 100% mortalities are reported. Anecdotal reports of a death in a discus *(Symphysodon discus)* have also been reported.[43] The authors recommend weekly treatment with praziquantel for 4 to 6 weeks followed by recheck wet-mount cytology after treatment. Formalin is the only US Food and Drug Administration (FDA)-approved treatment for finfish. For marine infections, a freshwater dip in quarantine may be helpful to both diagnose and remove monogeneans.[30,32] This can be done using a dark, five-gallon bucket for freshwater dips and dipping marine fish for 1 to 3 minutes in the bucket. When dips are completed, water in the bucket can be swirled and dislodged capsalid parasites will look like snowflakes swirling in the water. Biologic control has been reported using cleaner fish (French angelfish, neon gobies, and Pacific cleaner wrasse) in marine systems.[30]

### Digenean Trematodes of Clinical Importance

Digenetic trematodes are parasites with an indirect life cycle with larval forms (metacercariae) that can cause unsightly lesions on fish but are generally not pathogenic. Severe infections can cause deaths, larval migration may lead to secondary bacterial infections, and ocular lesions may lead to feeding problems. Examples include *Clinostomum* ("yellow grub"), *Neascus* ("black spot"), *Diplostomum* ("eye fluke"), and *Posthodiplostomum* ("white grub"). The problem appears in outdoor-raised pond fish such as koi and goldfish, but can be seen occasionally in tropical pet fish kept in aquaria. The life cycle does not typically continue in indoor aquaria unless snails (or other intermediate hosts) are present. **Fig. 19** shows a pond-raised perch with a severe *Clinostomum* infestation.

### Turbellarians of Clinical Importance

Turbellarians are a free-living flat worm from the group Platyhelminthes that have been implicated in causing disease in several species of marine tropical fish. Although most turbellarians are commensal organisms, several species have been implicated as pathogens for tropical marine species. The first evidence of pathology noted in Pacific and Caribbean fish, was dubbed "tang turbellarian" in 1981 by Cannon and Lester.[44] Two species were also identified as causing disease in Australian fishes.[44] These

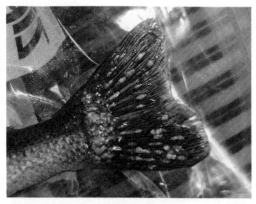

**Fig. 19.** A yellow perch with a severe "yellow grub" (*Clinostomum* sp) infestation on the caudal peduncle.

parasites look like small black spots on the skin that can cause damage through grazing on the epidermal surface, or by encysting in the gill filaments. They should not be confused with black spots associated with a Digenean infection. The life cycle for many Turbellarians is direct, with feeding stages on the fish and reproductive stages in the sediment. The most effective control has been through repeated treatments with organophosphates followed by thorough vacuuming of the sediment, and backwashing of the filters. Nonpathogenic free-living turbellarians are often seen in both freshwater and marine aquaria. The presence of large numbers of commensals often indicates a high nutrient load, and can be controlled by increasing water changes and improving environmental quality. Decreasing biologic waste is the key to controlling both pathogenic and nonpathogenic species of turbellarian.

### Nematodes of Clinical Importance

Pet fish can be either intermediate or final hosts of nematodes.[39] Nematodes in fish are similar to other animal species and appear as smooth, long worms. Most important are parasitic roundworms of pet fish species that affect the intestinal tract; these include *Camallanus*, *Capillaria*, and *Capillostrongyloides*. Clinical signs can range from none to anemia, lethargy, poor weight gain, failure to thrive, and reproductive problems.[32,45] Other species, such as *Eustrongyloides*, can cause cysts to form in the liver, muscles, and peritoneum.[28,29] *Camallanus* is an ovoviviparous nematode that affects cichlids, guppies and other liver bearers.[32,39] In *Camallanus* infections, the owner may a report a "red worm" protruding from the vent of their fish. *Capillaria* sp is most often diagnosed in angelfish, discus, and other cichlids, but can be found in many other tropical freshwater fish. It has a direct life cycle. In a closed aquarium, an infestation of *Capillaria* can spread very rapidly among susceptible fish. A wet-mount examination of fresh feces reveals a typical capillarid egg with bipolar plugs (**Fig. 20**). Diagnosis of nematodes in general is by fecal examination, cloacal wash, squash preps of affected organs, and histopathology. Treatment of nematodes can be accomplished by the use of fenbendazole (25–50 mg/kg in food) or levamisole (1–2 mg/L bath × 24h). Neither drug is FDA-approved for use in food fish.

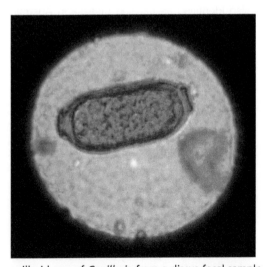

**Fig. 20.** The classic capillarid egg of *Capillaria* from a discus fecal sample.

## Cestodes of Clinical Importance

There are few important cestodes of pet fish. The most detrimental, the Asian tapeworm, *Bothriocephalus acheilognathi*, has been found in koi and other cyprinids (excluding goldfish), channel catfish, and aquarium fish such as discus, livebearers, killifishes, and angelfish.[27,32,39] Clinical signs range from none to lethargy, anorexia, weight loss, chronic intestinal inflammation, intestinal obstruction, and severe mucosal damage. Diagnosis is made by wet mounts of the feces, necropsy examination, and histopathology. Oral praziquantel (not FDA approved) can be used to treat at 50 mg/kg by mouth for one dose, or 5 to 12 gm/kg of feed every 24h × 2 to 3 days.[32] Treatment is recommended to be given in a separate tank to prevent the dispersion of eggs when the cestode dies.[32]

## Crustacean Parasites of Clinical Importance

Parasitic crustaceans are considered "macroparasites," visible to the naked eye. Three genera, *Argulus*, *Ergasilus*, and *Lernaea*, are commonly found in freshwater fish. In marine systems, *Gnathia* sp larval stages are parasitic isopods that can damage host tissue and even kill small fish.[32] *Argulus*, a branchiuran parasite also known as the "fish louse," is a circular, flattened, moving parasite that is commonly seen on koi and goldfish (**Fig. 21**). Fish lice can create damage by their feeding behavior and movement on the fish. *Argulus* may act as a vector for viral diseases such as Spring Viremia of Carp[32] and Koi Herpes Virus. Clinical signs include flashing, agitation, focal red skin lesions, and secondary cutaneous ulcers. Diagnosis is made by gross visualization or wet-mount examination. Anchor worms, *Lernaea* sp, are also easily seen on fish. Females attach under the skin of a fish with an anchoring apparatus; a characteristic forked tail is composed of egg sacs (**Fig. 22**). Anchor worms should be carefully removed manually and the remaining wound treated for any potential secondary bacterial infection. Treatment methods for all crustaceans include chitin inhibitors such as lufenuron (0.1–0.2 mg/L prolonged immersion) and dimilin, organophosphates, formalin dips, and potassium permanganate. The owner should be warned when using a chitin inhibitor that nontarget invertebrate species in the pond such as various insects may also be affected. Water should be carefully disposed of and not allowed into natural waterways.

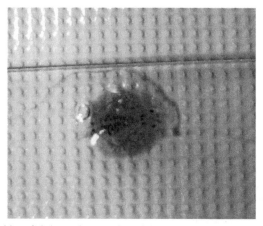

**Fig. 21.** *Argulus* sp (the "fish louse") on a glass slide.

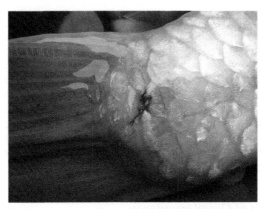

**Fig. 22.** *Lernaea* sp (the "anchor worm") on the body wall of a koi (*Cyprinus carpio*).

## SUMMARY

Bacterial and parasitic diseases are very common problems in pet fish. Shotgun treatment of fish should never be based simply on gross appearance of clinical signs and lesions without the benefit of diagnostics. Diagnostic testing for bacterial and parasitic diseases is simple to do; many tests can be done on ambulatory visits. Because of unique media requirements and incubation temperatures for some fish pathogens, it is vital to develop a relationship with a diagnostic laboratory that can provide these needs and correctly handle diagnostic samples from aquatic animal patients. When logical treatment strategies are initiated and supported by diagnostic testing, a successful outcome is possible. Identification of the correct pathogens also allows an educational opportunity for discussions on prevention and biosecurity practices with the owners and clients. Also, and, although fish are cold-blooded, there are some bacterial and parasitic pathogens that are zoonotic.

## REFERENCES

1. Palmeiro B, Roberts H. Bacterial disease in fish. In: Mayer J, editor. Clinical Veterinary Advisor: Exotic Medicine. Elsevier; 2009, in press.
2. Barker G. Bacterial diseases. In: Wildgoose WH, editor. BSAVA manual of ornamental fish. 2nd edition. Gloucester (UK): British Small Animal Veterinary Association; 2001. p. 185–93.
3. Noga EJ. Fish disease: diagnosis and treatment. St. Louis (MO): St. Mosby; 1996.
4. Hunt CJG. Ulcerative skin disease in a group of koi carp (*Cyprinus carpio*). Vet Clin North Am Exot Anim Pract 2006;9:723–8.
5. Goodwin A, Merry G. Are all koi and goldfish ulcers caused by Aeromonas salmonicida achromogenes? Western Fish Disease Workshop/American Fisheries Society. June 5, 2007.
6. Palmeiro BS, Rankin S. Culture and susceptibility characteristics of ulcerative dermatitis in koi. In press.
7. Palmeiro BS. Bacterial diseases. In: Roberts HR editor. Fundamentals of Ornamental Fish Health. Wiley-Blackwell, in press.
8. Francis-Floyd R, Klinger RE. Disease diagnosis in ornamental marine fish: a retrospective analysis of 129 cases. In: Cato JC, Brown CL, editors. Marine ornamental species: collection, culture and conservation. Iowa State Press; 2003. p. 92–100.

9. Austin B. Bacterial pathogens of marine fish. In: Belkin SS, Colwell RR, editors. Oceans and health: pathogens in the marine environment. New York: Springer; 2005. p. 391–413.

10. Humphrey JD, Lancaster C, Gudkovs N, et al. Exotic bacterial pathogens Edwardsiella tarda and Edwardsiella ictaluri from imported ornamental fish Betta splendens and Puntius conchonius, respectively: isolation and quarantine significance. Aust Vet J 1986;63(5):369–71.

11. Klinger RE, Francis-Floyd R, Riggs A, et al. Use of blood culture as a nonlethal method for isolating bacteria from fish. J Zoo Wildl Med 2003;34(2):206–7.

12. Russo R, Curtis EW, Yanong R. Preliminary investigations of hydrogen peroxide treatment of selected ornamental fishes and efficacy against external bacteria and parasites in green wwordtails. J Aquat Anim Health 2007;19(2):121–7.

13. Yanong RPE, Francis-Floyd R. Streptococcal infections in fish. University of Florida IFAS extension publication #57. 2006. Available at: http://edis.ifas.ufl.edu/pdffiles/FA/FA05700.pdf. Accessed January 10, 2008.

14. Russo R, Yanong RPE, Mitchell H. Dietary beta-glucans and nucleotides enhance resistance of red-tail black shark (*Epalzeorhynchos bicolor*, family Cyprinidae) to *Streptococcus iniae* infection. J World Aquac Soc 2006;37(3):298–306.

15. Francis-Floyd R, Yanong RP. Mycobacteriosis in fish. University of Florida IFAS extension publication # VM-96. 2006. Available at: http://edis.ifas.ufl.edu/VM055. Accessed January 10, 2008.

16. Decostere A, Hermans K, Haesebrouck F. Piscine mycobacteriosis: a literature review covering the agent and the disease it causes in fish and humans. Vet Microbiol 2004;99:159–66.

17. Harriff MJ, Bermudez LE, Kent ML. Experimental exposure of zebrafish, Danio rerio, to Mycobacterium marinum and Mycobacterium peregrinum reveals the gastrointestinal tract as the primary route of infection: a potential model for environmental mycobacterial infection. J Fish Dis 2007;30:587–600.

18. Beran V, Matlova L, Dvorska L, et al. Distribution of mycobacteria in clinically healthy ornamental fish and their aquarium environment. J Fish Dis 2006;9:383–93.

19. Marinous M, Smith S. Efficacy of common disinfectants against Mycobacterium marinum. J Aquat Anim Health 2005;17:284–8.

20. Fryer JL, Mauel MJ. The Rickettsia: an emerging group of pathogens in fish. Emerg Infect Dis 1997;3(2):137–44.

21. Khoo L, Dennis PM, Lewbart GA. Rickettsia-like organisms in the blue-eyed plecostomus, *Panaque suttoni* (Eigenmann & Eigenmann). J Fish Dis 1995;18: 157–64.

22. Hoffman GL. Parasites of North American freshwater fishes. 2nd edition. Ithaca (NY): Cornell University Press; 1999. p. 1–539.

23. Roberts RJ. The parasitology of teleosts. In: Roberts RJ, editor. Fish pathology. 3rd edition. London: Harcourt; 2001. p. 254–96.

24. Smith SA. Parasites of Fish. In: Roberts HE editor. Fundamentals of Ornamental Fish Health. Hoboken (NJ): Wiley-Blackwell, in press.

25. Roberts-Thomson A, Barnes A, Fielder DS, et al. Aerosol dispersal of the fish pathogen, *Amyloodinium ocellatum*. Aquaculture 2006;257:118–23.

26. Bishop TM, Smalls A, Wooster GA, et al. Aerobiological (airborne) dissemination of the fish pathogen Ichthyophthirius multifiliis and the implications in fish health management. In: Cheng-Sheng L, Patricia OB, editors. Biosecurity in aquaculture production systems: exclusion of pathogens and other undesirables. Baton Rouge (LA): The World Aquaculture Society; 2003. p. 51–64.

27. Baker DG, Kent ML, Fournie JL. Parasites of fishes. In: Baker DG, editor. Flynn's parasites of laboratory animals. 2nd edition. Hoboken (NJ): Blackwell; 2007. p. 69–116.

28. Stoskopf M. Fish medicine. Philadelphia: Harcourt Publishing; 1993.

29. Reavill D, Roberts HE. Diagnostic cytology of fish. Vet Clin Exot Anim 2007;10: 207–34.

30. Noga EJ. Problems 10–42. In: Noga EJ, editor. Fish disease: diagnosis and treatment. St Louis (MO): Mosby; 1996. p. 75–138.

31. Hadfield C, Whitaker BR, Clayton LA. Emergency and critical care of fish. Vet Clin Exot Anim 2007;10:647–75.

32. Longshaw M, Feist S. Parasitic diseases. In: Wildgoose WH, editor. BSAVA manual of ornamental fish health. 2nd edition. Gloucester: BSAVA; 2001. p. 167–83.

33. Speare DJ, Ferguson HW. Gills and pseudobranchs. In: Ferguson HW, editor. Systemic pathology of fish–a text and atlas of normal tissues in teleosts and their responses in disease. 2nd edition. London: Scotian Press; 2006. p. 24–63.

34. Govett PD, Rotstein DS, Lewbart GA. Gill metaplasia in a goldfish, *Carassius auratus auratus* (L). J Fish Dis 2004;27:419–23.

35. Ferguson HW. Skin. In: Ferguson HW, editor. Systemic pathology of fish—a text and atlas of normal tissues in teleosts and their responses in disease. 2nd edition. London: Scotian Press; 2006. p. 64–89.

36. Weber EPS, Govett P. Parasitology and necropsy of fish. Compendium on Continuing Education for the Practicing Veterinarian 2009;31(2). Available at: http://www.compendiumvet.com/Media/PublicationsArticle/PV0209_WEB_Weber_Parasitology.pdf. Accessed March 26, 2009.

37. Williams CR, Whitaker BR. The evaluation and treatment of common ocular disorders in teleosts. Journal of Exotic Pet Medicine 1997;6(3):160–9.

38. Lumsden JS. Gastrointestinal tract, swimbladder, pancreas, and peritoneum. In: Ferguson HW, editor. Systemic pathology of fish—a text and atlas of normal tissues in teleosts and their responses in disease. 2nd edition. London: Scotian Press; 2006. p. 168–99.

39. Noga EJ. Problems 55–72. In: Noga EJ, editor. Fish disease: diagnosis and treatment. St. Louis (MO): Mosby; 1996. p. 163–205.

40. Yanong RPE, Curtis E, Russo R, et al. Cryptobia iubilans infection in juvenile discus. JAVMA 2004;224(10):1644–50.

41. Ryan U, O'Hara, Xiao L. Molecular and biological characterization of a Cryptosporidium molnari- like isolate from a guppy (*Poecilia reticulata*). Appl Environ Microbiol 2004;70(6):3761–5.

42. Seng LT. Control of parasites in cultured marine finfishes in Southeast Asia—an overview. Int J Parasitol 1997;27(10):1177–84.

43. Marshall CJ. Use of Supaverm for the treatment of monogenean infestation in a koi carp (*Cyprinus carpio*). Fish Vet J 1999;(4):33–7.

44. Cannon LRG, Lester RJG. Two turbellarians parasitic in fish. Dis Aquat Org 1988; 5:15–22.

45. Weber ES. Gastroenterology for the piscine patient. Vet Clin Exot Anim 2005;8: 247–76.

# Bacterial and Parasitic Diseases of Selected Invertebrates

Eric Klaphake, DVM, DACZM, DABVP–Avian[a,b,*]

**KEYWORDS**

- Invertebrate • Bacteria • Parasite • Antibiotic
- Pathogen • Treatment

A common refrain by veterinarians regarding their physician colleagues is that "they see only one species, while we have to see X number of species and know all of their diseases." For many practitioners, "X" may constitute dogs, cats, cattle, horses, sheep, pigs, chickens, turkeys, goats, and a handful of exotic species. For those who see pet exotic animals exclusively or work as a zoo or wildlife veterinarian, most could comfortably say they regularly work with hundreds of species. Yet even a practitioner claiming to provide veterinary care for every vertebrate species would only be seeing 2% of the entire animal species known on the planet. There are at least 30 phyla of invertebrates, whereas all of the vertebrates are only one subphylum in the phylum Chordata with its two other subphyla categorized as invertebrates. To try to put parasitic and bacterial diseases of the other 98% known species into a single article would be like putting everything else we currently know about all aspects of veterinary medicine into an article. Yet a closer look shows how little we currently do know versus how much we could know on this topic. Drs. Greg Lewbart and Frederic Frye have both produced texts on the subject, Dr. Frye's 1992 *Captive Invertebrates—A Guide to their Biology and Husbandry* (135 pages) and Dr. Lewbart's 2006 *Invertebrate Medicine* (327 pages). Although both are excellent references, much of the focus is placed on husbandry (as with many exotic animal species initially) and the disease sections of each chapter are perhaps most glaring in the paucity of information. This lack of information is no fault of the editors and authors, but simply reflects that so little is known. Much of what is known is esoteric or derived from necropsies, which is not very helpful when faced with a deteriorating classroom pet Madagascar hissing cockroach.

Fossil evidence of insect pathogens has been found in amber ranging in age from 15 to 100 million years. They include viruses, fungi, and a trypanosomatid infection in an adult biting midge (Diptera: Ceratopogonidae).[1] One of the best studied invertebrate groups for

[a] Animal Medical Center, 216 8th Avenue, Bozeman, MT 59715, USA
[b] ZooMontana, 2100 South Shiloh Road, Billings, MT 59106, USA
* Animal Medical Center, 216 8th Avenue, Bozeman, MT 59715.
*E-mail address:* dreklaphake@msn.com

diseases are the bees and flies, and the level of literature available is so extensive that it is not included within this article because entire books are written on it. For a brief review of the diseases, the reader is referred to http://en.wikipedia.org/wiki/Bee_diseases.

Another aspect to consider is the "pass-through" parasites that are natural or pathogenic in an invertebrate but are incidental findings in the predator feeding on that invertebrate. Much like *Cryptosporidium muris* from mice being found in reptiles and incorrectly identified as *Cryptosporidium serpentis*, there are invertebrate parasites that can confuse and misdirect the results of a vertebrate fecal analysis.

Selecting which species of invertebrates to focus on can be a challenge. For this article, focus was placed more on invertebrates the author has been asked to work on, with minimal emphasis placed on aquatic species, particularly marine, although for some species, such as shrimp and lobsters, there is a greater amount of medical information because of their economic value.[2]

Complaining about what is not available serves no purpose. Much can be learned by trial and error. A can-do attitude and applying basic veterinary medicine concepts can go a long way in convincing a client who has contacted you for advice about parasitic and bacterial issues. Peer-reviewed papers are coming out more frequently on diseases of these creatures (many in non-veterinary journals), although most lack the information of what to do, instead remaining at the more rudimentary stage of what this might be, but it is nonetheless a step forward. In addition to the texts mentioned previously, the *Journal of Invertebrate Pathology* is an excellent source of information. As has been found with amphibians and reptiles, culture media and incubation temperatures for bacteria and fungi may not be reflective of the standards used with mammals and birds. Likewise, necropsies and collection of samples for pathologic examination can be quite different, especially regarding the chitinous exoskeleton. The author recommends reading the chapters in Dr. Lewbart's text for further information and specifics on these topics.

Once a disease is diagnosed, what to do then? Much of the treatment information in the literature, both for the layperson and the scientist, is geared toward species of economic value—honeybees and edible crustaceans. Applying an understanding of the dosage of a drug from a honeybee to a tarantula is a leap equivalent to saying the dosage of a drug is the same for a human as for a frog, yet this may be all there is to work from. How is such a drug to be administered? If that species is part of the food chain, what is the withdrawal time? Is a parasite or bacteria pathogenic or an endosymbiont? Or is it simply an opportunistic organism, and a deeper look into the true etiology of the disease is required? Do you sacrifice one from a collection for the good of many to get answers? And perhaps most important of all, how does one treat "bugs" on other "bugs" without killing the "bugs" one is trying to save in the first place? Often, there are no good answers at this time. It is hoped that this chapter supplements the previous literature to some small degree by reviewing the diverse information currently available, but likely the reader looking for answers will come away with a sense of frustration about the dearth of such answers. Convincing clients, be they private or a zoologic collection, to invest in advanced analysis of invertebrate problems rather than just throwing them in the trash may be the continuing step we can contribute as veterinary practitioners to improving our understanding of these diseases in these fascinating and diverse organisms.

## ENDOSYMBIONTS

Determining symbiotic status can be a challenging conundrum. If an organism is an endosymbiont in one species, is that consistent across all species? Does that endosymbiont cause disease in species other than its host species, or is it unable to survive in any other species? For bacteria, the genus *Wolbachia* has garnered attention for the great diversity of terrestrial invertebrates in which it has been identified and how ancient some of those symbiotic relationships are. At least 20% of all arthropods and some nematode species are infected with intracellular bacteria of the genus *Wolbachia*. This highly diverse genus has been subdivided into eight "supergroups" and emphasizes the high variability of the genus.[3] *Wolbachia* are the most prevalent and influential bacteria described among the insects to date. A review of the literature indicated that horizontal transfer is most successful when *Wolbachia* move between related hosts, suggesting that patterns of host association are driven by specialization on a common physiologic background. Both geographic and phylogenetic barriers have promoted evolutionary divergence among these influential symbionts.[4] *Wolbachia* is maternally inherited and may have an impact on reproductive success.[5] Other endosymbiont genuses described in arthropods, such as *Cardinium*, *Rickettsia*, and *Spiroplasma*, may also affect reproduction and potentially explain skewed sex ratios or cases of parthenogenesis. Another maternally acquired endosymbiont, *Cardinium* is found to be widespread in spiders, perhaps more so than in other arthropod groups.[5]

## ENVIRONMENTAL PSEUDOPARASITES

Some of the "ectoparasites" found on invertebrates are actually environmental in nature and are of no pathogenic concern to the invertebrate beyond momentary annoyance, much as a butterfly landing on a person. There are house dust mites (*Dermatophagoides* sp and *Euroglyphus maynei*) that feed on dead and decaying organic matter and survive well in the environments and at the temperatures that many invertebrates are kept.[6] The term "mold mites" refers to various mites (families Acaridae, Pyroglyphidae, Tarsonemidae) found in association with fungal growths, such as mildew, moldy grain, and spoiled food. Many of these mites also are common in house dust.[7] Dust and mold mites are controlled by good environmental control. Other mites may be ectoparasites of warm blooded vertebrates, such as mice, household pets, or even humans. These usually are not attracted to the relatively cool body temperature of invertebrates and can be controlled by controlling their access to their food source—the host species. Food items for invertebrates may also attract other invertebrates, from fruit flies (*Drosophila* sp) to domestic flies (*Musca* sp), if allowed to sit too long.

## CRUSTACEANS
### Bacterial

*Beneckia chitinovora* can cause an ulcerative shell disorder in hermit crabs (*Coenobita* spp).[8] They are likely susceptible to the *Vibrio* species reported to be problematic in other crustaceans, but no such cases have been reported.[8] As this indicates, much of the current information on diseases seen in these species is derived from human-consumed marine species. Chitinolytic bacteria are believed to be the primary etiologic agents of shell disease syndrome in marine crustaceans. The disease principally results from the breakdown of the chitinous exoskeletons by the shell disease pathogens, but pathogenicity may also manifest internally should a breach of the carapace occur from the genus *Vibrio* as septicemic effects or toxic extracellular bacterial products affecting the blood cells and nervous system of the crabs.[9] Epizootic shell disease (ESD) in American lobsters (*Homarus americanus*) is the bacterial degradation of the carapace resulting in extensive irregular, deep erosions and can have a major impact on their health and mortality. Although the onset and progression of ESD in

American lobsters is undoubtedly multifactorial, there is little understanding of the direct causality of this disease. The host susceptibility hypothesis states that although numerous environmental and pathologic factors may vary around a lobster, it is eventually the lobster's internal state that is permissive to or shields it from the final onset of the diseased state.[10] Lobsters are also susceptible to gaffkemia (Red Tail) caused by *Aerococcus viridans* var *homari*, which is highly virulent in impounded lobsters, manifesting as severe lethargy, tail drooping, and a red ventrum. Spiny lobsters (*Panulirus* sp) have also had Gram stain–positive bacterial infections.[11] For shrimp, *Vibrio* spp are of greatest concern, particularly with larval rearing. Pathophysiology can include septicemias secondary to shell damage.[11] Certain *Aeromonas* spp have been found to be pathogenic in laboratory settings in giant freshwater prawns (*Macrobrachium rosenbergii*).[12] Systemic Gram stain–negative bacterial infections have been reported to cause mortality in crawfish.[11] Spirochetes have been reported in brine shrimp (*Artemia* spp), an important food source for aquarium fish and also sold as Sea Monkeys.[11]

Therapeutic information for disease treatment in invertebrates is quite limited, as are pharmacokinetic studies, but is of particular concern when a food species is affected. Oxytetracycline is the only US Food and Drug Administration (FDA)–approved drug for use in food-source crustaceans to treat gaffkemia at 1 g/lb of food daily for 5 days.[11] The pharmacokinetics of enrofloxacin following a single oral gavage (10 mg/kg) in mud crab, (*Scylla serrata*) were studied at water temperatures of 19°C and 26°C. The mean hemolymph enrofloxacin concentration versus time was described by a two-compartment model with first-order absorption at two water temperatures. The peak concentrations of hemolymph enrofloxacin at 19°C and 26°C were 7.26 and 11.03 μg/mL at 6 and 2 hours, respectively. These results indicated that enrofloxacin was absorbed and eliminated more rapidly at 26°C than at 19°C.[13] Dosages for benzalkonium chloride, chloramphenicol, furacin, furanace, furazolidone, oxytetracycline, and ormetoprim-sulfamethoxazole have been described for use in penaeid shrimp, but obvious ethical and legal ramifications need to be considered for their use.[11]

### Parasitic

All crustaceans can be affected by fouling, a condition seen secondary to poor management or immunocompromised individuals. Severity of clinical signs can range from none to lethal. Because of the presence of chitin, the shell and even gills can become attachment sites for various normally nonpathogenic organisms. Eggs can also be affected.[11] Microsporidiosis (cotton disease) is the presence of obligate, intracellular microsporidia in the muscle, causing it to grossly appear white. Environmentally resistant spores are released on the death of the host.[11]

Plerocercoids of the dogfish (*Mustelus canis*) cestode, *Calliobothrium verticillatum*, can cause pathology in the midgut ceca of hermit crabs.[11] Hematodiniosis (bitter crab disease), caused by the dinoflagellate *Hematodinium*, causes degeneration of hepatopancreas and muscle in some crab species. Systemic manifestations also occur in blue crabs (*Callinectes sapidus*) from paramoebiasis (gray-crab disease) due to *Paramoeba perniciosa*. *Anophyroides haemophila* (bumper-car disease) is a pathogenic scuticociliate of lobsters and some crabs causing mortality secondary to chronic destruction hemocytes.[11] A rickettsia-like organism infecting the redclaw crayfish (*Cherax quadricarinatus*) proliferated inside hemocytes.[14] A suspected ectosymbiont has been seen by the author and described in crayfish (*Cambarus* spp) as appearing as lice; however, it is actually a branchiobdellid annelid, *Cambarincola ingens*, and therefore treatment is not recommended.[15]

Outside of the obvious environmental changes to improve parasite issues, the use of copper sulfate, formalin, potassium permanganate, and zeolite have been described for penaeid shrimp, but again legal and ethical considerations are necessary for food sources, because all of this use would be off-label and not approved by the FDA.[11]

## SNAILS AND SLUGS
### Bacterial

No reports could be found of bacterial infections in snails or slugs, although they have been reported in abalones (*Haliotis* spp), a marine gastropod, including a rickettsial-like organism treated with oxytetracycline.[16] Likely these infections occur and have simply not been studied and identified yet.

Bath treatments as for fish and injections into the hemocoel or foot have been described.[16]

### Parasitic

Nematode cysts and larvae were found in the giant African snail (*Achatina fulica*) in Brazil that had been introduced for escargot farming.[17] It is also a public health concern, because it is one of the natural intermediate host of *Angiostrongylus cantonensis*, the etiological agent of the meningoencephalitis in Asia. In Brazil, *Aelurostrongylus abstrusus* (a cat parasite), and other nematode larvae (*Strongyluris*-like) were found in the interior of the pallial cavity of *A fulica*.[18] Non-snail marine gastropods have been reported with coccidial, *Labyrinthula*, ciliate, copepod, and tubellarian infections. Many snails are the first intermediate host for numerous digenetic trematodes, which clinically manifest as gigantism (increase food intake compensation), orange/brown discoloration of the foot, castration, behavioral changes, tissue necrosis, or shell variation. *Polydora* sp is a polychaete annelid commonly found in snail shells that destroy the mineralized matrix, thus weakening the shell, particularly in the older uppermost shell whorls.[16]

Bath treatments as for fish and injections into the hemoceol or foot have been described.[16]

## EARTHWORMS
### Bacterial

Although various *Mycobacteria* spp have been isolated from *Lumbricus terrestris*, the risk for being a carrier species is considered minimal and earthworms protect themselves from pathogenic bacteria by way of phagocytosis and coelomic fluid lytic enzymes. The bacteria *Bacillus thuringiensis* has been used as a biologic insecticide against certain insects, and at high concentrations in the soil has contributed to a 100% mortality rate in earthworms. *Aeromonas hydrophila* has been isolated from the coelom, but is considered nonpathogenic.[19]

No reports could be found on therapeutic antibacterials in earthworms, likely for the lack of pathogenic bacterial disease.

### Parasitic

In other oligochaetes, microsporidian infection has been reported.[19] The author has commonly seen fecal samples of reptiles and amphibians fed earthworms contain the earthworm parasite *Monocystis* sp, a gregarine sporozoite. The life cycle occurs primarily within the seminal vesicles and seems to be of no pathogenic concern to the earthworm hosts or their predators.[20] Attempts to use the earthworm to introduce beneficial nematodes for agricultural benefit have met with mixed success.[21] The oligochaete *Tubifex tubifex* is notorious as the intermediate host of the myxozoan,

*Myxobolus cerebralis*, which is responsible for whirling disease in fish. Tubifex worms are commonly provided in aquaculture to feed aquarium fish, but *M cerebralis* is excreted from the worm in the feces and does not seem to induce any pathology in the worm.[19]

There were no reports of recommendations for or need for antiparasitic administration in earthworms at this time.

## SPIDERS
### Bacterial

As is usually the case, little is known about the normal microflora of arachnids. If bacteria is cultured from correctly collected hemolymph (collect from leg to avoid accidental gastrointestinal microflora contamination), it is likely abnormal. *Bacillus* spp are likely normal gastrointestinal flora but have been implicated as a mortality cause secondary to low humidity.[21]

Enrofloxacin at 10 to 20 mg/kg by mouth every 24 hours has been used, with the recommendation of holding the spider upside down to encourage ingestion. Various uses of tetracyclines and topical trimethoprim-sulfonamides have been described also.[21]

### Parasitic

A more newly described condition in wild-caught and captive tarantulas is the oral nematode *Panagrolaimidae* spp. The clinical signs are anorexia, gradual lethargy progressing to a huddled posture, and finally death after several weeks. Nematodes may be observed in samples collected from a thick white discharge between the mouth and chelicerae. *Phoridae* spp flies have been a suggested vector. No treatment has been reliably successful in managing this condition and there is a zoonotic potential, especially secondary to bites. Both fenbendazole and oxfenbendazole have been used at various doses in attempt to treat this parasite with no permanent success.[21]

Mermithidae nematodes have been described in wild-caught spiders and have even been found in fossils from millions of years ago.[22] These are ingested in a paratenic host. Clinical signs include a swollen opisthosoma that may also be asymmetrical, malformed palps, shorter legs, stunted male secondary sex characteristic development, lethargic behavior, and sometime wandering toward a water source. They can completely fill the opisthosoma before the spider dies and they are released into the environment.[22–25]

Mites are a commonly reported problem in tarantulas; however, most are saprophytic and their presence directly on the spider is considered incidental (see environmental mites section elsewhere in this article). In high numbers, they may occlude the book lungs. Excessive humidity and poor environmental sanitation likely contribute. Baking substrate at low temperatures (200°F) for 6 hours often eliminates the mites and eggs. Another recommendation is the use of the predatory mite *Hypoaspis miles* that is sold to control fungus gnats, with a half teaspoon added to each enclosure. These mites die once their saprophytic mite food is gone. Quick water dips of spiders or a focal topical treatment with petroleum jelly may help reduce numbers but does not eliminate them.[22]

The previously mentioned Phoridae flies suspected in the transmission of *Panagrolaimidae* oral nematodes can also directly kill adult tarantulas through occlusion of book lungs and penetration of the opisthosoma/internal organs by high numbers of larvae. Spiderlings and their high humidity requirements are extremely susceptible to this problem and good quarantine and manual elimination of adult flies is recommended. In North America, *Megaselia scalaris* is the most common species.[22]

Several parasitic wasps are natural predators, particularly of tarantulas but also of other spiders. They rely on the spider to serve as a host for their larvae, causing abnormal behavior or paralysis of the spider, and usually end with the death of the spider. These are minimal consequence in spiders kept indoors, however.[22,26]

## CENTIPEDES, MILLIPEDES
### Bacterial

There are numerous studies discussing the normal gastrointestinal microflora of the millipede because of its significant role in leaf litter composting in forests. A *Pseudomonas* infection associated with a fungal infection was reported in a centipede.[27] Poor husbandry and the presence of mites (see later discussion) have been implicated as potential sequelae.

### Parasitic

Protozoa and a nematode indistinguishable from *Strongyloides stercoralis* have been identified in millipede feces, both of unknown significance because the animals were healthy.[28] Unlike most mites, mobile ones commonly seen on millipedes may actually be symbiotic, because they remove debris and microorganisms from between plates or at leg articulations. Other mites have been reported to cause apparent irritation. In those cases, a gentle warm rinse followed by a flour coating, followed by a second rinse after an hour seems to at least reduce their numbers.[28]

Centipede mites and nematodes have been described as being associated with limb loss, which may have been secondary to overall poor health and lack of normal meticulous grooming to remove such problems.[28]

## NON-BEE INSECTS
### Bacterial

Bacteria tend to enter the body of insects and affect primarily the gastrointestinal tract, particularly the midgut epithelium, with secondary septicemia possible.[29] *Bacillus thuringiensis* has played an important role in biocontrol of invertebrate pests, including locusts.[30] It is highly pathogenic but has low infectivity, so natural infections are rare but artificially induced infection leads to high mortality.[29] *Pseudomonas* spp can cause disease in insects, much like vertebrates. Various bacterial organisms have been implicated in larval disease of both Lepidoptera (butterflies/moths) and Hymenoptera (beetles), manifesting as loose feces, dehydration and death. *Serratia marcescens* can cause a septicemia, indicated by body reddening and liquefaction.[29] An infection with *Rickettsiella* sp was responsible for an illness causing heavy body swelling in the Oriental cockroach *Blatta orientalis*. Reproduction of the colony stagnated. Vacuoles with parasitic bacteria occurred mainly in the fat body, but also in nearly all other organs, such as gut epithelium, malpighian tubules, blood cells, and ovarioles. The parasites clearly differed from the symbiotic bacteria *Blattabacterium* spp, which regularly occurs in the mycetocytes of *B orientalis* and was provisionally named *Rickettsiella crassificans*.[31]

Treatment of these infections usually focuses on good quarantine, selective culling, and potentially antibiotics. Much of the published research on antibiotic use in insects has been performed in honeybees or other insects of agricultural or economic value. Many of these medications are strictly limited to avoid undesired ramifications in humans. Sulfonamides have been used orally in honeybees, grasshoppers, and crickets.

Oral and topical applications of several tetracyclines have been used in bees, although toxicity must be considered.[29] Several references to antibiotic use for microsporidia are noted later in this article.

## Parasitic

It is important to remember the potential of an ecto- or endosymbiont relationship with parasites. Eugregarines have been found in numerous cockroach species. Experimental infections were produced in all homologous host–parasite combinations. With the exception of one host–gregarine combination, no infection was produced in heterologous reciprocal combinations. Excystation occurred in all instances when oocysts were placed in homologous host gut homogenate but excystation was never observed in heterologous host gut homogenate, suggesting species specificity and possible endosymbiosis.[32] *Gregarina* sp in cockroaches (*Blattella germanica*) caused swollen abdomens, slower movement at high incidences of the protozoan, and short antennas. Dead cockroaches showed darkened body and putrid smell, indicating septicemia.[33]

As mentioned with spiders, Mermithidae nematodes are a problem, with signs including weakness/lethargy, weight changes, and worms in the body cavity. In a die-off in a captive colony of blue-winged grasshoppers (*Tropidacris collaris*), one fourth of the colony died within a year because of infection with worms initially mistaken for nematomorphs but later identified as nematodes belonging to the Mermithidae, genus *Mermis*. Mortality persisted and the grasshopper population dwindled over the following years. Mermithid larvae developed in the hemocoel of the insects until they eventually emerged from a hollowed-out exoskeleton. Circumstantial evidence suggests that the parasites were introduced with raspberry browse that was grown on site and contaminated with mermithid eggs.[34] Management includes culling and careful selection of vegetation provided for food.[29] Nematodes tend to affect particular organs and cause stunting or reproductive issues.[29]

Microsporidiosis causes locomotion stiffness and colored cysts under the skin. Management focuses on hygiene and antibiotics.[29] Long-term persistence was reported of *Paranosema locustae* in grasshoppers of Argentina. The pathogen was introduced from North America. This persistence highlights the ability of *P locustae* to recycle in local grasshopper communities by parasitizing susceptible species other than the natural hosts.[35] Thiabendazole, quinine, albendazole, and fumagillin significantly reduced but did not eliminate microsporidia spore counts in the grasshopper host. Among these four drugs, thiabendazole was most effective in reducing the microsporidia spore level up to 90%, followed by quinine (70%), albendazole (62%), and fumagillin (59%). No control or quinine-treated animals died, whereas 45% of albendazole animals died. Despite the high mortality induced by albendazole, this drug significantly reduced spore counts, a result not seen in previous per os trials. Among the treatment groups, grasshoppers injected with thiabendazole lost significant mass.[36] Oral treatment with fumagillin or thiabendazole significantly reduced pathogen spore counts, whereas grasshoppers fed with albendazole, ampicillin, chloramphenicol, griseofulvin, metronidazole, sulfadimethoxine, quinine, streptomycin, or tetracycline show no reduction in spore counts. In no case was the pathogen totally eliminated.[37,38] Benomyl, a benzimidazole with toxicity concerns, has been used as an antiprotozoal treatment by way of diet or as a spray in Lepidoptera, although is currently difficult to obtain.[29]

As with spiders, there are several parasitic wasps that rely on insects for their offspring's development.[29]

## SUMMARY

There is still much more unknown with invertebrates than known. Practitioners need to try to assist these fascinating creatures medically and surgically. It is hoped that further research and anecdotal information will continue to provide guidance to a starting point, and that in the years to come invertebrate medicine will continue to advance, much in the same manner as reptile, amphibian, and avian medicine have over the last 30 years.

## REFERENCES

1. Poinar G, Poinar R. Fossil evidence of insect pathogens. J Invertebr Pathol 2005; 89:243–50.
2. Sparks A. Observations on the history of non-insect invertebrate pathology from the perspective of a participant. J Invertebr Pathol 2005;89:67–77.
3. Ros V, Fleming V, Feil E, et al. How diverse is the genus Wolbachia? Multiple-gene sequencing reveals a putatively new Wolbachia supergroup recovered from spider mites (Acari: Tetranychidae). Appl Environ Microbiol 2009;75:1036–43.
4. Russell J, Golman-Huertas B, Moreau C, et al. Specialization and geographic isolation among *Wolbachia* symbionts from ants and lycaenid butterflies. Evolution 2009;63:624–40.
5. Martin O, Goodacre S. Widespread infections by the bacterial endosymbiont *Cardinium* in Arachnids. J Arachnol 2009;37:106–8.
6. House dust mite. Available at: http://en.wikipedia.org/wiki/Dust_mite. Accessed May 31, 2009.
7. Mold mite. Available at: http://en.wikipedia.org/wiki/Mold_mite. Accessed May 31, 2009.
8. Frye F. Crustaceans. In: Frye F, editor. Captive invertebrates: a guide to their biology and husbandry. Malabar (FL): Krieger Publishing; 1992. p. 65–73.
9. Vogan C, Costa-Ramos C, Rowley A. Shell disease syndrome in the edible crab, *Cancer pagurus* – isolation, characterization and pathogenicity of chitinolytic bacteria. Microbiology 2002;148:743–54.
10. Tlusty MF, Smolowitz RM, Halvorson HO, et al. Host susceptibility hypothesis for shell disease in American lobsters. J Aquat Anim Health 2007;19:215–25.
11. Noga E, Hancock A, Bullis R. Crustaceans. In: Lewbart G, editor. Invertebrate medicine. Ames (IA): Blackwell Publishing; 2006. p. 179–93.
12. Sung HH, Hwang SF, Tasi FM. Responses of giant freshwater prawn (Macrobrachium rosenbergii) to challenge by two strains of Aeromonas spp. J Invertebr Pathol 2000;76:278–84.
13. Fang WH, Hu LL, Yang XL, et al. Effect of temperature on pharmacokinetics of enrofloxacin in mud crab, Scylla serrata (Forsskal), following oral administration. J Fish Dis 2008;31:171–6.
14. Romero X, Turnbull JF, Jimenez R. Ultrastructure and cytopathology of a rickettsia-like organism causing systemic infection in the redclaw crayfish, Cherax quadricarinatus (Crustacea: decapoda), in Ecuador. J Invertebr Pathol 2000; 76:95–104.
15. Brown B, Creed R. Host preference by an aquatic ectosymbiotic annelid on 2 sympatric species of host crayfishes. J North Am Benthol Soc 2004;23:90–100.
16. Smolowitz R. Gastropods. In: Lewbart G, editor. Invertebrate medicine. Ames (IA): Blackwell Publishing; 2006. p. 65–78.
17. Franco-Acuña D, Pinheiro J, Torres E, et al. Nematode cysts and larvae found in *Achatina fulica* Bowdich, 1822. J Invertebr Pathol 2009;100:106–10.

18. Thiengo S, Fernandez M, Torres E, et al. First record of a nematode Metastrongyloidea (*Aelurostrongylus abstrusus* larvae) in *Achatina* (*Lissachatina*) *fulica* (Mollusca, Achatinidae) in Brazil. J Invertebr Pathol 2008;98:34–9.
19. Lewbart G. Annelids. In: Lewbart G, editor. Invertebrate medicine. Ames (IA): Blackwell Publishing; 2006. p. 115–31.
20. Morgan M. Monocystis. Available at: http://www.microscopy-uk.org.uk/mag/artmar99/cystis.html. Accessed May 31, 2009.
21. Campos-Herrera R, Trigo D, Gutierrez C. Phoresy of the entomopathogenic nematode Steinernema feltiae by the earthworm Eisenia fetida. J Invertebr Pathol 2006;92:50–4.
22. Pizzi R. Spiders. In: Lewbart G, editor. Invertebrate medicine. Ames (IA): Blackwell Publishing; 2006. p. 143–68.
23. Poinar G. Heydenius araneus n.sp (Nematoda: Mermithidae), a parasite of a fossil spider, with an examination of helminths from extant spiders (Arachnida: Araneae). Invertebr Biol 2000;119:388–93.
24. Penney D, Bennett SP. First unequivocal Mermithid-Linyphiid (Araneae) parasite-host association. J Arachnol 2006;34:273–8.
25. Vandergast AG, Roderick GK. Mermithid parasitism of Hawaiian Tetragnatha spiders in a fragmented landscape. J Invertebr Pathol 2003;84:128–36.
26. Allard C, Robertson MW. Nematode and dipteran endoparasites of the wolf spider Pardosa milvina (Araneae, Lycosidae). J Arachnol 2003;31:139–41.
27. Eberhard W. Under the influence: webs and building behavior of Plesiometa argyra (Araneae, Tetragnathidae) when parasitized by Hymenoepimecis argyraphaga (Hymenoptera, Ichneumonidae). J Arachnol 2001;29:354–66.
28. Frye F. Scorpions. In: Lewbart G, editor. Invertebrate medicine. Ames (IA): Blackwell Publishing; 2006. p. 169–77.
29. Chitty J. Myriapods (centipedes and millipedes). In: Lewbart G, editor. Invertebrate medicine. Ames (IA): Blackwell Publishing; 2006. p. 195–203.
30. Cooper J. Insects. In: Lewbart G, editor. Invertebrate medicine. Ames (IA): Blackwell Publishing; 2006. p. 208–19.
31. Song LL, Gao MY, Dai SY, et al. Specific activity of a Bacillus thuringiensis strain against Locusta migratoria manilensis. J Invertebr Pathol 2008;98:169–76.
32. Radek R. Light and electron microscopic study of a Rickettsiella species from the cockroach Blatta orientalis. J Invertebr Pathol 2000;76:249–56.
33. Smith AJ, Cook TJ. Host specificity of five species of Eugregarinida among six species of cockroaches (Insecta: Blattodea). Comp Parasitol 2008;75:288–91.
34. Lopes RB, Alves SB. Effect of Gregarina sp parasitism on the susceptibility of Blattella germanica to some control agents. J Invertebr Pathol 2005;88:261–4.
35. Attard LM, Carreno RA, Pare JA, et al. Mermithid nematode infection in a colony of blue-winged grasshoppers (Tropidacris collaris). J Zoo Wildl Med 2008;39:488–92.
36. Lange CE, Azzaro FG. New case of long-term persistence of Paranosema locustae (Microsporidia) in melanopline grasshoppers (Orthoptera: Acrididae: Melanoplinae) of Argentina. J Invertebr Pathol 2008;99:357–9.
37. Johny S, Nimmo AS, Fisher MA, et al. Testing intra-hemocelic injection of antimicrobials against Encephalitozoon sp (Microsporidia) in an insect host. Parasitol Res 2009;104:419–24.
38. Johny S, Lange CE, Solter LF, et al. New insect system for testing antibiotics. J Parasitol 2007;93:1505–11.

# Index

*Note:* Page numbers of article titles are in **boldface** type.

### A

Abscesses, bacterial, in ferrets, 543–544
    in turtles, aural, 592
  crop, in columbiformes, 464–465
*Acanthocephalus* spp., in amphibians, 605
  in anseriformes, 484
  in nonhuman primates, 574
  in raptors, 500
Acid-fast bacteria, slow-growing, in pet fish, 615, 618–620
*Acuaria skrjabini,* in passerines, 447
Adenovirus, in columbiformes, 454
Aeromonad septicemia, motile, in pet fish, 610
*Aeromonas hydrophilia,* in reptiles, 591
*Aeromonas salmonicida,* in pet fish, 612
*Aeromonas* spp., in parrots, 422
  in passerines, 435–436
Air sac mites, in parrots, 429
  in passerines, 449
Alkali poisoning, in anseriformes, 482
*Ambiphyra* spp., in pet fish, 626
Amoebiasis, in amphibians, 601
Amphibians, bacterial diseases of, **597–608**
    chlamydiosis as, 600
    chlamydophilosis as, 600
    fungal infections vs., 597–598
    gram-negative, 600
    mycobacteriosis as, 600–601
    normal microflora vs., 599
      antimicrobial effects of, 599–600
    summary overview of, 597, 606
    viral infections vs., 597–598
    zoonoses as, 601
  parasitic diseases of, **597–608**
    acanthocephala as, 605
    cestodes as, 604–605
    external, 605–606
    fungal infections vs., 597–598
    nematodes as, 603–604
    protozoa as, 601–603
    summary overview of, 597, 606
    trematodes as, 604–605

Vet Clin Exot Anim 12 (2009) 649–672
doi:10.1016/S1094-9194(09)00056-5
1094-9194/09/$ – see front matter © 2009 Elsevier Inc. All rights reserved.

# *Our* issues help you manage *yours.*

## Every year brings you new clinical challenges.

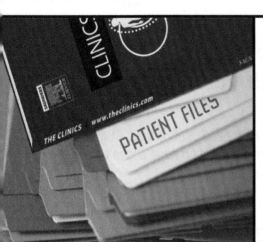

Every **Clinics** issue brings you **today's best thinking** on the challenges you face.

Whether you purchase these issues individually, or order an annual subscription (which includes searchable access to past issues online), the **Clinics** offer you an efficient way to update your know how…one issue at a time.

## DISCOVER THE CLINICS IN YOUR SPECIALTY!

**Veterinary Clinics of North America: Equine Practice.**
Publishes three times a year.
ISSN 0749-0739.

**Veterinary Clinics of North America: Exotic Animal Practice.**
Publishes three times a year.
ISSN 1094-9194.

**Veterinary Clinics of North America: Food Animal Practice.**
Publishes three times a year.
ISSN 0749-0720.

**Veterinary Clinics of North America: Small Animal Practice.**
Publishes bimonthly.
ISSN 0195-5616.

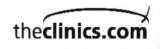

# Moving?

## Make sure your subscription moves with you!

To notify us of your new address, find your **Clinics Account Number** (located on your mailing label above your name), and contact customer service at:

Email: **journalscustomerservice-usa@elsevier.com**

**800-654-2452** (subscribers in the U.S. & Canada)
**314-447-8871** (subscribers outside of the U.S. & Canada)

Fax number: **314-447-8029**

**Elsevier Health Sciences Division**
**Subscription Customer Service**
**3251 Riverport Lane**
**Maryland Heights, MO 63043**

*To ensure uninterrupted delivery of your subscription, please notify us at least 4 weeks in advance of move.